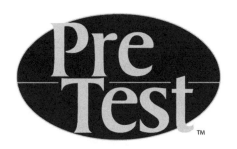

Physical Diagnosis

PreTest™ Self-Assessment and Review

D1114381

Notice

Medicine is an ever-changing science. As new research and clinical experience broaden our knowledge, changes in treatment and drug therapy are required. The authors and the publisher of this work have checked with sources believed to be reliable in their efforts to provide information that is complete and generally in accord with the standards accepted at the time of publication. However, in view of the possibility of human error or changes in medical sciences, neither the authors nor the publisher nor any other party who has been involved in the preparation or publication of this work warrants that the information contained herein is in every respect accurate or complete, and they disclaim all responsibility for any errors or omissions or for the results obtained from use of the information contained in this work. Readers are encouraged to confirm the information contained herein with other sources. For example and in particular, readers are advised to check the product information sheet included in the package of each drug they plan to administer to be certain that the information contained in this work is accurate and that changes have not been made in the recommended dose or in the contraindications for administration. This recommendation is of particular importance in connection with new or infrequently used drugs.

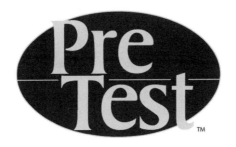

Physical Diagnosis
PreTest™ Self-Assessment and Review
Sixth Edition

Jo-Ann Reteguiz, M.D., F.A.C.P.
Associate Professor of Medicine
Vice-Chair for Education
UMDNJ—New Jersey Medical School
Newark, New Jersey

McGraw-Hill
Medical Publishing Division

New York   Chicago   San Francisco   Lisbon   London   Madrid   Mexico City
Milan   New Delhi   San Juan   Seoul   Singapore   Sydney   Toronto

The *McGraw·Hill* Companies

Physical Diagnosis: PreTest™ Self-Assessment and Review, Sixth Edition

Copyright © 2006 by The McGraw-Hill Companies, Inc. All rights reserved. Printed in the United States of America. Except as permitted under the United States Copyright Act of 1976, no part of this publication may be reproduced or distributed in any form or by any means, or stored in a data base or retrieval system, without the prior written permission of the publisher.

PreTest is a trademark of The McGraw-Hill Companies, Inc.

2 3 4 5 6 7 8 9 0 DOC/DOC 0 9 8 7 6

ISBN 0-07-145551-5

This book was set in Berkeley by North Market Street Graphics.
The editor was Catherine A. Johnson.
The production supervisor was Sherri Souffrance.
Project management was provided by North Market Street Graphics.
The cover designer was Mary McKeon.
RR Donnelley was printer and binder.

This book is printed on acid-free paper.

Library of Congress Cataloging-in-Publication Data

Reteguiz, Jo-Ann.
Physical diagnosis : pretest, self-assessment, and review / Jo-Ann Reteguiz.—6th ed.
p. cm.
Includes bibliographical references and index.
ISBN 0-07-145551-5
1. Physical diagnosis—Examinations, questions, etc. I. Title.
RC76.R47 2006
616.07'54076—dc22
2005054361

To the faculty, residents, and students in the Department of Medicine at the New Jersey Medical School for their commitment to bedside teaching and bedside learning.

Student Reviewers

Robert Boykin
Vanderbilt University School of Medicine
Class of 2006

Mona Karimullah
University of Texas—Houston Medical School
Class of 2006

Contents

Obstetrics and Gynecology

Pediatrics and Neonatology

Bonus Chapter: The TEN Toughest Physical Diagnosis Questions Ever Written

High-Yield Facts

Introduction

A good doctor must be able to solve problems by performing a careful history and physical examination. This skill is learned and mastered at the bedside. If you understand the normal and abnormal characteristics of each organ system, you will recognize the pattern of the syndrome and reach the correct diagnosis. Skills in physical diagnosis are instrumental if you desire to become an astute and competent physician.

The purpose of this book is to provide medical students and physicians with a comprehensive and convenient method for review and self-assessment of their pattern recognition skills in physical diagnosis. The more than 500 revised and updated questions cover the most relevant and pertinent topics in medicine.

The questions have been designed to parallel the format and degree of difficulty of the questions contained in medical school physical diagnosis courses as well as the United States Licensing Examination (USMLE) Step 1 and Step 2 CK examinations. Students and physicians preparing for an OSCE or the USMLE Step 2 CS will find this book to be an excellent resource. This will be a true test of your mastery of physical diagnosis from beginning to end. Each chapter of the book is based on a specific organ system, so students can assess and target their specific weaknesses and strengths. There is a section on important miscellaneous subjects, such as geriatrics, infectious diseases, obstetrics and gynecology, and pediatrics. A new bonus chapter of 10 master-level physical diagnosis questions will challenge and strengthen your knowledge in the Oslerian method of bedside diagnosis.

Each question in this book is accompanied by an answer that contains a thorough explanation of the question's learning objectives and a specific page reference to a current textbook (see below). All high-yield information in the explanations is set in boldface type for easy reference and access. A special High-Yield Facts section filled with meaningful mnemonics is included in the back of the book for quick review before examinations.

Perhaps the most effective way to use this book is to allow yourself one minute to answer each question in a given chapter; as you proceed, indicate your answer beside each question. By following this suggestion, you will be approximating the time limits imposed by the board examinations.

When you have finished answering the questions in a chapter, you should then spend as much time as you need verifying your answers by carefully reading the explanations. Although you should pay special attention to the explanations for the questions you answered incorrectly, you should read every single explanation. Even a question you answer effortlessly is followed with a unique collection of physical diagnosis pearls. Each question and explanation has several important learning objectives, and the explanations have been designed to reinforce and supplement the information tested by the questions. If, after reading the explanations for a given chapter, you feel you need more information about the material covered, you should consult and study the reference indicated. For your convenience, I have limited the number of references to five:

Behrman RE et al: *Nelson's Book of Pediatrics,* 17/e. Philadelphia, Saunders, 2004.

Fitzpatrick TB et al: *Color Atlas and Synopsis of Clinical Dermatology,* 4/e. New York, McGraw-Hill, 2001.

Goldman L: *Cecil Textbook of Medicine,* 22/e. Philadelphia, Saunders, 2004.

Seidel HM et al: *Mosby's Guide to Physical Examination,* 5/e. St. Louis, MO, Mosby, 2003.

Tierney LM Jr et al: *Current Medical Diagnosis and Treatment,* 44/e. New York, McGraw-Hill, 2005.

It is my hope that after completion of this book you will be better able to recognize and understand the clinical characteristics of many important medical syndromes. You are on the road to becoming a master diagnostician if you take the appropriate history and skillfully perform the proper physical examination. Good luck with physical diagnosis at the bedside!

Acknowledgments

I wish to acknowledge the University of Medicine and Dentistry of New Jersey—New Jersey Medical School, Newark, and in particular, the Department of Medicine, for its exceptional commitment to patient care and medical education. I also wish to acknowledge the residents and medical students of UMDNJ—New Jersey Medical School for contributing some of the mnemonics found in this review book.

The publisher would like to acknowledge the contributions of the two student reviewers, whose comments and suggestions helped make this sixth edition even better than the previous one: Robert Boykin, Vanderbilt University School of Medicine (Class of 2006), and Mona Karimullah, University of Texas—Houston Medical School (Class of 2006).

General Principles of Disease

Questions

DIRECTIONS: Each item below contains a question followed by suggested responses. Select the **one best** response to each question.

1. A 37-year-old postal worker from Atlantic City, New Jersey, presents to the emergency room with the chief complaint of dry cough for several days. He has fever, malaise, dyspnea on exertion, and pleuritic chest pain. He has experienced mild nausea and diffuse abdominal pain. He has been in good health otherwise and has no recent travel history. No contacts have been ill. Physical examination is remarkable for a temperature of 38.5°C (101.4°F) and decreased breath sounds at the lung bases bilaterally. Chest radiograph reveals pleural effusions and a widened mediastinum. Which of the following is the most likely diagnosis?

a. Pneumonic plague
b. Tularemia
c. Hemorrhagic fever
d. Inhalation anthrax
e. Hantavirus pulmonary syndrome

2. A 47-year-old nurse presents to your office complaining of a poorly healing ulcer of her left second digit. The ulcer started a week ago and is painless. The patient has tried using over-the-counter antibacterial and hydrocortisone creams without improvement. She denies trauma to the hand. The patient has a temperature of 38.4°C (101.1°F) and left-sided epitrochlear and axillary adenopathy. She has a 4-cm ulcer on the dorsal side of the left second digit covered by a black eschar and surrounded by an extensive amount of nonpitting edema. Which of the following is the most likely diagnosis?

a. Smallpox infection
b. Cutaneous anthrax
c. Cat-scratch disease
d. Leprosy infection
e. Brown recluse spider bite

3. A 79-year-old woman presents to the emergency room with a one-week history of fever, myalgias, nausea, vomiting, and diarrhea. Her symptoms started shortly after she ate at a Mexican restaurant with her daughter and son-in-law. She did not eat raw foods, and her family members did not become ill. She has no past medical history and takes no medications. She has a temperature of 39.5°C (103.2°F) and appears extremely ill. She is awake and oriented to person and place but not to time. Heart and lung examinations are normal, and she has no focal neurologic deficits. Computed tomography (CT) scan of the head is normal. Lumbar puncture reveals pleocytosis, increased protein concentration, and normal glucose. Blood and cerebrospinal fluid cultures identify a gram-positive rod organism. Which of the following is the most likely diagnosis?

a. *Actinomyces* infection
b. *Bacillus cereus* infection
c. Invasive *Listeria* infection
d. Inhalation anthrax infection
e. *Clostridium* botulism infection

4. An 81-year-old man is admitted to the hospital with a one-month history of generalized weakness, lethargy, and a 10-lb weight loss. He states that recently his dietary intake has decreased secondary to poor dentition. Physical examination reveals an emaciated man with bitemporal wasting. He has no peripheral edema. Serum albumin level is 3.5 mg/dL (normal = 3.5 to 5.7 mg/dL). Which of the following is the most likely diagnosis?

a. Kwashiorkor
b. Hypothyroidism
c. Zinc deficiency
d. Riboflavin deficiency
e. Protein-energy malnutrition

5. A 21-year-old man presents to your office for a preemployment physical examination. He is 6 ft 3 in. tall and weighs 70 kg. Heart examination is remarkable for a midsystolic click and a grade 2 systolic murmur that increases with Valsalva maneuver. The patient has an arm span that exceeds his height and has long, slender fingers. The thumb sign (Steinberg's sign) is positive. Which of the following is the most likely diagnosis?

a. Lesch-Nyhan syndrome
b. Turner's syndrome
c. Ehlers-Danlos syndrome
d. Marfan's syndrome
e. Noonan's syndrome

6. A 22-year-old college student with a seven-year history of Crohn's disease presents to her gastroenterologist with a two-month history of numbness and tingling of her feet and fingertips. Her past surgical history is significant for several previous bowel resections. On physical examination, there is loss of vibration and position sense of the hands and feet. Motor and cerebellar examinations are normal. Deep tendon reflexes are intact. Which of the following is the most likely diagnosis?

a. Vitamin D deficiency
b. Vitamin E deficiency
c. Vitamin A deficiency
d. Vitamin B_{12} deficiency
e. Vitamin K deficiency

7. A 29-year-old woman was an unbelted passenger in a motor vehicle accident. On arrival at the hospital, the paramedics inform you that her calculated Glasgow Coma Scale (GCS) score is 5. Vital signs reveal a blood pressure of 100/60 mmHg, a pulse of 50, and a respiratory rate of 6 breaths per minute. Pupils are 5 mm bilaterally and poorly reactive to light. Heart and lung examinations are normal. Electrocardiogram reveals a sinus bradycardia, and oximetry shows an oxygen saturation of 88%. Which of the following is the most appropriate next step in the management of this patient?

a. MRI of the head
b. Airway intubation
c. Intravenous fluids
d. CT scan of the head
e. Chest tube insertion
f. Intravenous naloxone
g. Repeat GCS in one hour

8. A 59-year-old patient presents with fever and agitation. On physical examination, his temperature is 39.5°C (103.2°F). His respirations are 26 breaths per minute, pulse is 126 beats per minute, and blood pressure is 100/70 mmHg. He appears warm and flushed. A Swan-Ganz catheter is inserted that demonstrates increased cardiac output, decreased peripheral vascular resistance, and normal pulmonary capillary wedge pressure (PCWP). The patient's urine Gram stain reveals pyuria and gram-negative rods. Which of the following is the most likely diagnosis?

a. Late septic shock
b. Early septic shock
c. Cardiogenic shock
d. Hypovolemic shock
e. Neurogenic shock

9. A 23-year-old medical student presents with the chief complaint of palpitations while playing basketball. The episode lasted 15 minutes. He denies dizziness, syncope, chest pain, and shortness of breath. He admits to a sedentary lifestyle but tries to eat three healthy meals per day. He is adopted, and a family history of heart disease is unknown. Physical examination is remarkable for a *reverse* pulsus paradoxus. Which of the following is the most likely diagnosis?

a. Hypertrophic cardiomyopathy
b. Pulmonary embolism
c. Right ventricular failure
d. Right ventricular infarction
e. Atrial septal defect
f. Aortic regurgitation

10. An 11-year-old girl with cystic fibrosis presents to her pediatrician with the chief complaint of weakness. Her mother states that the child has been lethargic and has lost 6 lb over a period of two weeks. Her bowel movements have increased and are foul smelling. Physical examination reveals a cachectic child. Abdominal examination is normal. Laboratory results reveal a prolonged prothrombin time (PT). Which of the following in the most likely cause of these findings?

a. Pseudocyst
b. Malabsorption
c. Iron-deficiency anemia
d. Underlying malignancy
e. *Pseudomonas* abscess
f. Phlegmon

11. A 39-year-old man is the recipient of a lung transplant for primary pulmonary hypertension. He was extubated soon after surgery, and his hospital course was unremarkable. On discharge, his lung and heart exams are normal. His triceps skinfold measurement is in the fiftieth percentile, and his body mass index (BMI) is 23 kg/m^2. He is discharged on cyclosporine. Which of the following is the most appropriate diet for this patient?

a. Regular diet
b. Low-calorie diet
c. Low-salt diet
d. Low-carbohydrate diet
e. Low-potassium, low-fat diet
f. Low-fat, low-calorie, low-sodium diet

12. A 47-year-old woman is referred to your office for two consecutive blood pressure readings of 139/89 mmHg. She has no complaints, and physical examination is normal. Which of the following best describes her stage of hypertension?

a. Stage 1 hypertension
b. Stage 2 hypertension
c. Stage 3 hypertension
d. Stage 4 hypertension
e. Prehypertension
f. High normal blood pressure
g. Normal blood pressure

13. A woman with a history of left mastectomy and subsequent radiation therapy for breast cancer two years ago presents with a 3-cm mass along the edge of the surgical suture line. She denies fever, chills, night sweats, and weight loss. Physical examination reveals some generalized induration and a tanned appearance of the skin overlying the mastectomy secondary to radiation therapy. There is a nonmobile nontender mass along the suture line that is not warm or fluctuant. She has no axillary lymphadenopathy. A biopsy specimen of the breast mass is most likely to show which of the following?

a. Fibroadenoma
b. Malignancy
c. Benign cyst
d. Abscess
e. Lipoma

14. A 52-year-old man is 48 hours post-laryngectomy for malignancy. On physical examination, he has inflammation around the surgical incision, which prevents him from swallowing easily. He has no abdominal pain, nausea, vomiting, or diarrhea. Abdominal examination reveals normal bowel sounds and no tenderness. Which of the following is the most appropriate method of feeding this patient?

a. Enteral formula nutrition
b. Pureed soft food diet
c. Total parenteral nutrition
d. Intravenous dextrose
e. Peripheral alimentation

15. A 67-year-old woman presents to your office complaining of "losing her taste buds." She cooks with table salt and adds it to meals but has difficulty tasting the salt. On physical examination, her tongue is normal in size, consistency, and color. The patient fails to sense stimulation of the anterior two-thirds of the tongue with sugar or salt. Bitter and sour taste sensations are intact. Which of the following cranial nerves is most likely responsible for the lack of sensation?

a. Ophthalmic branch of the trigeminal nerve
b. Vagus nerve
c. Facial nerve
d. Maxillary branch of the maxillary nerve
e. Mandibular branch of the trigeminal nerve

16. A 39-year-old man with a 12-year history of human immunodeficiency virus (HIV) presents with 3+ pitting edema of the lower extremities. He denies fever, polyuria, frequency, nocturia, and hematuria. He does not drink alcohol, smoke cigarettes, or use illicit drugs. He has no past medical history of hypertension or diabetes mellitus. He is compliant with his HIV medication. Blood pressure is 120/80 mmHg; heart, lung, and abdominal examinations are normal. Serum albumin is 2.8 mg/dL (normal = 3.5 to 5.7 mg/dL), and 24-hour urine protein is 3800 mg/dL (normal < 150 mg/dL). The patient has significantly elevated lipid (predominantly LDL) levels. Which of the following is the most likely cause for the lipid abnormalities?

a. A defect in the LDL receptor resulting in an increase in lipid levels
b. A defect in the VLDL receptor resulting in an increase in lipid levels
c. Increased lipoprotein clearance of lipids from the blood by lipoprotein lipase
d. Decreased lipoprotein clearance of lipids from the blood by lipoprotein lipase
e. Decreased hepatic synthesis of proteins

17. A 45-year-old woman presents to the emergency room with altered mental status. On physical examination, her temperature is 38.9°C (102°F), pulse is 120 beats per minute, and respirations are 24 breaths per minute. She has increased fremitus and bronchial breath sounds at the left base. Neurologic exam reveals no focal deficits, but the patient is disoriented to place and time. Chest radiograph confirms the diagnosis of pneumonia. The patient's $PaCO_2$ is 30 mmHg. Which of the following best categorizes this patient's illness?

a. The patient has bacteremia
b. The patient has systemic inflammatory response syndrome (SIRS)
c. The patient has sepsis
d. The patient has severe sepsis
e. The patient has septic shock
f. The patient has sepsis-induced hypotension
g. The patient has multiple organ dysfunction syndrome (MODS)

18. A 56-year-old woman complains of a 10-lb weight loss over a two-month period. She has generalized malaise and anorexia. She does not smoke cigarettes or drink alcohol. She has no past medical history and takes no medications. Three years ago, her colonoscopy, mammogram, and Papanicolaou smear were negative. Physical examination reveals a temperature of 38°C (100.4°F). Heart, lung, and abdominal examinations are normal. A 2-cm fixed, hard, nontender node is palpable in the right supraclavicular area. Which of the following is the most appropriate next step?

a. Chest radiograph
b. Colonoscopy
c. Mammography
d. CT scan of the chest
e. Papanicolaou smear

19. A 28-year-old woman is brought to the emergency room in a coma. Her respiratory rate is 6 breaths per minute and shallow. Blood pressure is 90/60 mmHg, heart rate is 50 beats per minute, and temperature is 35.5°C (96°F). Her pupils are pinpoint but reactive to light and accommodation. She has no focal neurologic deficits. Which of the following is the most likely diagnosis?

a. Carbon monoxide poisoning
b. Opiate overdose
c. Ethylene glycol poisoning
d. Methanol poisoning
e. Mercury poisoning

20. A 41-year-old man presents to the emergency room complaining of itchiness and difficulty breathing. He states that his symptoms started after attending a party where he ate some fish and peanuts. On physical examination, the patient is anxious, tachypneic, and tachycardic. He has urticaria over his chest, neck, and extremities. Lung examination reveals inspiratory and expiratory wheezes. Heart examination is normal. Which of the following is the most likely diagnosis?

a. Angioedema
b. Exacerbation of asthma
c. Pulmonary embolus
d. Toxic shock syndrome
e. Allergic reaction

21. A 16-year-old student has recurrent episodes of facial swelling without urticaria. Family history reveals that two siblings and both parents have similar symptoms. Which of the following is the most likely diagnosis?

a. Familial C1 inhibitor deficiency
b. Cystic fibrosis
c. Exacerbation of asthma
d. Acquired C1 inhibitor deficiency
e. Serum sickness

22. A 6-year-old girl with spina bifida is admitted to the intensive care unit because of rapidly progressive swelling of her lips, wheezing, and stridor. She had been playing with balloons at a birthday party. Which of the following is the most likely diagnosis?

a. Food anaphylaxis
b. Latex anaphylaxis
c. Severe drug allergy
d. Exercise-related anaphylaxis
e. Idiopathic anaphylaxis

23. A 23-year-old Japanese man attends a party where he drinks three glasses of wine. In a short period of time, he develops facial erythema and experiences severe facial flushing. Which of the following is the most likely diagnosis?

a. Alcohol dehydrogenase deficiency
b. Glucoronyl transferase deficiency
c. Aldehyde dehydrogenase deficiency
d. Angioedema
e. Photosensitivity reaction

24. A 46-year-old man presents to your office because of the recent onset of blackouts. He has no past medical history and admits to smoking cigarettes and drinking beer socially. His blackouts usually occur on weekends, when he is out with his friends relaxing at the neighborhood bar. The patient has recently divorced. Which of the following is the best next diagnostic step for this patient?

a. CAGE questionnaire
b. Liver function tests
c. Percussion of the liver for hepatomegaly
d. Mini–mental status examination (MMSE)
e. Check for macrocytic anemia

25. A 36-year-old woman, accompanied by her attentive husband, presents to the emergency room complaining of right wrist pain. She states that she fell down a flight of stairs and is concerned the wrist may be fractured. On physical examination, the wrist has minimal swelling and is nontender, with a full range of motion. There is a bruise over the right forearm above the wrist, which appears to be several days old. Which of the following is the most likely diagnosis?

a. Recurrent falls
b. Alcohol intoxication
c. Opiate use
d. Benzodiazepam abuse
e. Domestic violence victim

26. A 22-year-old man develops shortness of breath and difficulty breathing while mountain climbing at an altitude of 12,000 ft. His temperature is 36.1°C (97°F). He has a blood pressure of 120/80 mmHg, respirations of 24 breaths per minute, and a heart rate of 114 beats per minute. He has retinal hemorrhages on funduscopy exam. He has no heart murmur. Bilateral crackles are audible on lung examination. Which of the following is the most likely diagnosis?

a. Carbon monoxide poisoning
b. Acute mountain sickness
c. Hypothermia
d. Exhaustion
e. Dehydration

27. A 47-year-old man admits that he has a problem with cigarettes. He is committed to stopping smoking and has come to your office to seek help. Which of the following best describes the stage of behavior change in this addicted patient?

a. Precontemplation
b. Contemplation
c. Preparation
d. Action
e. Maintenance
f. Termination

28. A 17-year-old high school student presents to your office with a six-month history of menstrual irregularities. She has no past medical history and does not smoke cigarettes, drink alcohol, or use illicit drugs. She is not sexually active. Her menarche was at the age of 12 years. The patient is 66 in. tall and has weighed 115 lb for nearly three years. Mouth examination reveals dental enamel erosion. She has enlarged parotid glands bilaterally. Examination of the extremities reveals scars on the dorsal surfaces of the hands. Which of the following is the most likely diagnosis?

a. Bulimia
b. Premature menopause
c. Substance dependence
d. Anorexia nervosa
e. Personality disorder

29. A 71-year-old man with end-stage renal disease secondary to hypertension presents for his dialysis session complaining of "funny fingernails" for several months. Physical examination reveals left unilateral clubbing of the fingers. Clubbing of the right fingers and right and left toes is absent. Lovibond's angle of each left digit is greater than 180°. Schamroth's sign was not attempted. Which of the following best explains the etiology of the unilateral clubbing?

a. Aneurysm of the aorta
b. Aneurysm of the subclavian artery
c. Aneurysm of the innominate artery
d. Congenital heart disease
e. Bacterial endocarditis
f. Arteriovenous fistula
g. Hodgkin's disease

30. A 41-year-old woman is brought to the emergency room after sustaining a burn in a house fire. She shows some evidence of smoke inhalation but is improving with oxygen. Her heart and lung examinations are normal. Her left arm has a 12-cm burn that extends to the papillary layer of the dermis. Which of the following best describes the degree of the burn?

a. First-degree burn
b. Second-degree burn
c. Third-degree burn
d. Fourth-degree burn

31. Paramedics bring a 41-year-old man to the emergency room. He is complaining of headache, dizziness, nausea, and abdominal pain. The paramedics state that the patient's apartment has a coal furnace. His blood pressure is 110/70 mmHg, respirations are 20 breaths per minute, and pulse is 100 beats per minute. The patient has a cherry red appearance most noticeable around the lips and nail beds. Neurologic examination reveals a disoriented and confused man without focal deficits. Oxygen saturation by pulse oximetry is normal. Which of the following is the most likely diagnosis?

a. Drug overdose
b. Carbon monoxide poisoning
c. Alcohol intoxication
d. Methemoglobinemia
e. Dysbarism

32. A 34-year-old woman presents with left-sided chest pain for eight months. She describes the pain as sharp, intermittent, and associated with palpitations, dizziness, trembling, nausea, paresthesias, and diaphoresis. She experiences three episodes per week. The episodes last 15 minutes each and may occur at rest or with exertion. The episodes are unpredictable, and the patient often feels as if she is going to die because of the chest pain. The patient does not smoke cigarettes, drink alcohol, or use drugs. She has no family history of heart disease. Her blood pressure and pulse are normal. Physical examination is normal. Electrocardiogram is normal. Which of the following is the most likely diagnosis?

a. Acute myocardial infarction (AMI)
b. Unstable angina
c. Mitral valve prolapse (MVP)
d. Panic disorder
e. Malingering
f. Hyperthyroidism
g. Posttraumatic stress disorder (PTSD)

33. A 61-year-old man presents to a New York City emergency room in the summertime with a three-day history of fever, malaise, sore throat, nausea, and vomiting. While being examined by a medical student, the patient becomes lethargic, then convulses, requiring intravenous benzodiazepam administration. Physical examination is remarkable for a temperature of 38.3°C (101.0°F). There is bilateral papilledema and neck stiffness. Deep tendon reflexes are exaggerated, and spastic paralysis is evident. Which of the following is the most likely diagnosis?

a. Mollaret's meningitis
b. Neurosyphilis
c. Herpes simplex virus
d. Cerebrovascular accident
e. Brain abscess
f. West Nile virus
g. Heatstroke

34. A 51-year-old homeless man presents to the emergency room in winter complaining of numbness of his feet. Physical examination of the feet reveals erythema, edema, and the presence of several clear blisters. Peripheral pulses are palpable. Which of the following is the most likely diagnosis?

a. Frostnip
b. First-degree frostbite injury
c. Second-degree frostbite injury
d. Third-degree frostbite injury
e. Fourth-degree frostbite injury

35. A 66-year-old nursing home resident was recently started on haloperidol for behavioral problems. One week later, the patient develops a temperature of 40.3°C (104.5°F) and is transferred to the hospital. The patient is awake but not responsive. His heart rate is 110 beats per minute, his respiratory rate is 24 breaths per minute, and he is diaphoretic. Neurologic examination reveals a rigid muscle tone and catatonia. Which of the following is the most likely diagnosis?

a. Tardive dyskinesia
b. Neuroleptic malignant syndrome
c. Acute schizophrenia
d. Dystonic reaction
e. Drug-induced parkinsonism

DIRECTIONS: Each group of questions below consists of lettered options followed by a set of numbered items. For each numbered item, select the **one** lettered option with which it is **most** closely associated. Each lettered option may be used once, more than once, or not at all.

Questions 36–37

For each patient with an allergic reaction, select the most likely type of allergic reaction.

a. Type I allergic reaction
b. Type II allergic reaction
c. Type III allergic reaction
d. Type IV allergic reaction

36. A 26-year-old graduate student presents with a photosensitive cutaneous facial rash after starting a two-week course of tetracycline.

37. A 61-year-old woman develops hemolysis and thrombocytopenia after receiving a blood transfusion prior to elective surgery.

Questions 38–41

For each patient with head trauma, select the most likely diagnosis.

a. Cerebellar tonsillar herniation
b. Uncal herniation
c. Basilar skull fracture
d. Subdural hematoma
e. Epidural hematoma
f. Cerebral concussion
g. Postconcussion syndrome
h. Contusion

38. A 49-year-old man presents after a fall from a platform that is 15 ft high. On physical examination, the patient has blood in the soft tissue overlying the left mastoid bone and has cerebrospinal fluid (CSF) otorrhea.

39. A woman survives a motor vehicle accident and is alert, oriented, and neurologically intact on arrival at the emergency room. Within one hour she becomes less arousable, and she expires while being transported to the radiology department for imaging studies.

40. A 9-year-old boy falls off a skateboard and strikes his head. He momentarily loses consciousness but subsequently has no neurological deficit and appears fine. He complains of a slight headache but no dizziness or personality changes.

41. A 55-year-old man is the victim of a mugging in which he was hit on the head repeatedly with a baseball bat. On arrival at the emergency room, his right pupil is dilated and nonreactive. The patient rapidly progresses to coma and expires.

Questions 42–44

For each patient with a specific breath odor, select the most likely etiology.

a. Diabetic ketoacidosis
b. Cyanide poisoning
c. Marijuana use
d. Mercaptan poisoning
e. Arsenic poisoning
f. Naphthalene ingestion

42. A 30-year-old man presents to the emergency room with headache, dizziness, abdominal pain, nausea, vomiting, and confusion. The odor of bitter almonds is detected on his breath. Venous oxygen saturation is more than 90%.

43. A 19-year-old college student is brought to the emergency room by ambulance. She has no past medical history and takes no medications. She does not smoke cigarettes, drink alcohol, or use illicit drugs. She is unresponsive and hyperpneic. Her breath has a fruity odor.

44. A 44-year-old factory worker presents with a 12-hour history of abdominal pain, vomiting, watery diarrhea, and muscle cramps. An odor of garlic is detected on his breath. He has diminished vibration sensation of the lower extremities.

Questions 45–47

For each patient with an abnormal level of consciousness, select the most appropriate description of the level of consciousness.

a. Confusion
b. Lethargy
c. Delirium
d. Stupor
e. Decorticate
f. Decerebrate

45. A 67-year-old man, who has recently been resuscitated after a motor vehicle accident, is arousable for short periods of time to visual, verbal, or painful stimuli. He responds by moving slowly or by moaning.

46. A 73-year-old woman is admitted to the cardiac unit for elective placement of a pacemaker. While in the hospital, she becomes confused and experiences hallucinations. She has a diminished attention span, is anxious, and reacts inappropriately to stimuli.

47. A patient with urosepsis presents drowsy and falls asleep several times during physical examination. Once aroused, the patient is cooperative and responds to questions and commands appropriately.

General Principles of Disease

Answers

1. The answer is d. (*Tierney, pp 1361–1363.*) The postal worker from New Jersey is presenting with symptoms most consistent with **inhalation anthrax.** Sentinel clues include chest pain, shortness of breath, malaise, headache, fever, dry cough, abdominal pain, and nausea. Chest radiograph may show a **widened mediastinum** (mediastinitis) and pleural effusions (thoracentesis will show these to be hemorrhagic). This presentation rapidly leads to sepsis, shock, and respiratory failure. Although anthrax was previously rare except among high-risk groups such as farmers, tannery workers, wool workers, and veterinarians, bioterroristic use has resulted in cases. Patients with **pneumonic plague** present with mucopurulent sputum, chest pain, and hemoptysis. **Tularemia** is a gram-negative coccobacillus that causes pneumonia accompanied by bilateral hilar adenopathy. Patients with hemorrhagic fever present with generalized mucous membrane hemorrhage and evidence of pulmonary, renal, neurologic, and hematopoietic dysfunction. **Hantavirus** is a rodent-borne RNA virus more common in the southwestern United States; patients present in a shocklike state with thrombocytopenia and leukocytosis.

2. The answer is b. (*Tierney, p 1362.*) Fever, regional adenopathy, and a painless ulcer covered by a black eschar and surrounded by extensive non-pitting edema is a presentation most consistent with **cutaneous anthrax.** Patients with **leprosy** present with pale, anesthetic, and erythematous macular or nodular skin lesions. **Cat-scratch disease** is an acute infection of children and young adults transmitted by cats through a scratch or bite. Patients develop a papule or ulcer at the site of the inoculation and weeks later develop fever, malaise, headache, and regional lymphadenopathy. Patients with **smallpox** present with generalized macular or papular-vesicular-pustular eruptions, with the greatest concentration of the rash being on the face and the distal extremities, especially the palms. Although spider bites are rare, the bite of the **brown recluse spider** may cause a severe necrotic reaction and death due to intravascular hemolysis.

3. The answer is c. *(Tierney, pp 1360–1361.)* The patient is presenting with **Listeria,** an intracellular pathogen with a predilection for causing illness in immunocompromised persons, including the elderly. Transmission is food-borne; implicated foods include coleslaws, soft cheeses such as **Mexican cheeses,** pasteurized milk, undercooked hot dogs, and deli meats. Patients typically present with bacteremia and central nervous system (CNS) infection. **Botulism** bacillus is usually found in canned, smoked, or vacuum-packed foods. Patients present with dysphagia, dysphonia, visual disturbances, diplopia, ptosis, and fixed and dilated pupils. Patients with **anthrax** present with cough, dyspnea, and evidence of mediastinitis and pneumonia. Fried rice consumption is associated with *B. cereus* infection; patients present with a noninflammatory diarrhea. *Actinomyces* species are gram-positive organisms that may branch out into bacillary forms. Infection typically follows trauma, such as a **dental extraction.**

4. The answer is e. *(Tierney, pp 1222–1224.)* **Protein-energy malnutrition (PEM)** or **marasmus** results when the body's requirement for calories and protein is not met by the diet. It is characterized by wasting, loss of lean body mass, weight loss, and loss of subcutaneous fat stores. **Kwashiorkor** or severe deficiency of protein is characterized by edema, skin changes, change in hair pigmentation, and hypoalbuminemia. Although the elderly are at risk for hypothyroidism, patients usually present with weight gain. Patients with **zinc deficiency** present with a psoriasiform rash, eczematous scaling, and hypogeusia. Patients with **riboflavin deficiency** present with scrotal dermatosis, photophobia, conjunctival inflammation, glossitis, angular stomatitis, and tongue atrophy.

5. The answer is d. *(Goldman, p 1636.)* Persons with **Marfan's syndrome** have arm spans that are greater than their height and above-average crown-to-heel height. Joints are hyperextensible, and patients have long, spiderlike, slender fingers (**arachnodactyly**). **Steinberg's sign** or the **thumb sign** is positive when the fingers are clenched over the thumb and the thumb protrudes beyond the ulnar margin of the hand. Patients often have a high-arched palate, kyphoscoliosis, subluxation of the lens, and a murmur of mitral valve prolapse. Aortic regurgitation and dissection of the aorta may complicate Marfan's syndrome. Patients with **Lesch-Nyhan syndrome** (X-linked disorder) present with self-mutilation, choreoathetosis, spasticity, gout, and mental retardation. Patients with gonadal dysgenesis or **Turner's syndrome** are 45,X; the syndrome is characterized by primary amenorrhea, short stature, webbed neck with low posterior hairline, and multiple congenital abnormalities. Patients with **Ehlers-Danlos syndrome (EDS)** present with hyperelasticity of the skin ("rubber man" syndrome) and hypermobile joints. **Noonan's syndrome** is an autosomal dominant disorder characterized by webbed neck, short stature, and congenital heart disease. Patients have normal karyotypes and normal gonads.

6. The answer is d. (*Tierney, pp 582–583.*) Patients with a history of previous bowel resection are susceptible to malabsorption of the essential nutrients. Ileal resections cause deficiency in bile salts, which are essential for the absorption of the fat-soluble vitamins (**A, D, E, and K**). Since the vitamin B_{12}–intrinsic factor complex is absorbed in the ileum, vitamin B_{12} must be replaced in patients with terminal ileum resection. The patient in the question presents with symptoms consistent with **vitamin B_{12} deficiency.** Other signs of vitamin B_{12} deficiency include megaloblastic anemia, altered cerebral function, neuropsychiatric changes, and difficulty with balance (posterior columns). Patients with **vitamin A deficiency** present with night blindness, keratomalacia, scaling of the skin, increased intracranial pressure, and depressed immunity. **Osteomalacia** and **rickets** are a result of vitamin D deficiency. **Vitamin E deficiency** is rare; patients may present with neuropathy, ophthalmoplegia, and ataxia; hemolysis may occur in infants. Clotting times are prolonged in patients with vitamin K deficiency.

7. The answer is b. (*Seidel, p 93.*) The best next step in the management of this patient is intubation. She has a respiratory rate of 6 breaths per minute and a pulse oximetry reading of less than 90% (**90% correlates with a P_{O_2} of 60 mmHg**). Although intravenous fluids might be given, her blood pressure and heart rate appear stable. Her pupils are not constricted, and naloxone for opiate overdose is probably not indicated. A CT scan of the head should be done in the future after vital signs (including airway and breathing) have been stabilized. MRI of the head detects structural lesions of the brain and is rarely used to evaluate head trauma. Chest tube placement is not indicated in a patient with bilateral breath sounds. The **Glasgow Coma Scale (GCS)** is often used to quantify consciousness and assess cerebral cortex and brainstem function by assessing the patient's verbal response, motor response, and eye opening response to stimuli. It may be repeated at intervals to detect improvement or deterioration and is now widely used in coma assessment. The minimum score is 3 and the maximum score is 15. Three behaviors are assessed in the GCS:

Eye Opening Response	Verbal Response	Motor Response
4 = Spontaneous	5 = Oriented	6 = Obeys commands
3 = To verbal stimuli	4 = Confused	5 = Localizes pain
2 = To pain	3 = Inappropriate words	4 = Withdraws from pain
1 = None	2 = Incoherent	3 = Flexion to pain or decorticate
	1 = None	2 = Extension to pain or decerebrate
		1 = None

8. The answer is b. *(Tierney, pp 460–462.)* The **early phase of septic shock** is characterized by vasodilation resulting in a warm, flushed patient with a normal or elevated cardiac output (CO). Despite the elevation in CO, however, cardiac function is remarkably abnormal. Fever, agitation, or confusion is often present. In **late septic shock,** patients become obtunded with decreased cardiac output and hypotension that is not reversible by volume replacement. Patients with **cardiogenic shock** have signs of pulmonary vascular congestion (jugular venous distention, S_3 gallop, bilateral lung crackles), increased PCWP, and decreased cardiac output. **Neurogenic shock** follows a spinal cord injury (warm skin, bradycardia, neurologic deficits), and **hypovolemic shock** is characterized by a physical examination consistent with volume depletion (tachycardia; hypotension; cool, clammy skin; poor capillary refill) and decreased PCWP. A mnemonic to remember the causes of shock is **SHOCK: S**epsis, **H**ypovolemia, **O**ther (i.e., Addison's disease), **C**NS (neurogenic), and **K**ardiac causes.

9. The answer is a. *(Tierney, p 390.)* An increase in systolic blood pressure that coincides with inspiration rather than expiration is called a **reverse pulsus paradoxus.** Normally, inspiration causes a decrease in intrathoracic pressure and an increase in venous return to the right ventricle with a decrease in venous return to the left ventricle (due to pooling of blood in the pulmonary bed and a leftward shift of the septum into the left ventricle). This smaller left ventricular end-diastolic volume results in a lower stroke volume and a lower systolic blood pressure. If this drop is severe enough (>20 mmHg), the patient is said to have a **pulsus paradoxus.** This may be seen in constrictive pericarditis, lung disease, pulmonary embolism, shock, right ventricular infarction, and right ventricular failure. A **reverse pulsus paradoxus** occurs when a stiff ventricle is unable to fill adequately. This is typical of **hypertrophic obstructive cardiomyopathy.**

10. The answer is b. *(Tierney, pp 241–243.)* Patients with **cystic fibrosis** are at risk for developing various nutritional deficiencies due to malabsorption. These may include deficiencies of both the **fat-soluble** vitamins **(A, D, E, K)** and the **water-soluble** vitamins **(B_6 and B_{12}).** B_{12} deficiency occurs because pancreatic enzymes are not available to cleave R-protein and assist in B_{12} absorption. Patients with cystic fibrosis have high caloric, protein, and fat requirements. Vitamin therapy and appropriate enzyme therapy are needed to prevent nutritional complications.

11. The answer is e. *(Tierney, p 1220.)* The **triceps skinfold (TSF) measurement** is performed with a caliper that measures the thickness of the skin and fat at the middle of the nondominant arm over the triceps muscle. It represents the amount of calories stored as subcutaneous fat. A TSF measurement greater than the ninety-fifth percentile implies obesity. Patients who are post-transplantation require increased high-protein and high-calorie diets (regardless of TSF or BMI) to replete stores and to assist with wound healing during the catabolic state following surgery. Patients taking **cyclosporine** are susceptible to hyperkalemia, hypertriglyceridemia, and hypercholesterolemia. Dietary intake of potassium, saturated fats, and cholesterol should be limited. Assessment of **body mass index (BMI)** [weight in kg divided by height in m^2 or weight in pounds divided by (height in inches)^2 × 703.1] is useful in assessing both over- and undernutrition. It is a useful measure to predict the risk of certain diseases associated with obesity. For example, non-insulin-dependent diabetes mellitus (NIDDM) is rare in persons with a BMI below 22 kg/m^2.

Normal BMI is defined as 18.5 to 24.9 kg/m^2.
Overweight is a BMI of 25 to 29.9 kg/m^2.
Obesity is a BMI of 30 to 39.9 kg/m^2.

Morbid obesity is a BMI of more than 40 kg/m^2.
Mild malnutrition is defined as a BMI of 17 to 18.4 kg/m^2.
Moderate malnutrition is a BMI of 16 to 16.9 kg/m^2.
Severe malnutrition is a BMI of less than 16.0 kg/m^2.

12. The answer is e. *(Tierney, p 405.)* The classification of blood pressure is based on the average of two or more readings.

Category of BP	Systolic Blood Pressure (mmHg)	Diastolic Blood Pressure (mmHg)
Normal	<120	<80
Prehypertension	120–139	80–89
Stage 1	140–159	90–99
Stage 2	≥160	≥100

13. The answer is b. *(Tierney, pp 674–677.)* **Fibroadenomas** are the most common benign neoplasms of the breast. They are well demarcated, rubbery, mobile, and nontender. **Benign cysts** are the most common cause of breast lumps and tend to occur in association with other cysts. They are round, mobile, and soft, with a cystic consistency. They are tender premenstrually, become smaller immediately after menses, and regress after menopause. **Breast abscesses** are localized and are tender, swollen, erythematous, and fluctuant. **Malignant lesions** are painless, irregular in contour and shape, hard, nonmobile, and not well demarcated.

14. The answer is a. *(Tierney, pp 1237–1238.)* The indications for **enteral tube feeding** include poor appetite or anorexia, inability to ingest food due to dysphagia or injury to the head and neck, gastroparesis, and maldigestion. This patient has a clear indication for tube feeding. **Peripheral parenteral nutrition** (**PPN**) is reserved for patients who require short-term parenteral nutrition and are not hypermetabolic or fluid restricted. PPN patients must have suitable peripheral venous access. **Central total parenteral nutrition** (**TPN**) is indicated in patients with poor peripheral venous access or in those who require long-term nutrition (>7 days).

15. The answer is c. *(Seidel, pp 784–787.)* The **facial nerve** (**cranial nerve VII**) mediates taste (salty and sweet) on the anterior two-thirds of the tongue. The **glossopharyngeal nerve** (**cranial nerve IX**) mediates taste (bitter and sour) on the posterior one-third of the tongue.

16. The answer is d. *(Tierney, pp 891–893.)* The patient with edema, proteinuria, hypoalbuminemia, and hyperlipidemia has **nephrotic syndrome** secondary to HIV disease. Hyperlipidemia occurs because of increased hepatic protein synthesis and reduced lipoprotein clearance from the blood by lipoprotein lipase. Patients have elevations of low-density lipoprotein (LDL), very-low-density lipoprotein (VLDL), and triglycerides (TGL). High-density lipoprotein (HDL) may be normal or decreased. Dietary cholesterol should be limited in these patients (<300 mg/day); pharmacological therapy is often required. The **severity of edema** is characterized by a grading system, which is as follows:

1+: slight pitting edema (2 mm deep) with no distortion on release of finger

2+: a 4-mm-deep pit whose detectable distortion disappears in 10 to 15 seconds

3+: a 6-mm-deep pit that lasts more than 1 minute on release of finger

4+: an 8-mm-deep pit that lasts 2 to 5 minute on release of finger

17. The answer is d. *(Goldman, p 624.)* **Bacteremia** is the presence of bacteria in blood culture bottles. **SIRS** is not a diagnosis but a response to a variety of clinical situations (i.e., infection, burns, trauma, pancreatitis) and is characterized by two or more of the following: (1) temperature higher than 38°C (>100.5°F) or less than 36.1°C (<97°F), (2) heart rate more than 90 beats per minute, (3) respiratory rate more than 20 breaths per minute, (4) $PaCO_2$ of less than 32 mmHg, (5) white blood cell count of more than 12,000/μL or less than 4000/μL or more than 10% immature (band) forms. **Sepsis** is a systemic response to infection manifested by two of the five described conditions of SIRS. **Severe sepsis** is sepsis associated with organ dysfunction, hypoperfusion, or hypotension (i.e., lactic acidosis, oliguria, altered mental status). **Septic shock** is sepsis-induced hypotension despite adequate fluid resuscitation. **Sepsis-induced hypotension** is a systolic blood pressure of more than 90 mmHg or a reduction of less than 40 mmHg from baseline in the absence of other causes to explain the hypotension. **MODS** is the presence of organ dysfunction in an acutely ill patient such that homeostasis cannot be maintained without intervention.

18. The answer is c. *(Tierney, p 578.)* The finding of a palpable supraclavicular node, whether right or left, may indicate metastatic involvement due to ipsilateral breast or lung cancers. Additionally, if located on the left side, a palpable supraclavicular node may also represent intraabdominal or intrapelvic malignancies (**Trosier's node**). A large left supraclavicular node representing metastasis from a gastric carcinoma is specifically referred to as **Virchow's node**. In this patient, the best next step would be to order a mammogram, since her last study was three years ago.

19. The answer is b. (*Goldman, p 632.*) **Accidental overdose** of opiates may occur in drug addicts; patients present with pinpoint pupils, hypothermia, bradycardia, hypotension, and shallow breathing. Treatment involves the immediate reversal of the opiates with **naloxone.** During withdrawal, patients experience yawning, diaphoresis, rhinorrhea, restlessness, anxiety, muscular twitching, vomiting, diarrhea, hypertension, tachycardia, and tachypnea. **Methanol** (methyl alcohol or wood alcohol) is found in "moonshine"; patients present with blindness. **Ethylene glycol** is found in antifreeze; ingestion leads to seizures and coma. Patients develop oxalate crystals in the urine, and deposition may result in renal failure. Both methanol and ethylene glycol overdoses are treated with ethanol to prevent the formation of formic acid (toxic). Patients with **carbon monoxide** poisoning appear cherry red but are hypoxemic. Patients with poisoning due to **mercury** (found in thermometers, dental amalgams, and batteries) develop acrodynia (pink disease due to flushing and desquamation) and neurologic, gastrointestinal, and renal problems.

20. The answer is e. (*Tierney, p 767.*) **Anaphylaxis** may occur several minutes after the introduction of a specific antigen; presenting symptoms may include pruritus, urticaria, angioedema, abdominal pain, nausea, vomiting, diarrhea, respiratory distress, and shock. This life-threatening emergency requires immediate treatment with epinephrine (for α- and β-adrenergic effects resulting in vasoconstriction), antihistamines, β agonist inhaled treatments for bronchospasm, oxygen, steroids, and vascular and ventilatory support when needed. **Angioedema** may appear, with or without urticaria, and occurs at the mucosal surfaces of the upper respiratory tract. It is characterized by a nonpitting edema of the subcutaneous tissues, and patients are at risk for death due to airway obstruction from laryngeal edema.

21. The answer is a. (*Tierney, pp 767–769.*) **Hereditary angioedema** is an autosomal dominant disease due to a deficiency of **C1 inhibitor** (**C1INH**). The family history and the lack of urticaria suggest the diagnosis. Acquired C1 inhibitor deficiency has the same clinical manifestations as the inherited form but is associated with lymphoproliferative disorders and lacks the family history. **Serum sickness** is due to the deposition of drug-antibody complexes causing complement activation and subsequent urticaria, arthralgias, lymphadenopathy, glomerulonephritis, and cerebritis. **Most cases of serum sickness are due to penicillin.** Asthma and cystic fibrosis are not associated with facial swelling.

22. The answer is b. *(Goldman, p 1617.)* **Latex anaphylaxis** occurs in patients with spina bifida or congenital urologic defects who have undergone repetitive surgeries. Other groups at risk include employees of rubber manufacturers and health care workers. The diagnosis is confirmed by skin-prick testing for IgE to latex or by radioallergosorbent test (RAST) assay. Patients with latex-induced anaphylaxis must avoid latex during surgical procedures and live in a latex-free environment.

23. The answer is c. *(Tierney, p 1052.)* Fifty percent of Chinese and Japanese people lack **aldehyde dehydrogenase (ALDH)** and develop facial flushing and erythema after ingestion of alcohol. The lack of this enzyme results in accumulation of acetaldehyde after ingestion of alcohol.

24. The answer is a. *(Tierney, pp 17–19.)* Although liver function tests (LFTs), macrocytic red blood cell changes, and hepatomegaly are good tests for establishing whether the patient has complications of alcoholism, the **CAGE questionnaire** is the best screening tool for alcohol dependence. If patients respond "yes" to more than one question, alcoholism is likely. There are four CAGE questions:

1. Have you felt the need to **C**ut down on your drinking?
2. Have you ever felt **A**nnoyed by criticisms of your drinking?
3. Have you ever felt **G**uilty about your drinking?
4. Have you ever needed an **E**ye-opener in the morning?

25. The answer is e. *(Tierney, pp 16–17.)* The patient most likely is a victim of **domestic violence.** Patients may present to a physician with a poorly explained injury, an obvious injury, or a subtle, pain-related complaint (headache, chest pain, or abdominal pain). One in five patients presenting to a primary care practice is involved in a relationship where abuse exists, and all physicians should screen for this problem. The **SAFE questionnaire** may be used to screen for domestic violence:

S = Do you feel **S**afe or **S**tressed in a relationship?
A = Have you ever been **A**bused or **A**fraid in a relationship?
F = Are your **F**riends and **F**amily aware of your relationship problem?
E = Do you have an **E**mergency plan if needed?

26. The answer is b. *(Goldman, p 545.)* **High-altitude sickness** can occur at altitudes greater than 9500 ft, and mountain climbers at extreme altitudes (over 18,000 ft) are susceptible to hypoxemia and physiologic deterioration. Allowing sufficient time to acclimate and avoiding rapid ascent may prevent **acute mountain sickness (AMS)**. AMS is characterized by headache, breathlessness, nausea, vomiting, weakness, and lassitude, but may progress to ataxia, altered mental status, pulmonary edema, cerebral edema, and coma. Funduscopy examination may reveal retinal hemorrhages and venous tortuosity. Descent is the definitive treatment for all forms of AMS. **Hypothermia** is defined as core body temperature of less than 35°C (95°F).

27. The answer is c. *(Goldman, p 60.)* There are **six stages of behavior change in addicted personalities:**

1. Precontemplation = denies problem; no intention of changing
2. Contemplation = acknowledges problem; seriously thinks about solving it
3. Preparation = committed to action; needs to plan
4. Action = modifies behavior and surroundings
5. Maintenance = at risk for relapse if not committed to following through with changes
6. Termination = no continuing effort needed; addiction no longer a threat

28. The answer is a. *(Tierney, pp 1227–1229.)* The patient most likely has **bulimia** (more common than anorexia nervosa). Patients typically maintain their body weight by induced vomiting or the use of laxatives or diuretics. Patients present with dental enamel erosion, excessive dental caries, parotid enlargement, and scars on the dorsal surfaces of the hands from inducing vomiting. Electrolytes may reveal abnormalities from chronic use of laxatives, diuretics, and enemas. Patients with **anorexia nervosa** present below their ideal body weight. Characteristics of anorexia nervosa include cold intolerance, emaciated appearance, hypothermia, hypotension, and bradycardia. Irregularities in the menstrual cycle may be a presenting sign in both bulimia and anorexia nervosa.

29. The answer is f. (*Seidel, p 189.*) The causes of **unilateral clubbing** include aneurysm of the aorta, innominate artery, or subclavian artery; Pancoast's tumor; and placement of an arteriovenous fistula for dialysis. The causes of **bilateral clubbing** may be intrathoracic (bronchogenic carcinoma, metastatic lung cancer, Hodgkin's disease, mesothelioma, bronchiectasis, empyema, lung abscess, cystic fibrosis, pulmonary interstitial fibrosis, pneumoconiosis), cardiovascular (congenital cyanotic heart disease, subacute bacterial endocarditis), or gastrointestinal (cirrhosis, inflammatory bowel disease, carcinoma of the colon or esophagus). **Schamroth's sign** is a maneuver to confirm the loss of the subungual angle in patients with bilateral clubbing. When the terminal phalanges of paired digits are juxtaposed, the diamond-shaped window that is normally present disappears with clubbing. Lovibond's angle (between the base of the nail and its surrounding skin) is greater than 180° in patients with clubbing (<180° is normal).

30. The answer is b. (*Tierney, p 1546.*) A first-degree burn involves the epidermis. **Second-degree burns** may be superficial (papillary layer) partial thickness and deep (reticular layer) partial thickness. **Third-degree burns** are full-thickness burns that involve the entire thickness of the skin. **Fourth-degree burns** extend through the skin to subcutaneous fat, muscle, and bone. The **rule of 9's** is often used to calculate burn surface area in adults: 9% for each arm and the head and 18% for each leg and each side of the torso.

31. The answer is b. (*Tierney, p 1572.*) Gasoline engines, paint removers, and the incomplete combustion of wood, coal, or natural gas produce **carbon monoxide** (**CO**), which binds preferentially to hemoglobin and decreases the release of oxygen to tissues. It is especially important to exclude this poisoning in the winter because of the furnaces used in heating. Patients develop a cherry red appearance, headache, dizziness, confusion, visual field defects, blindness, nausea, abdominal pain, syncope, chest pain, heart arrhythmias, seizures, and coma. Pulse oximetry reveals a falsely elevated saturation; therefore, the diagnosis must be confirmed by determining the actual carboxyhemoglobin fraction in an arterial blood gas. **Methemoglobinemia** (from chemicals, antimalarials, and sulfonamides) results in **cyanosis that is unresponsive to oxygen.** Patients have **chocolate-colored blood,** a gray appearance, and a falsely normal saturation.

32. The answer is d. *(Tierney, p 1013.)* The patient has no risk factors for coronary artery disease, such as family history or tobacco or cocaine use, and her ECG is normal. Hyperthyroidism is unlikely without tachycardia and other physical examination findings. A click and murmur are often found on heart auscultation in patients with MVP. The patient has no previous traumatic event in her life to have caused PTSD. The patient has symptomatology consistent with **panic disorder.** Four of five criteria are needed for the diagnosis of panic disorder: **PANIC** = **P**alpitations; **A**bdominal pain; **N**ausea; **I**ncreased perspiration; and **C**hest pain, **C**hills, or **C**hoking.

33. The answer is f. *(Tierney, pp 1324–1325.)* Identified in 1999, the **West Nile virus** is an arbovirus (anthropod-borne agent) that causes malaise, lethargy, sore throat, stiff neck, nausea, and vomiting. It progresses to stupor, convulsions, cranial nerve palsies, paralysis of extremities, and exaggerated deep tendon reflexes (signs of upper motor neuron disease). Specific antiviral therapy is not available for West Nile virus infection, and prognosis is almost always guarded. **Neurosyphilis** has a progressive course and patients may present with signs of a chronic meningitis (headache, irritability, unequal reflexes, and irregular pupils) or **tabes dorsalis** (hyporeflexia, hypotonia, and impairment of proprioception and vibration sense). Patients with heatstroke typically have core body temperatures above 40.5°C (105°F). **Mollaret's meningitis** is a benign recurrent lymphocytic meningitis. **Herpes simplex virus** has been implicated as a major cause of Mollaret's meningitis; it is associated with headache, flulike symptoms, behavioral and speech disturbances, and seizures (often, temporal lobe). Patients with brain abscesses and cerebrovascular accidents typically present with more focal findings.

34. The answer is c. *(Tierney, p 1542.)* **Frostnip** is a superficial freeze injury that causes no tissue loss. Patients complain of some discomfort, and the involved area is pale; rewarming quickly reverses the symptoms. **First-degree frostbite** is characterized by partial skin freezing, erythema, edema, no blisters, and desquamation several days later. **Second-degree frostbite** is characterized by full-thickness skin freezing, erythema, edema, and the presence of clear blisters. Patients complain of throbbing and numbness. **Third-degree frostbite** injuries are characterized by damage that extends into the subdermal plexis. The skin is blue or gray, and there are hemorrhagic blisters. Patients complain of burning, shooting pains, and the feeling that the involved area feels like a block of wood. Prognosis is poor. **Fourth-degree frostbite** injuries extend into the subcutaneous tissue, muscle, and bone. There is typically no edema, and the skin is mottled and cyanotic; eventually these injuries form a mummified eschar.

35. The answer is b. *(Tierney, pp 1032–1033.)* **Neuroleptic malignant syndrome** is a complication of neuroleptic medications (especially haloperidol). Patients present with hyperthermia, rigidity, catatonia, labile blood pressure, autonomic dysfunction, tachycardia, and tachypnea. It usually occurs within 30 days of starting the neuroleptic drug but may occur at any time during medication use. **Tardive dyskinesia** is a common complication of neuroleptics; patients present with choreoathetoid movements of the face and mouth (lip smacking). **Dystonic reaction** may also complicate neuroleptic use; patients present with torticollis, rigidity of the back muscles, carpopedal spasm, blepharospasm, or chorea. Symptoms usually resolve with anticholinergic medication. **Drug-induced parkinsonism** may be due to dopamine antagonists (i.e., reserpine, phenothiazines, or butyrophenones). Although the etiology for all of these neuroleptic complications is unclear, dopamine antagonism probably plays some role in all of these disorders.

36–37. The answers are 36-d, 37-b. *(Goldman, p 224.)* **Type I allergic reactions** cause urticaria and anaphylaxis and are seen with penicillin, insulin, sulfonamides, morphine, and contrast media. **Type II allergic reactions** are due to transfusions (ABO mismatch) or use of medications (quinidine, heparin, phenacetin, sulfonamides) and typically cause hemolysis, thrombocytopenia, and nephritis. **Type III allergic reactions** are seen with penicillin, propylthiouracil, hydralazine, and procainamide and cause serum sickness. **Type IV allergic reactions** are seen with tetracyclines, nitrofurantoin, neomycin, parabens, and sulfonamides. These medications cause a contact dermatitis, pulmonary fibrosis, photosensitivity, and toxic epidermal necrolysis.

38–41. The answers are 38-c, 39-e, 40-f, 41-b. *(Tierney, pp 988–989.)* Patients with basilar skull fracture may present with **Battle's sign** (subcutaneous blood over the mastoid due to fracture of the petrous bone) and **raccoon eyes** (subcutaneous blood around the eyes due to fractures through the cranial fossa). These fractures are associated with CSF otorrhea and CSF rhinorrhea. Patients with epidural hematoma typically present after a lucid period. These are arterial hemorrhages from tears of the middle meningeal artery from temporal bone fractures, and death occurs if the bleeding is not controlled. **Epidural hematomas** appear as **convEx (Epidural = EE)** hyperdensities on CT scan. **Subdural hematomas (SDHs)** are venous hemorrhages; patients may present with headache, confusion, and hemiparesis. An SDH appears as a **concave** hyperdensity on CT scan. A **concussion** is a temporary impairment of cerebral function without structural cerebral damage. **Postconcussion syndrome** follows a concussion; patients complain of personality changes, dizziness, and headache. A **contusion** is due to bruising of the brain tissue and may be **coup** (at the site of impact) or **contracoup** (at the opposite side of the impact). **Uncal herniation** causes compression of cranial nerve III and results in a blown pupil (dilated and nonreactive). **Cerebellar tonsillar herniation** results in compression of the pons and medulla; patients present with severe hypertension, dizziness, ataxia, drowsiness, weakness, spasticity, and, if left untreated, coma and death.

42–44. The answers are 42-b, 43-a, 44-e. *(Seidel, p 894.)* **Cyanide poisoning** is associated with a **bitter almond** odor, and diabetic acidosis is associated with a **fruity** odor. Hyperpnea refers to respiration, which is deep (increase in tidal volume) as well as rapid (**Kussmaul breathing**). Venous oxygen saturation may be elevated in cyanide poisoning because tissues fail to take up arterial oxygen. **Arsenic ingestion** and **parathion poisoning** are associated with a **garlic** odor. Marijuana odor is that of **burned rope**, and **rotten egg odor** is associated with poisoning due to hydrogen sulfide mercaptans. The odor of **camphor** is associated with ingestion of naphthalene (mothballs).

45–47. The answers are 45-d, 46-c, 47-b. *(Seidel, p 94.)* Stuporous patients are arousable for short periods of time to visual, verbal, or painful stimuli. They often moan or have slow motor movements in response to stimuli. **Delirious** patients are confused and hallucinate. They are anxious and demonstrate motor and sensory excitement. **Lethargic** patients are drowsy and fall asleep easily but, once aroused, respond appropriately. Confused patients have poor memory and decreased attention span and respond inappropriately to questions. Comatose patients are neither aware nor awake. **DecErebrate** patients **Extend (EE)** to painful stimuli, and **decorticate** patients **flex** to painful stimuli.

The Systems

Dermatology

Questions

DIRECTIONS: Each item below contains a question followed by suggested responses. Select the **one best** response to each question.

48. A 10-year-old girl presents with multiple pigmented macules on the vermilion border of her lower lip. The dark brown lesions are 2 to 5 mm in size and are arranged in a cluster. The patient's older brother has similar lesions. The patient complains of recurrent bouts of abdominal pain. Which of the following is the most likely diagnosis?

a. Gardner's syndrome
b. Herpes simplex virus infection
c. Freckles
d. Peutz-Jeghers syndrome
e. Hand-foot-and-mouth disease

49. A 16-year-old student with a history of herpetic gingivostomatitis develops a generalized and symmetric rash. The lesions are 1 to 2 cm in diameter and look like round patches. They consist of two concentric rings surrounding a central disk. The rash is burning and pruritic. A few erosive lesions are visible in the oral mucosa. Which of the following is the most likely diagnosis?

a. Erythema multiforme
b. Secondary syphilis
c. Systemic lupus erythematosus
d. Pemphigus vulgaris
e. Urticaria

50. A 17-year-old patient presents with severe pruritus that is worse at night. On examination of the skin, areas of excoriated papules are observed in the interdigital area. Family members report similar symptoms. Which of the following is the most likely diagnosis?

a. Scabies
b. Cutaneous larva migrans
c. Contact dermatitis
d. Dermatitis herpetiformis
e. Impetigo

51. A 35-year-old woman who had been camping in Wisconsin two weeks ago develops an erythematous rash on her inner thigh. The macular lesion is 10 cm in diameter and has a distinct red border with central clearing. Two days ago, a second, similar lesion developed. The patient reports no fever, chills, or other symptoms. She has no medical problems or allergies and takes no medications. She does not recall any spider or tick bites. The rest of the physical examination is normal. Which of the following is the most likely diagnosis?

a. Brown recluse spider bite
b. *Borrelia burgdorferi* infection
c. *Bartonella henselae* infection
d. *Mycobacterium marinum* infection
e. *Rickettsia rickettsii* infection

52. A 31-year-old man presents to the emergency room three days after undergoing a hernia repair operation. He is febrile and hypotensive. The symptoms began with the sudden onset of a diffuse maculopapular rash that was pruritic and erythematous. Cutaneous examination reveals that the erythroderma involves the palms and soles and is beginning to desquamate. The patient has no other illnesses and takes no medications. Which of the following is the most likely diagnosis?

a. Toxic epidermal necrolysis
b. Toxic shock syndrome
c. Necrotizing fasciitis
d. Scarlet fever
e. Cellulitis

53. A 6-year-old child presents with patchy hair loss on the back of the scalp. Examination reveals well-demarcated areas of erythema and scaling, and although there are still some hairs in the area, they are extremely short and broken in appearance. Which of the following is the most likely diagnosis?

a. Androgenic hair loss
b. Psoriasis of the scalp
c. Seborrheic dermatitis
d. Tinea capitis
e. Carbuncle

54. A 37-year-old man who works in a fish market presents with a burning pain in his right hand for one week. Physical examination reveals a large violaceous plaque on his finger. Gram stain reveals no organism. Which of the following is the most likely diagnosis?

a. Erythrasma
b. Ecthyma
c. Erysipelas
d. Erysipeloid
e. Nummular eczema

55. Five days after going on a nature walk, a 13-year-old boy develops well-demarcated erythematous plaques and vesicles over his arms and face. The plaques are arranged in a linear fashion and are crusting. The boy has some facial edema. He has no history of fever or chills but complains of pruritus. Which of the following is the most likely diagnosis?

a. Rubeola
b. Atopic dermatitis
c. Acute contact dermatitis
d. Impetigo
e. Erythema infectiosum

56. A 6-year-old child presents with flesh-colored papules on the hand that are not pruritic. Examination reveals lesions that are approximately 4 mm in diameter with central umbilication. A halo is seen around those lesions undergoing regression. Which of the following is the most likely diagnosis?

a. Verruca vulgaris
b. Molluscum contagiosum
c. Keratoacanthoma
d. Herpetic whitlow
e. Hemangioma

57. A 42-year-old man presents with blisters and erosions of his hands for six months. He has noticed excessive hair growth on his temples lateral to his eyebrows. On physical examination of the skin, vesicles, bullae, and milia are visible on the dorsa of the hands. The patient complains of generalized malaise but has no other symptoms. Which of the following is the most likely diagnosis?

a. Porphyria cutanea tarda
b. Acute intermittent porphyria
c. Variegate porphyria
d. Pemphigus
e. Tinea versicolor
f. Pemphigoid

58. A 59-year-old man has fine, scaly plaques over his abdomen that have been recurrent for 15 years. Several skin biopsies have been nondiagnostic (lymphocytic epidermal infiltrate), and the lesions respond poorly to topical steroids. The rest of the physical examination is remarkable for a small axillary lymph node. Which of the following is the most likely diagnosis?

a. Lichen planus
b. Pityriasis rosea
c. Mycosis fungoides
d. Kaposi's sarcoma
e. Seborrheic keratosis

DIRECTIONS: Each group of questions below consists of lettered options followed by a set of numbered items. For each numbered item, select the **one** lettered option with which it is **most** closely associated. Each lettered option may be used once, more than once, or not at all.

Questions 59–61

For each patient with skin abnormalities, select the most likely diagnosis.

a. Discoid lupus
b. Melasma
c. Acne vulgaris
d. Red man syndrome
e. Spider angioma
f. Petechiae
g. Rosacea
h. Ecchymoses
i. Purpura
j. Telangiectasia

59. A 15-year-old presents with inflammatory papules, pustules, and crusting on the forehead and cheeks.

60. A 51-year-old woman presents with pustules and papules around the central parts of her face. She complains of facial flushing after drinking alcohol or hot fluids.

61. A 22-year-old woman in her fifth month of pregnancy presents with well-demarcated, hyperpigmented macules on her cheek, nose, and forehead.

Questions 62–64

For each patient with ulcer formation, select the most likely diagnosis.

a. Venous ulcer
b. Arterial ulcer
c. Neuropathic ulcer
d. Aphthous ulcer
e. Pressure ulcer

62. A 64-year-old patient with a history of previous strokes is chronically bedridden. Her nutritional intake is poor, and she has fecal and urinary incontinence. She complains of pain in her lower back and has a low-grade fever.

63. A 67-year-old woman presents with a long history of aching and swelling of her legs, relieved by elevation. Over the last several weeks, she has developed two blue-red, irregular, punched-out patches over the medial malleolus of her left leg.

64. A 55-year-old diabetic patient presents with complaints of a painful right leg when walking and at rest. The pain is worse at night and improves with dependency. His distal leg is porcelain white and cool to the touch. No dorsalis pedis pulse is palpable. A sharply demarcated, punched-out ulcer is visible over the supramalleolar area.

Questions 65–69

For each patient with abnormal nail findings, select the most likely nail finding.

a. Leukonychia
b. Koilonychia
c. Muehrcke's nails
d. Terry's nails
e. Blue nails
f. Beau's lines
g. Pitting nails
h. Brown nails
i. Mees's lines
j. Splinter hemorrhages
k. Yellow nail syndrome
l. Brittle nails

65. A 34-year-old woman presents with concavity of the outer surfaces of her fingernails. When a drop of water is placed on the nail bed surface, it does not roll off. Her past medical history is significant for menorrhagia.

66. A 61-year-old man has early nephrotic syndrome secondary to diabetes mellitus; he presents with fingernails containing two white lines parallel to the lunula. The lines do not appear to progress with the growth of the nail.

67. A 16-year-old boy with a four-year history of psychiatric illness presents with signs of portal hypertension. The lunulae of his fingernails are light blue instead of white.

68. A 62-year-old man is recovering from a myocardial infarction. Transverse grooves are visible on each fingernail.

69. A 41-year-old woman presents with fingernails that are half white (proximally) and half brown (distally). She has a history of hypotension, hyponatremia, hyperkalemia, and eosinophilia.

Questions 70–71

For each patient with skin abnormalities, select the most likely vitamin deficiency.

a. Zinc deficiency
b. Niacin deficiency
c. Vitamin C deficiency

70. A 71-year-old woman presents with ecchymoses and perifollicular hemorrhage on her legs in a saddle distribution (how a rider would touch the saddle). She is edentulous with bleeding gums and is anemic. She lives alone and eats a diet with no added fruits or vegetables.

71. A bottle-fed infant presents with the triad of acral dermatitis, alopecia, and diarrhea.

Questions 72–73

For each patient with skin abnormalities, select the most likely lymphoma.

a. Adult T cell leukemia/lymphoma
b. Sézary's syndrome (cutaneous T cell lymphoma)
c. Cutaneous B cell lymphoma

72. A 65-year-old man presents with intractable pruritus and diffuse erythroderma. He has generalized lymphadenopathy and leukocytosis. Examination of buffy coat smear reveals abnormal circulating T cells.

73. A 57-year-old woman presents with a large red nodular lesion on her abdomen. She has lymphadenopathy and hepatosplenomegaly. Her leukocyte count is over 500,000/μL and her serum calcium level is elevated.

Questions 74–76

For each patient with skin abnormalities, select the most likely disorder.

a. Superficial spreading melanoma
b. Basal cell carcinoma
c. Squamous cell carcinoma
d. Bowen's disease
e. Actinic keratoses
f. Seborrheic keratoses
g. Leukoplakia
h. Erythroplasia of Queyrat

74. A 50-year-old construction worker presents with a slow-growing eroded papule on his lower lip. He has a history of leukoplakia and was a heavy smoker. He has a small, tender supraclavicular node.

75. A 46-year-old man presents with a large, well-demarcated, erythematous, glistening plaque on his glans penis.

76. A 42-year-old man presents with a single shiny, red nodule on his nose that appears to glisten and shine.

Dermatology

Answers

48. The answer is d. *(Fitzpatrick, p 492.)* The most likely diagnosis in this patient is **Peutz-Jeghers syndrome** (**PJS**). This is an autosomal dominant polyposis characterized by multiple small macules (lentigines) on the lips and oral membranes. Abdominal symptoms occur because of multiple benign hamartomatous polyps in the small and large bowel and in the stomach. Freckles (ephelides) are lighter lesions due to increased epidermal pigment in the distribution of sun-exposed areas. **Gardner's syndrome** is an autosomal dominant disease characterized by facial cysts and adenomatous polyps in the small and large intestines. **Herpes simplex virus** is characterized by painful vesicles, which are grouped and confluent. **Hand-foot-and-mouth** disease is a highly contagious systemic infection caused by coxsackievirus A16 and characterized by ulcerative oral lesions and a vesicular exanthem on the distal extremities.

49. The answer is a. *(Fitzpatrick, pp 136–139.)* **Erythema multiforme** (**EM**) minor due to herpes infection is the most likely diagnosis in this patient. The lesions of EM are classically target lesions; they are burning and pruritic. They are generalized and often involve the oral mucosa. Etiologies of EM major include drugs such as phenytoin, sulfonamides, barbiturates, and allopurinol. Finger pressure in the vicinity of a lesion in EM major leads to a sheetlike removal of the epidermis (**Nikolsky's sign**). **Pemphigus vulgaris** is a chronic bullous autoimmune disease usually seen in middle-aged adults. The Nikolsky's sign is positive in pemphigus vulgaris. **Secondary syphilis** appears a few weeks or up to six months after a primary infection and consists of round to oval maculopapular lesions 0.5 to 1.0 cm in diameter. The eruptions typically involve the palms and soles. Secondary syphilis lesions that are flat and soft with a predilection for the mouth, perineum, and perianal areas are called condylomata lata. The skin lesions of **systemic lupus erythematosus** (**SLE**) range from the classic butterfly malar rash to the discoid plaques of **chronic cutaneous lupus erythematosus** (**CCLE**). **Urticaria** is characterized by pruritic wheals typically lasting several hours.

50. The answer is a. *(Fitzpatrick, pp 834–837.)* The history is classic for **scabies,** an infestation by the mite *Sarcoptes scabiei* that is spread by skin-to-skin contact. Although there are few skin findings on physical examination, patients usually complain of intense pruritus. Contact dermatitis is unlikely in this location, and **cutaneous larva migrans** (most commonly from *Ancylostoma brasiliense* due to the dog and cat hookworm) typically has large, erythematous, serpiginous tracks. **Dermatitis herpetiformis** is associated with a gluten-sensitive enteropathy and is characterized by tiny papules, vesicles, and urticarial wheals. **Impetigo** is an infectious skin disease due to either *Staphylococcus aureus* or *Streptococcus pyogenes,* seen typically on the face and characterized by discrete vesicles that rupture to form a yellowish crust.

51. The answer is b. *(Fitzpatrick, p 675.)* The rash described is **erythema migrans (EM),** the early pathognomonic eruption of Lyme disease, a spirochetal infection transmitted to humans by the bite of an infected ixodid deer tick. Most cases in the United States involve the northeastern or northcentral areas of the country. The rash typically occurs one to two weeks after the bite, but less than 20% of patients recall a bite. *R. rickettsii,* transmitted by dog or wood ticks, is the etiologic agent of **Rocky Mountain spotted fever.** The characteristic maculopapular rash begins peripherally and often involves the palms and soles. *B. henselae* (formerly *Rochalimaea henselae*) is the etiologic agent responsible for **cat-scratch disease (CSD).** *M. marinum* infections follow a traumatic inoculation in aquariums and swimming pools. The bite of the **brown recluse spider** (*Loxosceles*) begins as an area of erythema. In some cases, the bite progresses to become a painful bulla and deep necrotic ulcer.

52. The answer is b. *(Fitzpatrick, pp 624–625.)* **Toxic shock syndrome (TSS)** is the most likely diagnosis in this patient. This disease is a toxin-mediated multisystem infection caused by *Staphylococcus aureus.* Risk factors for TSS include surgical wounds, nasal packs, burns, skin ulcers, postpartum infections, eye injuries, and use of vaginal tampons. The rash is typically generalized and macular and involves the mucous membranes. Desquamation of the epithelium of the palms and soles and subsequent multisystem failure occur in TSS. **Cellulitis** is an acute infection of the dermal and subcutaneous tissues characterized by erythema, warmth, and tenderness of the skin at the site of the entry of the bacteria. **Necrotizing**

fasciitis begins as a painful induration of the underlying soft tissues with rapid development of an eschar and necrotic mass. **Scarlet fever** is seen in children and is due to an exotoxin-producing strain of group A *Streptococcus*. It has a characteristic confluent (scarlatiniform) erythema, which begins centrally, spreads to the extremities, and then desquamates. **Toxic epidermal necrolysis (TEN)** is a mucocutaneous, primarily drug-induced eruption characterized by a generalized erythema and exfoliation that may lead to multisystem failure. Drugs that have been implicated include sulfa derivatives, allopurinol, and hydantoins. TEN is a more severe variant of **Stevens-Johnson syndrome (SJS)** and begins one to three weeks after drug exposure.

53. The answer is d. (*Fitzpatrick, pp 700–705.*) The history is most consistent with **tinea capitis** due to either *Trichophyton tonsurans* or *Microsporum canis*. It is usually seen in school-age children and may be transmitted from person to person. **Psoriasis** is a hereditary disorder characterized by scaling patches and plaques appearing in specific areas of the body, such as the scalp, elbows, lumbosacral region, and knees. The lesions are salmon pink with a silver-colored scale that, on removal, produces blood (**Auspitz's sign**). The **Koebner phenomenon** (with trauma, the lesion jumps to a new location) is also elicited in patients with psoriasis. **Seborrheic dermatitis** is a common chronic dermatosis occurring in areas with active sebaceous glands (face, scalp, and body folds) and may be seen either in infancy or in people over the age of 20. The eczematous plaques of seborrheic dermatitis are yellowish red and are often greasy with a sticky crust. Androgenic hair loss is a progressive hereditary bitemporal, frontal, or vertex balding that may begin any time after puberty. A **carbuncle** is a deep infectious collection of interconnecting abscesses (**furuncles**) arising from several hair follicles.

54. The answer is d. (*Fitzpatrick, pp 606–611.*) **Erysipeloid** occurs in persons employed as handlers of fish, poultry, or dead meat. It is a slowly evolving, painful cellulitis due to the gram-positive organism *Erysipelothrix rhusiopathiae*. **Erysipelas** is a cellulitis due to group A β-hemolytic streptococci. **Ecthyma** is impetigo that extends into the dermis. **Erythrasma** is often seen in patients with diabetes and consists of large, well-demarcated macules affecting the intertriginous areas of the body, especially the groin. The lesions are brownish red and are due to *Corynebacterium minutissimum*, a gram-positive rod that is a part of normal skin flora. **Nummular eczema** is a chronic pruritic dermatitis composed of plaques of papules and vesicles. The lesions are coin-shaped (nummular) and often occur on the lower extremities of older men in the winter months, when dryness of the skin is common. Nummular eczema is often associated with a history of atopy.

55. The answer is c. (*Fitzpatrick, pp 18–25.*) **Contact dermatitis** can be due to an allergen causing a type IV cell-mediated delayed hypersensitivity reaction. It may also be due to a nonallergen such as a chemical irritant. This patient presents with typical symptoms of acute contact dermatitis due to poison ivy resin. This results in sensitization within a week of exposure. Contact dermatitis due to poison ivy is usually pruritic, localized to one region, and often linear. **Impetigo** is an epidermal bacterial infection seen on the face and characterized by vesicles that rupture and crust. **Erythema infectiosum,** or **fifth disease,** is a childhood disease due to parvovirus B19 and is characterized by edematous, erythematous plaques on the cheeks ("**slapped cheek**" **disease**). **Atopic dermatitis,** or **eczema,** is an autosomal dominant pruritic inflammation with a predilection for the neck, face, flexor areas, feet, wrists, and hands. Usually there is a personal or family history of asthma, allergic rhinitis, or hay fever. **Rubeola** (**measles**) is a viral infection characterized by conjunctivitis, coryza, and cough (**the three C's**) and a confluent erythematous maculopapular rash that spreads centrifugally. **Koplik spots** (bright red spots with blue-white specks in the center), which appear on the buccal mucosa opposite the premolar teeth, are pathognomonic for rubeola.

56. The answer is b. (*Fitzpatrick, pp 754–757.*) The description of the skin lesions is most consistent with **molluscum contagiosum.** This is a self-limited viral infection due to a poxvirus (molluscum contagiosum virus) seen in children, sexually active adults, and HIV-infected patients. These lesions characteristically have a central keratotic plug that gives them the appearance of being dimpled (umbilication). The lesions resolve spontaneously. Common warts, or **verrucae vulgaris,** are due to human papillomavirus (HPV). Warts are firm, hyperkeratotic, round papules 1 to 10 mm in diameter. They have no umbilication but have a predilection for sites of trauma including hands, fingers, and knees. A **keratoacanthoma** is a skin-colored, isolated dome-shaped nodule with a central hyperkeratotic core usually found on the face. A **herpetic whitlow,** due to herpes simplex virus, consists of a painful group of vesicles on the volar finger.

Capillary **hemangiomas** are bright red or purple nodules or plaques that develop at birth and spontaneously disappear by the fifth year.

57. The answer is a. *(Fitzpatrick, pp 238–247.)* **Porphyria cutanea tarda (PCT)** is a disease of adults and is found equally in males and females. Although the disease is often hereditary, drugs (estrogens including oral contraceptives, chloroquine, and alcohol), chemicals, and illnesses (**hepatitis C virus**) may induce PCT. It occurs gradually, with formation of tense bullae on the dorsae of the hands, feet, and nose and hypertrichosis. Eliciting an **orange-red fluorescence in the urine with a Wood's lamp** makes the diagnosis. Patients with **variegate porphyria** and **acute intermittent porphyria** have life-threatening attacks of abdominal pain and may present with a peripheral neuropathy or respiratory failure. **Pemphigus** is a serious autoimmune bullous disorder of the skin and mucous membranes that may be fatal without treatment. **Pemphigoid** is a chronic bullous autoimmune disorder seen mostly in patients older than 60 years. Mucous membrane involvement is less common in pemphigoid than pemphigus. **Tinea versicolor, or pityriasis versicolor (PV)**, is an asymptomatic dermatosis characterized by scaling macules with sharply marginated borders distributed throughout the trunk. A Wood's lamp will demonstrate the presence of a fungal infection (green fluorescence).

58. The answer is c. *(Fitzpatrick, pp 528–538.)* **Mycosis fungoides,** also called cutaneous T cell lymphoma (CTCL), is a neoplastic disease of the helper T cells that first manifests in the skin but eventually spreads to the lymph nodes and internal organs. The scaly plaques of this disease disappear with sun exposure, mimicking psoriasis. Multiple biopsies and a careful examination for adenopathy are required to make the diagnosis. **Lichen planus** is an inflammatory dermatosis with unknown etiology that involves the skin and mucous membranes. **Pityriasis rosea** is seen in patients under the age of 40 and is more common in the spring and fall months. Its characteristic course begins with a single bright red **herald,** or primary patch, usually on the trunk, followed one to two weeks later by similar nonpruritic (may be mildly itchy) plaques distributed in a **Christmas tree** pattern. The disorder is self-limited and remits within six weeks. **Seborrheic keratosis** is a benign epithelial tumor seen in individuals over the age of 30. It typically appears as brown plaques, papules, or nodules with a stuck-on appearance and has a predilection for the face, trunk, and upper extremities. **Kaposi's sarcoma (KS)** is a multisystem vascular neoplasm that may be seen in elderly males of eastern European heritage (Mediterranean and Ashkenazi Jewish) and predominantly arises in the legs. The papules and nodules of KS are usually violaceous. The disease is also seen in patients who are immunocompromised due to transplant, chemotherapy, or HIV and is thought to be due to herpesvirus type 8 (HHV-8).

59–61. The answers are 59-c, 60-g, 61-b. (*Fitzpatrick, pp 2–11.*) **Acne** is an inflammation of the pilosebaceous units of the face and trunk occurring usually in adolescence. It manifests itself as comedones, papulopustules, or nodules and cysts. **Rosacea** is a chronic acneform disorder of the facial pilosebaceous units coupled with an increased reactivity of capillaries to heat, leading to flushing and the formation of telangiectasia. **Melasma** is an acquired hyperpigmentation that occurs in sun-exposed areas, especially the face. It is common in women with brown and black skin color and may occur in pregnancy or with oral contraceptive use. **Discoid lupus** presents with facial plaques that may result in dyspigmentation and scarring. **Red man (neck) syndrome** is due to histamine release and occurs in patients who receive a rapid infusion of vancomycin. A **spider angioma** is a pulsatile arteriolar lesion that blanches with pressure and is seen in patients with cirrhosis (hyperestrogenism). Petechiae are hemorrhages less than 1 mm in size, and ecchymoses are larger hemorrhages. Purpura is a general term for a collection of red blood cell deposition in the skin and, when palpable, represents antigen-antibody immune complex. A **telangiectasia** is a fine, irregular line due to a dilated capillary.

62–64. The answers are 62-e, 63-a, 64-b. (*Fitzpatrick, pp 474–476.*) **Pressure ulcers** are common in patients who are chronically ill and bedridden. Risk factors for development of pressure ulcers include immobility, incontinence, poor nutritional status, and hypoalbuminemia. Sixty percent of pressure ulcers occur over the sacrum. Prevention is possible by turning immobile patients (every one to two hours) to prevent skin compression and subsequent ischemic necrosis. **Venous ulcers** usually develop in the medial calf or over the malleolus (both lateral and medial). Minor trauma may precipitate venous ulcer formation. **Arterial ulcers** are typically painful at night and improve with dependency. Patients present with complaints of claudication. Arterial insufficiency may lead to atrophic skin changes (shiny and white) and loss of hair on the feet and legs. **Neuropathic ulcers** occur in diabetics; early symptoms may include paresthesias of the leg and foot. Trauma usually precedes the formation of the neuropathic ulcers of the toe, heel, or metatarsal areas (**Charcot joint**). **Aphthous ulcers** are painful, gray-based ulcers with erythematous rims occurring in the oropharynx.

65–69. The answers are 65-b, 66-c, 67-e, 68-f, 69-h. *(Fitzpatrick, pp 968–973.)* White lines parallel to the lunula, separated by normal nail, that remain immobile as the nail grows (they are located in the nail bed, not the nail plate) are called **Muehrcke's nails.** They are seen in patients with severe hypoalbuminemia, such as those with nephrotic syndrome. **Blue nails** (azure half-moons) may be due to Wilson's disease, hemochromatosis, use of antimalarial drugs, or exposure to silver nitrate. Times of severe stress (i.e., myocardial infarction) may cause a temporary growth arrest and horizontal depressions across the nail plate that constitute **Beau's lines.** **Koilonychia,** also called **spoon nails** (due to a thin and soft nail plate), is seen in iron-deficiency anemia and may be demonstrated when a drop of water on the nail does not roll off. Multiple **brown nails** occur with Addison's disease, hemochromatosis, gold therapy, and arsenic intoxication. **Mees's lines** are transverse white lines distal to the cuticle seen with arsenic poisoning, chemotherapy, and Hodgkin's lymphoma; they may also be seen with severe cardiac and renal disease. **Terry's nails** is a nail abnormality seen in patients with cirrhosis, non-insulin-dependent diabetes mellitus, chronic renal failure, or congestive heart failure whereby the proximal four-fifths of the nail is white and the distal rim is pink. **Pitting** of the nails is seen in psoriasis. **Splinter hemorrhages** are brown or red streaks in the midportion of the nail and may be seen in patients with endocarditis or trichinosis; splinter hemorrhages are commonly the result of trauma. **Yellow nails** are characterized by a yellowish color of the nail plates due to poor lymphatic circulation. **Leukonychia** occurs when there are white patches (subungual air bubbles) between the nail and its bed; it may be congenital or a result of trauma. **Brittle nails** (frayed and irregular) may be seen with hyperthyroidism, malnutrition, or calcium or iron deficiency.

70–71. The answers are 70-c, 71-a. *(Fitzpatrick, pp 428–429.)* **Scurvy,** or vitamin C deficiency, is seen in infants under one year of age or in older adults. Perifollicular hemorrhage and areas of ecchymosis are common, especially on the back of the lower legs, arms, and inner thighs (**saddle distribution**). Older patients' diets usually lack fruits and vegetables. Loose teeth and bleeding gums are seen with scurvy. Genetic **zinc deficiency** causes **acrodermatitis enteropathica** in infancy, characterized by the classic triad of acral dermatitis, alopecia, and diarrhea. Adults may also develop zinc deficiency. **Niacin deficiency** is seen in alcoholic patients and causes **pellagra**, which is characterized by a triad of dementia, diarrhea, and dermatitis.

72–73. **The answers are 72-b, 73-a.** (*Fitzpatrick, pp 535–542.*) **Sézary's syndrome** is a cutaneous T cell lymphoma (also called **mycosis fungoides**) characterized by an erythroderma (a generalized erythema, scaling, and thickening of the skin) and leukocytosis. Abnormal circulating T cells (**Sézary type**) are seen on **buffy coat.** **Adult T cell leukemia/ lymphoma** is a neoplasm caused by the retrovirus human T cell lymphotrophic virus 1 (HTLV-1) and manifested by skin lesions, lymphadenopathy, hypercalcemia, lytic bone lesions, internal organ involvement, and abnormal lymphocytes on peripheral blood smear (polylobulated lymphocytes). It is transmitted through blood products and through sexual intercourse and may occur 20 years after exposure. Skin lesions may be single, multiple, or generalized. **Cutaneous B cell lymphoma** is a rare clonal proliferation of B lymphocytes often associated with systemic B cell lymphoma.

74–76. **The answers are 74-c, 75-h, 76-b.** (*Fitzpatrick, pp 983–987.*) Oral **leukoplakia** is a white macular lesion found in the buccal mucosa. Predisposing factors include tobacco use, alcohol use, human papillomavirus, and syphilis. It may lead to squamous cell carcinoma. **Actinic** (**solar**) **keratoses** are dry, rough, adherent, scaly lesions occurring in sun-exposed areas of adults. These lesions are premalignant and may develop into squamous cell carcinoma. **Bowen's disease** or **squamous cell carcinoma in situ** is a solitary, well-demarcated plaque. When Bowen's disease occurs on the glans penis, it is called **erythroplasia of Queyrat.** Both Bowen's disease and erythroplasia of Queyrat may lead to a fungating and ulcerating squamous cell carcinoma. **Seborrheic keratosis** is the most common benign epithelial tumor. **Basal cell carcinoma** (**BCC**) is the most common type of skin cancer. It is invasive and aggressive but rarely metastasizes. These lesions are usually round, firm, glistening (pearly), and shiny. Histologically, basal cell carcinomas have **palisading nuclei. Superficial spreading melanomas** (**SSMs**) have five cardinal features: **A**symmetry, **B**order that is irregular, **C**olor that is mottled and haphazard, **D**iameter that is large, and **E**nlargement/**E**levation (ABCDE).

Head, Ears, Eyes, Nose, and Throat

Questions

DIRECTIONS: Each item below contains a question followed by suggested responses. Select the **one best** response to each question.

77. A 71-year-old woman presents to your office complaining of unilateral hearing loss. She denies vertigo and tinnitus. A Weber test lateralizes to the deaf ear, and a Rinne test is negative. The tympanic membranes are bilaterally normal. Which of the following best explains her hearing loss?

a. Conductive hearing loss
b. Sensorineural hearing loss
c. Electrical hearing loss
d. Hysterical hearing loss
e. Semantic hearing loss

78. A 61-year-old man comes to your office complaining of a popping sensation in his left ear for nearly two weeks. He also complains of impaired hearing. Recently, another physician treated him for an acute otitis media with antibiotics. Physical examination reveals a normal right ear canal and tympanic membrane. The left tympanic membrane is gray, retracted, and immobile. Which of the following is the most likely diagnosis?

a. Otitis media with effusion
b. Acute otitis media
c. Mastoiditis
d. Otitis externa
e. Malignant otitis externa

79. A 48-year-old man presents complaining of bilateral vision loss. He has noticed that his vision has been deteriorating over the last several months. His pupils are equal and reactive to light and accommodation. Extraocular muscle movements and visual field examinations are intact. He has decreased visual acuity as determined by a Snellen chart. Funduscopic examination is normal. Which of the following is the most appropriate next step in diagnosis?

a. Slit-lamp examination
b. Pinhole test
c. Pseudochromatic plate test
d. Schiötz tonometry
e. Amsler grid test
f. Fluorescein stain

80. A 52-year-old man comes to your office complaining of an itchy feeling in his right ear. He has been trying to scratch the itchiness using a cotton swab applicator. He denies tinnitus or hearing loss. On physical examination, the patient is afebrile and complains of pain when the pinna is pulled for the examination. The ear canal is red and swollen with some areas of white debris. Because of the debris, you cannot visualize the tympanic membrane. There is no adenopathy. Which of the following is the most likely diagnosis?

a. Otitis media
b. Serous otitis
c. Otitis externa
d. Cerumen blockage
e. Malignant otitis

81. A 74-year-old man with a history of previous myocardial infarction and stroke presents with the sudden onset of left-sided vision loss. Blood pressure is 135/85 mmHg. Heart rate is 80 beats per minute and regular. Heart and lungs are normal. Funduscopic examination of the left eye reveals a bright yellow refractile deposit wedged at the bifurcation of a peripheral arteriole. The deposit appears to be migrating down the vessel. Which of the following is the most appropriate next step in diagnosis?

a. Holter monitor
b. Cardiac isoenzymes
c. Carotid dopplers
d. Echocardiogram
e. Electrocardiogram
f. CT scan of the head

82. A 14-year-old boy presents to your office after being hit in the face by a soccer ball. He complains of left eye pain, and on physical examination you see blood in the anterior chamber. Pupils are equal and reactive to light, and extraocular muscles are intact. Which of the following is the most likely diagnosis?

a. Hyphema
b. Esotropia
c. Amblyopia
d. Subconjunctival hemorrhage
e. Strabismus

83. A 31-year-old man is brought into the emergency room after blunt trauma to the right eye. He complains of diplopia on upward gaze. A step-off is felt at the inferior rim of the orbit. Palpation of the surrounding tissue reveals subcutaneous crepitus. Subconjunctival air bubbles are obvious with a penlight. Extraocular muscle movement examination reveals that the patient is unable to gaze upward. Which of the following is the most likely diagnosis?

a. Blowout fracture
b. Preseptal cellulitis
c. Dyschromatopsia
d. Hypopyon
e. Pseudostrabismus

84. A 70-year-old man complains of the sudden onset of visual loss in his right eye, accompanied by a headache. He has a history of hypertension and diabetes mellitus. On physical examination, visual acuity in the left eye is 20/20 while visual acuity in the right eye is 20/90. Funduscopic exam shows the right disc to be pale and swollen, with some hemorrhages. Which of the following is the most likely diagnosis?

a. Diabetic retinopathy
b. Retinal vein occlusion
c. Retinal artery occlusion
d. Ischemic optic neuropathy
e. Hypertensive retinopathy
f. Retinal detachment

85. A 43-year-old woman who is positive for HIV presents with painful vesicles of the right ear canal and eardrum. Physical examination reveals right facial paralysis, hyperacusia, and unilateral loss of taste. Which of the following is the most likely diagnosis?

a. Sweet syndrome
b. Bullous myringitis
c. Sturge-Weber disease
d. Ramsay Hunt's syndrome
e. Behçet syndrome

86. A 41-year-old man with a 10-year history of sarcoidosis presents with the chief complaint of nose disfiguration. His nose is not enlarged, but he has a nonblanching purple discoloration of the skin of the external nose. There is no history of trauma, and he denies epistaxis. He has no other skin lesions. Which of the following best describes the nose abnormality?

a. Rhinophyma
b. Nasal fracture
c. Septal hematoma
d. Lupus pernio
e. Saddle nose deformity
f. Polychondritis

87. A 73-year-old man presents to the emergency room with chest pain. He denies shortness of breath, dyspnea on exertion, palpitations, nausea, vomiting, and dizziness. His past medical history is significant for hypertension for which he takes a diuretic. His blood pressure is 170/110 mmHg; heart rate is 100 beats per minute. Heart and lungs are normal. Examination of the neck reveals a downward displacement of the cricoid cartilage with each ventricular contraction. Cardarelli's sign is positive. Which of the following is the most appropriate next step in diagnosis?

a. Electrocardiogram
b. Transthoracic echocardiogram
c. Transesophageal echocardiogram
d. Serial cardiac isoenzymes
e. Holter monitor

88. A 30-year-old man presents complaining of facial pain and nasal congestion with a yellow nasal discharge after an upper respiratory tract infection 10 days ago. Physical examination reveals a temperature of 38.2°C (100.8°F). The patient has maxillary sinus tenderness with palpation, and the nasal mucosa are pale with some yellowish drainage. Clouding of the maxillary sinus is seen with transillumination. Which of the following is the most likely diagnosis?

a. Acute sinusitis
b. Chronic sinusitis
c. Vincent's angina
d. Ludwig's angina
e. Orbital cellulitis

89. A 66-year-old woman presents for her annual eye examination. She has been seeing floaters recently but has no other complaints. Intraocular pressure measurement by Schiötz tonometry is 15 mmHg. Red reflex is visible and normal. Pupils are equal and reactive to light; extraocular muscles are intact. Examination of the fundi reveals the presence of white, indistinct opaque areas in the superficial retina. They occasionally obscure nearby vessels. There is a positive and normal light reflex. There are no hard exudates, hemorrhages, bony spicule formation, or microaneurysms. The optic cup constitutes 25% of the optic disc, and there is no papilledema. Which of the following is the most likely diagnosis?

a. Glaucoma
b. Early cataract
c. Macular degeneration
d. Hypertensive retinopathy
e. Retinitis pigmentosa
f. Early retinal detachment

90. A 32-year-old woman presents with a two-day history of "the room spinning." She states that this occurs when she suddenly moves her head from one position to another. She complains of nausea and vomiting accompanying the spinning sensation but has no other symptoms. On physical examination, she is afebrile and her tympanic membranes are bilaterally normal. Nystagmus to the left is produced when the patient is lying on her left side. Which of the following is the most likely diagnosis?

a. Cerebellopontine tumor
b. Viral labyrinthitis
c. Benign paroxysmal positional vertigo
d. Ménière's disease
e. Trismus

91. A 48-year-old man presents with inability to move the right side of his mouth. On physical examination, the patient has difficulty raising his right eyebrow, puffing out his right cheek, and smiling using the right side of his mouth. His nasolabial fold on the right is absent. Blinking is sparse on the right compared to the left, but extraocular muscles are intact and pupils are equal and reactive. The patient's tongue is midline. Which of the following is the most likely diagnosis?

a. Paralysis of cranial nerve V
b. Paralysis of cranial nerve VII
c. Paralysis of cranial nerve XII
d. Horner's syndrome
e. Pancoast's tumor

92. A 71-year-old man complains of difficulty in seeing street signs when driving and some difficulty with vision when reading. The patient's vision is 20/100 in his right eye and 20/80 in his left eye. The vision in neither eye improves with the pinhole test. There is dullness of the red reflex bilaterally; fundi are difficult to visualize with the funduscope. Intraocular pressure is measured to be 15 mmHg in both eyes. Which of the following is the most likely diagnosis?

a. Glaucoma
b. Macular degeneration
c. Presbyopia
d. Cataract
e. Arcus senilis

93. A 27-year-old man presents with hoarseness for six months. He has no other symptoms or complaints. He has no past medical history, takes no medications, and does not smoke cigarettes or drink alcohol. He uses no illicit drugs. He has been employed as a telephone operator for the last eight months. Which of the following is the most likely diagnosis?

a. Postnasal drip syndrome
b. Cancer of the larynx
c. Reflux esophagitis
d. Voice strain
e. Kallman's syndrome

94. A 22-year-old woman presents with complaints of runny nose, itchy throat, and sneezing that seem to occur every year in the springtime. She has no history of known allergies, but her mother and sister have similar symptoms. Physical examination reveals swollen nasal turbinates. There is a transverse crease across the nose, and Dennie-Morgan lines are visible below the inferior eyelids. The posterior pharynx does not have a cobblestone appearance. Lung examination is normal. Which of the following is the most appropriate next step in diagnosis?

a. Nasal cytology
b. Skin testing for food allergies
c. Multiallergen screening tests
d. Serum IgE levels
e. Serum eosinophil count
f. Radioallergosorbent test (RAST)

95. A 21-year-old man presents with a sore throat. He also complains of dysphagia, odynophagia, and otalgia. His temperature is 39.2°C (102.5°F). The patient speaks with a hot potato voice and is drooling. Examination of the throat reveals a hypertrophied right tonsil that appears to be displaced inferiorly and medially. There is contralateral deflection of the uvula. The patient has trismus and cervical lymphadenopathy. Which of the following is the most likely diagnosis?

a. Retropharyngeal abscess
b. Peritonsillar abscess
c. Exudative pharyngitis
d. Cancer of the right tonsil
e. Mononucleosis

DIRECTIONS: Each group of questions below consists of lettered options followed by a set of numbered items. For each numbered item, select the **one** lettered option with which it is **most** closely associated. Each lettered option may be used once, more than once, or not at all.

Questions 96–98

For each patient with ear complaints, select the most likely diagnosis.

a. *Mycoplasma* infection
b. Nasopharyngeal carcinoma
c. Acoustic neuroma
d. Cholesteatoma
e. Ramsay Hunt's syndrome

96. A 30-year-old woman complains of severe left ear pain. On physical examination, there is hemorrhagic blistering of the left eardrum.

97. A 47-year-old man complains of hearing loss and otorrhea. On physical examination, there is a perforation of the tympanic membrane.

98. A 51-year-old man complains of vertigo, hearing loss, and tinnitus of the left ear.

Questions 99–100

For each patient with eye complaints, select the most likely diagnosis.

a. Adenoviral conjunctivitis
b. Bacterial conjunctivitis
c. Blepharitis
d. Hordeolum
e. Keratitis
f. Iritis
g. Allergic conjunctivitis

99. A 17-year-old student complains of bilateral red eyes with a watery discharge. Physical examination reveals some preauricular lymphadenopathy.

100. A 22-year-old man with a history of hilar adenopathy and lung disease presents with eye pain and photophobia. Eye exam reveals an irregular pupil and ciliary flush.

Questions 101–102

For each patient with pupil abnormalities, select the most appropriate pupillary description.

a. Argyll Robertson pupil
b. Adie tonic pupil
c. Marcus Gunn pupil
d. Anisocoria

101. A 59-year-old woman presents with a history of several untreated sexually transmitted diseases in the past. Pupils are small and irregular and do not respond to light but respond to accommodation.

102. A 25-year-old woman presents with a hyperemic and swollen left optic disc. The swinging flashlight test is positive.

Questions 103–104

For each patient with nystagmus, select the most likely kind of nystagmus.

a. Up-beating nystagmus
b. Down-beating nystagmus
c. Nystagmus that disappears with convergence
d. Rotary nystagmus
e. Asymmetric lateral nystagmus
f. End-point nystagmus
g. Pendular nystagmus

103. A newborn has congenital nystagmus.

104. A 19-year-old man presents for his precollege medical clearance and is found to have nystagmus when asked to gaze to the extreme far left.

Head, Ears, Eyes, Nose, and Throat

Answers

77. The answer is a. (*Seidel, pp 330–331.*) The **Weber test** is performed by placing a tuning fork on the midline vertex of the head. In **conductive hearing loss** the Weber lateralizes to the deaf ear, while in sensorineural hearing loss the Weber lateralizes to the better ear. The **Rinne test** is performed by placing a 512-Hz tuning fork over the mastoid process. When the vibration is no longer heard via bone conduction, the tuning fork is placed near the ear to determine whether the vibration is heard. If the vibration is heard, then **air conduction is greater than bone conduction and the test is considered positive or normal.** If the vibration is not heard, then bone conduction is greater than air conduction and this **negative Rinne test denotes conductive hearing loss. Sensorineural hearing loss** occurs when a positive or normal Rinne test is complemented by a Weber test that lateralizes to the better ear.

78. The answer is a. (*Tierney, pp 181–183.*) **Otitis media with effusion** may follow an episode of acute respiratory tract infection or acute otitis media. Symptoms include hearing loss, ear fullness, ear pain, dizziness, and tinnitus. The eardrum appears retracted or scarred and a clear fluid is visible in the middle ear. Pain and fever are usually absent in otitis media with effusion. Treatment measures are aimed at facilitating drainage of the effusion, and antibiotics are generally not necessary.

79. The answer is b. (*Seidel, p 285.*) A **pinhole test** allows only paraxial parallel light rays through and improves visual acuity if refractory errors are present (most commonly myopia). The **slit-lamp examination** is a direct visualization of the eye and its components. The **pseudochromatic plate test** detects color blindness, and **Schiötz tonometry** measures intraocular pressure. **Visual field testing** determines whether the patient has any blind spots. The **Amsler grid test** screens for macular degeneration. **Fluorescein staining** is used to detect abrasions of the cornea. A **cobalt blue light** is used to detect foreign bodies after the fluorescein is instilled into the affected eye.

80. The answer is c. *(Tierney, p 179.)* **Otitis externa,** an infection of the external ear canal, may be due to trauma or water in the ear canal (**swimmer's ear**). Either of these may lead to maceration of the epithelium and subsequent colonization by bacteria or fungi. Diabetic patients are especially at risk for this ear infection. Physical examination often reveals a tender, erythematous ear occluded with debris. Patients complain of pain when the examiner pulls on the pinna or tragus. The treatment is removal of debris with antibiotic otic drops or the placement of a wick to facilitate drainage. **Malignant otitis** (often seen in diabetic patients and usually due to *Pseudomonas*) causes severe, unrelenting otorrhea and otalgia and a foul-smelling discharge. Malignant otitis requires the use of systemic antibiotics for nearly two months. Patients with acute otitis media rarely complain of discomfort when the pinna is moved. Cerumen blockage is the leading cause of conduction hearing loss.

81. The answer is c. *(Tierney, p 440.)* The patient described has a **Hollenhorst plaque.** A Hollenhorst plaque or cholesterol embolus represents an arterial embolus that originates from an atheromatous plaque in a more proximal vessel, usually the internal carotid. It is a sign of severe atherosclerosis. These plaques are bright, refractile, and yellow. They appear to migrate down the vessel; carefully massaging the eyeball can actually facilitate migration.

82. The answer is a. *(Tierney, p 169.)* A common sequela of blunt trauma to the eye is a **hyphema** (blood in the anterior chamber). This is caused by rupture of the small blood vessels lying close to the cornea. **Strabismus** is a misalignment of the eyes. **Esotropia** is a kind of strabismus in which one eye is deviated inward. **Amblyopia** (lazy eye) is loss of visual acuity in an otherwise healthy eye. This happens because the healthy eye closes to compensate for the deviating eye to avoid the discomfort of diplopia. This is treatable if discovered early. A **subconjunctival hemorrhage** (between the conjunctiva and sclera) causes the sudden appearance of a bright red spot.

83. The answer is a. *(Tierney, p 168.)* The signs are consistent with **blowout fracture** of the floor of the orbit. Crepitus and air bubbles are due to air escaping from the fractured sinus. The inability to gaze upward and diplopia are due to entrapment of the inferior rectus muscle. **Preseptal cellulitis** is cellulitis that involves only the eyelids; ocular motility remains normal. **Hypopyon** is pus in the anterior chamber. The eyes appear to be misaligned in pseudostrabismus, when in reality they are straight. **Dyschromatopsia** is acquired color blindness (instead of congenital color blindness) due to optic nerve disease or degenerative disease of the macula.

84. The answer is d. *(Tierney, pp 163–166.)* Visual acuity is recorded as a fraction in which the numerator is the distance of the patient from the chart (usually 20 ft) and the denominator is the distance at which the average person can read the same line (20 ft). **Ischemic optic neuropathy** usually occurs in patients with a history of diabetes or hypertension (underlying vascular disease). The disc is pale and swollen, with splinter hemorrhages. This disorder is due to occlusion of the posterior ciliary arteries, with subsequent production of edema. **Central artery occlusion** is sudden and painless. It is usually due to infarction from a thrombus or embolus and causes the retina to become pale. The thin tissue of the macula area appears like a **cherry red spot. Occlusion of the retinal vein** occurs from slow venous blood flow and thrombosis, which results in a slowly progressive loss of vision. The funduscopic image of retinal vein occlusion is so dramatic that it is often described as "**blood and thunder.**" In **retinal detachment,** the fundus appears elevated and often has folds. Patients complain of acute vision loss after noticing flashing lights, floaters, and then a shade over the eye. **Diabetic retinopathy** may be proliferative or nonproliferative. In **nonproliferative** (background) disease, retinal findings include microaneurysms, dot-and-blot hemorrhages, hard exudates, and macular edema. **Proliferative diabetic retinopathy** (neovascularization with the formation of fragile vessels) is a response to continuous retinal ischemia and is responsible for most of the blindness seen in diabetes mellitus. **Hypertensive retinopathy** is classified by the **Keith-Wagener-Barker classification:**

Grade 1: arteriolar narrowing and copper wiring
Grade 2: grade 1 changes and arteriovenous nicking
Grade 3: grade 2 changes with the addition of hemorrhages and exudates
Grade 4: grade 3 changes with the addition of papilledema

85. The answer is d. *(Tierney, p 1309.)* **Ramsay Hunt's syndrome** is involvement of the geniculate ganglion by herpes zoster. Patients may present with facial paresis, hyperacusia, unilateral loss of taste, reduced tear formation, reduced salivation, pain in the ear, and vesicles in the ear canal and eardrum. **Bullous myringitis** is an inflammation of the tympanic membrane due to the presence of vesicles; patients complain of earache, hearing loss, and bloody discharge. It occurs in several viral and bacterial infections (i.e., *Mycoplasma pneumoniae*). **Sturge-Weber disease** is characterized by a port-wine nevus on the scalp and vascular abnormalities that may lead to seizures and cerebellar calcifications; examination of the ear may reveal auricle ecchymoses. **Sweet syndrome** is characterized by dark red nodules that are often ulcerated, located over the hands, face, arms, and legs; it is seen in patients with leukemias or other proliferative disorders. **Behçet syndrome** is characterized by the presence of aphthous ulcers of the mouth and genitalia; the ulcers are associated with arthritis, uveitis, and neurological disorders.

86. The answer is d. (*Tierney, p 116.*) **Rhinophyma** is thickening of the nasal skin; the nose may appear mildly erythematous and is covered with multiple telangiectasias. It may be due to excessive alcohol intake or to cold exposure. The best example of rhinophyma is the nose of comedian W.C. Fields. **Lupus pernio** is a chronic, nonblanching purple discoloration of the nose seen in active **sarcoidosis;** this lesion may be seen with **erythema nodosum. Septal hematoma** is a result of trauma; a red, painful nodule is visible in the nasal septum. **Saddle nose deformity** (destruction of the bony nose) may be acquired or congenital; it may be a complication of Wegener's granulomatosis or congenital syphilis. **Polychondritis** can cause **pseudo–saddle nose deformity,** but cartilage is destroyed rather than bone. Nasal fractures follow trauma; patients present with severe pain and significant anterior bilateral epistaxis. Periorbital ecchymoses, septal hematoma, and septal deviation are complications of septal fractures. **All nasal fractures require antibiotics to prevent osteomyelitis.**

87. The answer is c. (*Goldman, p 460.*) The patient described has a **positive tracheal tug sign** (**Oliver's sign**). It can be elicited by asking the patient to sit with the head extended while grasping the cricoid cartilage and applying upward pressure. A downward tug of the trachea synchronous with each systole reveals the presence of an aortic arch aneurysm. This occurs due to the anatomic position of the aortic arch, which overrides the left main bronchus. **Cardarelli's sign** is elicited by pressing on the thyroid cartilage and displacing it to the patient's left; this increases contact between the left bronchus and the aorta, making a tracheal pulsation palpable. The best next step would be a **transesophageal echocardiogram,** which would visualize an aortic arch aneurysm better than a transthoracic echocardiogram.

88. The answer is a. *(Tierney, pp 192–194.)* **Acute sinusitis** is predominantly due to *Streptococcus pneumoniae, Haemophilus influenzae,* or *Moraxella catarrhalis* infection that occurs when the cleaning mechanism—namely, the ciliary activity through the sinuses into the nasal passages—fails. Patients often complain of headache, facial pain, nasal congestion, and purulent discharge. Facial pain is worsened with percussion of the affected sinus, and cloudiness of the sinus may be seen with transillumination. CT films of the sinuses (air-fluid levels) are the best method of making a definitive diagnosis, but should be done only if the patient fails to respond to a two-week course of antibiotic therapy aimed at the common bacteria. **Chronic sinusitis** occurs after adequate treatment of an acute sinusitis has failed to eradicate the symptoms. Common organisms for chronic sinusitis include anaerobes and *Staphylococcus aureus.* **Ludwig's angina** is a rare accumulation of pus in the floor of the mouth (cellulitis) and causes induration of the neck. **Orbital cellulitis** may follow ethmoid or maxillary sinusitis and causes the upper eyelid to become swollen, red, and tender. **Vincent's angina** is a necrotizing ulcerative gingivitis (**trench mouth**).

89. The answer is d. *(Seidel, pp 295–297.)* **Normal intraocular pressure (IOP)** is in the range of 10 to 21.5 mmHg. IOP is determined by the outflow of aqueous humor from the eye; the greater the resistance to outflow, the higher the IOP. IOP is important in the diagnosis of glaucoma. A **Schiötz tonometer** is used to measure IOP. The **red reflex** represents the light reflected from the retina; it means that all of the light-transmitting media of the eye will be transparent and visible. Cataracts and retinal detachment obscure the presence of a red reflex. The **light reflex** is emitted from the retinal arterioles; their walls are transparent and the bright light occupies approximately 25% of the diameter of the arterial column of blood. Changes in the light reflex occur with hypertension or with aging (walls thicken and more light is reflected, resembling copper wires). **Cotton-wool spots** (these are misnamed soft exudates) are white, indistinct, opaque areas of the inner or superficial retina. They represent microinfarctions and are due to hypertension, diabetes mellitus, infections, collagen vascular diseases, AIDS, and severe anemia. **Hard exudates** are yellowish, well-demarcated, deep retinal lesions. They are the result of **leaky and damaged vessels, not of microinfarcts;** they are most commonly due to hypertension and diabetes. **Drusen bodies** are yellow, deep epithelial pigment deposits located in the macula; they are the earliest sign of macular degeneration. The optic cup is enlarged to more than 30% of the disc in glaucoma. **Retinal hemorrhages** are due to leaky and damaged retinal capillaries. Depending on their retinal layer location, they may be **blot-and-dot** (due to diabetes and hypertension), **flame-and-splinter** (due to intracranial hemorrhage, papilledema, and glaucoma), or white-centered (**Roth spots** seen in endocarditis, leukemia, and diabetes). **Microaneurysms** are outpouchings of the retinal capillaries and are almost always associated with diabetes mellitus. In **retinitis pigmentosa,** the fundi are covered with a bony spicule formation.

90. The answer is c. (*Tierney, pp 187–191.*) **Vertigo** is an illusion of movement that gives the sensation of spinning and is most commonly due to **benign paroxysmal positional vertigo (BPPV).** Each attack lasts several seconds and is provoked by head movements. It is caused by the detachment of calcium carbonate crystals from the affected side into the semicircular canal. The **Nylen-Bárány maneuver** (reproducing the vertigo by having the patient go from a sitting to supine position while quickly turning the head to the side) will reproduce the vertigo of BPPV. **Ménière's disease** (hydrops) is a disorder of endolymph control; patients often complain of vertigo and tinnitus and have **sensorineural hearing loss. Viral labyrinthitis** is due to a viral infection; patients present within weeks of the illness. The cerebellopontine angle may house tumors, such as **schwannomas** (**acoustic neuromas**); patients complain of vertigo, tinnitus, hearing loss, and facial numbness and weakness as the tumor compresses on the adjacent cranial nerves (VII and VIII) and brainstem. **Trismus,** or **lockjaw,** is a sustained spasm of the jaw muscles and is seen in tetanus and other infectious diseases.

91. The answer is b. (*Seidel, p 786.*) **Bell's palsy,** or paralysis of cranial nerve VII (lower motor neuron), causes ipsilateral drooping of the mouth and facial muscles, inability to close the ipsilateral eye, and difficulty eating and speaking (due to the mouth droop or weakness). Bell's palsy may be idiopathic or due to trauma, multiple sclerosis, or infections such as herpes zoster (**Ramsay Hunt's syndrome**) and Lyme disease. **Horner's syndrome** is caused by a lack of sympathetic innervation to one side of the face and neck. With loss of this innervation, the pupil becomes constricted, the eyelid droops, and there is loss of sweating on the ipsilateral side of sympathetic loss. Horner's syndrome is often secondary to a Pancoast's tumor. Cranial nerve V controls the muscles of mastication, and cranial nerve XII innervates the muscles of the tongue.

92. The answer is d. (*Tierney, pp 157–161.*) A **cataract** is opacity of the lens; patients often present complaining of a disturbance in vision. When the lens has a cataract, the red reflex is diminished and it becomes difficult to see the fundus through the opacity. Patients with **macular degeneration** present with central vision loss, and **drusen bodies** (yellow-white lesions), retinal atrophy, and neovascularization are often found on funduscopic examination. **Presbyopia** is a decreased ability to focus on near objects (because of loss of accommodation) that occurs with aging. **Glaucoma** is an insidious disease, and symptoms occur late in the disease. Patients complain of peripheral vision loss (central vision is spared until late in the disease) and scotomas. Intraocular pressure may be elevated.

93. The answer is d. (*Tierney, p 208.*) **Hoarseness** may be due to edema or swelling of the larynx or vocal cords or to external compression of the larynx or the recurrent laryngeal nerve. Certain occupations, such as being a singer or a telephone operator, place people at risk for **voice strain** (**chronic laryngitis**) due to overuse. Medications, such as inhaled corticosteroids, may contribute to the problem. Viral infections are a common cause of laryngitis, but the patient would have other signs of a viral syndrome. Laryngeal carcinoma must be considered in patients with a history of heavy tobacco use. Reflux disease may cause hoarseness, but the patient would also complain of heartburn, nocturnal cough, chronic sore throat, and excess phlegm production. **Postnasal drip** syndrome leads to chronic throat clearing, and physical examination reveals **cobblestoning** of the posterior pharynx. **Kallmann's syndrome** is bilateral loss of smell with gonadotropin deficiency, micropenis, and cryptorchism. Bilateral loss of smell may be seen with asthma, sarcoidosis, diabetes, chronic renal failure, cirrhosis, multiple sclerosis, and Parkinson's disease. A mnemonic for hoarseness is **VINDICATE: V**ascular (thoracic aneurysm), **I**nflammation,

Neoplasm, Degenerative (i.e., amyotrophic lateral sclerosis), Intoxication (smoking, alcohol), Congenital (laryngeal web), Allergies, Trauma, and Endocrine (thyroiditis).

94. The answer is c. (*Tierney, pp 195–196.*) The patient has symptoms consistent with **seasonal allergic rhinitis (AR)**. Fifty percent of patients have a family history of seasonal rhinitis. Symptoms include runny nose, pruritus, sneezing, itchy throat, congestion, stuffiness, conjunctival erythema, tearing, and frequent throat clearing. Physical examination may reveal a nasal mucosa that is **boggy (pale and swollen)** or **blue-gray (severe AR)**. Turbinates may be swollen; polyps may be visible. A **nasal salute** (a transverse crease across the nose resulting from repeated rubbing), **allergic shiners** (dark circles under the eyes), and **Dennie-Morgan lines** (folds below the margin of the inferior eyelids) may be visible. The pharynx may have a **cobblestone** appearance (due to lymphoid tissue hypertrophy), and postnasal drip may be visible. Multiallergen screening tests are the most sensitive and specific of all the screening options.

95. The answer is b. (*Tierney, pp 204–205.*) The patient has a **peritonsillar abscess,** which is an accumulation of pus between the tonsillar capsule and the superior constrictor muscle of the pharynx. Patients present with a **hot potato voice,** fever, cervical lymphadenopathy, **trismus** (inability to open the mouth), and a displaced uvula due to a unilaterally enlarged tonsil. Patients complain of dysphagia, odynophagia, and otalgia. A **retropharyngeal abscess** is an infection of the deep spaces of the neck (from the base of the skull to the tracheal bifurcation); patients are often young children who present with fever, cervical lymphadenopathy, neck pain, neck swelling, **torticollis** (rotation to the affected side), difficulty breathing, and stridor. Patients with an **exudative pharyngitis** have fever, cervical lymphadenopathy, bilateral tonsillar enlargement, erythema, edema of the midline uvula, and discrete tonsillar exudate.

96–98. The answers are 96-a, 97-d, 98-c. (*Tierney, pp 182, 246.*) **Bullous myringitis** is associated with *Mycoplasma pneumoniae* infection but may be seen with viral infections as well. **Cholesteatomas** (sacs) are a complication of chronic otitis media and consist of keratinized squamous epithelium that has entered the middle ear through a perforation from the external canal. These form in relationship to a perforation and can become infected, leading to bone (ossicular chain) destruction. **Acoustic neuromas** or **schwannomas** arise from cranial nerve VIII (vestibular division), and their growth within the internal auditory canal produces tinnitus and hearing loss. **Ramsay Hunt's syndrome** is due to herpes zoster (shingles) infection of the face that involves the seventh nerve and causes paralysis of the facial muscles.

99–100. The answers are 99-a, 100-f. *(Tierney, pp 153–155.)* The most common cause of **red eye** is **viral conjunctivitis** due to **adenovirus.** This is a highly contagious keratoconjunctivitis usually accompanied by preauricular adenopathy. **Bacterial conjunctivitis** is usually associated with a purulent discharge but no adenopathy. Allergic insults may cause itching and watery discharge of the eyes, but usually the patient complains of hypersensitivity to a specific agent. **Iritis (uveitis** or **iridocyclitis)** is an inflammation of the iris and ciliary muscle. It may be a systemic marker for ankylosing spondylitis, Reiter's syndrome, or sarcoidosis. The patient complains of eye pain and photophobia, and eye examination reveals a **ciliary flush** (engorgement of the deep pericorneal blood vessels, which is never seen in a superficial infection) and an irregular pupil. **Keratitis,** or **corneal inflammation,** may be due to trauma, including overuse of contact lenses. Patients complain of diminished visual acuity, photophobia, and a sensation of a foreign body in the eye. They are at risk for further vision loss. A **hordeolum** is an infection (pustule) of the eyelid gland, usually due to *S. aureus,* which causes pain and swelling of the lid margin **(stye). Blepharitis** is a chronic inflammation of the eyelid margins that causes burning, itching, and irritation of the lids. Patients often complain of sticky eyelids on awakening in the morning.

101–102. The answers are 101-a, 102-c. *(Seidel, p 305.)* **Argyll Robertson pupil** is usually miotic and almost always bilateral. The pupil does not react to light but will react to accommodation. It is suggestive of a neurosyphilis infection that affects the light reflex pathway. The description of a hyperemic and swollen disc is consistent with **optic neuritis,** which is an inflammation of the optic nerve sometimes seen in patients with multiple sclerosis. A **Marcus Gunn pupil** (afferent pupillary defect) requires the swinging flashlight test. Bright light is moved from one eye to the other, and pupillary reactions are observed. In lesions of the optic nerve (optic neuritis), the brainstem center perceives the light as being brighter in the normal eye and the affected pupil will dilate continuously. An **Adie tonic pupil** is a dysfunction of the constrictor muscle in which the pupil does not respond to direct light or accommodation. Often, the patient has **absent deep tendon reflexes. Anisocoria** implies pupils of unequal size and is found in up to 20% of normal subjects.

103–104. The answers are 103-c, 104-f. (*Seidel, p 290.*) **Nystagmus** is an abnormal involuntary rhythmic eye movement that may be induced by having the patient follow a rapid finger movement or can occur at rest. It consists of a **slow** component (**vestibular**) as the eye deviates in one direction, followed by a **rapid** corrective movement (**cerebral**) in the opposite direction. **Nystagmus is usually named for the rapid component. End-point nystagmus** occurs when a person is asked to gaze too far laterally. **Asymmetric lateral nystagmus** occurs in only one direction of lateral gaze and is seen in patients with vestibular disease. **Up-beating, down-beating,** and **rotary nystagmus** are seen in patients with brainstem disease, and congenital nystagmus that typically disappears with convergence is seen in newborns. **Pendular nystagmus** is nystagmus in which the eye moves at equal speeds in both directions.

Respiratory System

Questions

DIRECTIONS: Each item below contains a question followed by suggested responses. Select the **one best** response to each question.

105. A 59-year-old woman presents complaining of a cough productive of sputum for nearly 10 years. Her cough occurs during the day, and she produces sputum daily. The woman states that as a child, she had several episodes of pneumonia requiring hospital admissions and antibiotics. Several times a year, her sputum becomes purulent and she requires antibiotic therapy. She denies smoking cigarettes and has worked as a seamstress all of her life. On physical examination, the lungs are clear without wheezes, rhonchi, or crackles. A chest radiograph reveals tram-track markings at the bases. Which of the following is the most likely diagnosis?

a. Asthma
b. Cystic fibrosis
c. Chronic bronchitis
d. Emphysema
e. Bronchiectasis

106. A 71-year-old woman has been in the hospital for four days after suffering a stroke in the distribution of the middle cerebral artery. She is not ambulating but is able to eat a pureed diet with assistance from hospital personnel. On the fifth hospital day, she develops a fever and a cough productive of purulent sputum. Lung examination reveals increased fremitus and crackles at the right base. Chest radiograph reveals a right lower lobe patchy infiltrate. Which of the following is the most likely causal organism?

a. *Pseudomonas aeruginosa*
b. *Chlamydia pneumoniae*
c. Atypical mycobacterium
d. Influenza virus
e. Parainfluenza virus
f. *Moraxella catarrhalis*

107. An 80-year-old woman is transferred from a nursing home to the hospital for management of right lung collapse secondary to an endobronchial obstructing lesion. On physical examination she has decreased breath sounds and dullness over the right posterior hemithorax. Her respiratory rate is 24 breaths per minute, and she is afebrile. Pulse oximetry reveals a saturation of 90% on 4 L of nasal cannula. Which of the following is the most appropriate next step in management?

a. Laying the patient in the right lateral decubitus position
b. Laying the patient in the left lateral decubitus position
c. Laying the patient in the prone position
d. Laying the patient in the supine position
e. Immediate bronchoscopy

108. A healthy 50-year-old man presents with a one-month history of low-grade fever, exertional dyspnea, and cough productive of clear phlegm. He denies hemoptysis and hematuria. He has been taking two antibiotics for the symptoms without relief. He does not smoke cigarettes and works as an accountant. On physical examination, his temperature is 38.3°C (101.0°F) and his lung examination is normal. A chest radiograph reveals bibasilar fibrosis and air space densities in the lower lobes. Which of the following is the most likely diagnosis?

a. Bronchiolitis obliterans
b. Sarcoidosis
c. Allergic bronchopulmonary aspergillosis
d. Wegener's granulomatosis
e. Goodpasture's syndrome

109. A 39-year-old man presents to the emergency room after having a seizure. On physical examination he is comatose and cyanotic. Vital signs reveal a temperature of 38°C (100.5°F), heart rate of 110 beats per minute, and blood pressure of 150/85 mmHg. Lung examination reveals decreased breath sounds bilaterally. Heart examination is normal. Pulse oximetry reveals a hemoglobin saturation of 80% on 100% oxygen. Which of the following is the most appropriate next step in management?

a. Chest tube placement
b. Endotracheal intubation
c. Arterial blood gas analysis
d. Stat portable chest radiograph
e. Head tilt–chin lift maneuver

110. A 39-year-old woman presents with the sudden onset of pleuritic chest pain and shortness of breath. She has been in good health until three days ago, when she noticed some swelling of her left lower extremity. She is not a smoker and denies any recent trauma. On physical examination, she is afebrile but has a respiratory rate of 32 breaths per minute. Her heart rate is 120 beats per minute and her blood pressure is normal. An accentuated (loud) S_2 is heard on heart auscultation. The left lower extremity is swollen, tender to palpation, and erythematous. Dorsiflexion of the left foot (Homan's sign) causes severe calf discomfort. Lung examination and chest radiograph are normal. Arterial blood analysis on room air shows a P_{CO_2} of 30 mmHg and a P_{O_2} of 58 mmHg. Which of the following is the most appropriate next diagnostic step?

a. Transesophageal echocardiogram
b. Transthoracic echocardiogram
c. Cardiac catheterization
d. Ventilation-perfusion scan
e. D-dimer assay

111. A thin 35-year-old woman presents with a two-day history of cough. She complains of some mild dyspnea and chest pain. On physical examination, her temperature is 38.5°C (101.4°F) and her respiratory rate is 26 breaths per minute. Her blood pressure is 110/65 mmHg and her heart rate is 125 beats per minute. Examination of the lungs reveals increased fremitus and bronchial breath sounds at the right base. There are no crackles, egophony, or pectoriloquy in the area. Which of the following is the most likely diagnosis?

a. Right lower lobe emphysema
b. Right lower lobe pneumonia
c. Right lower lobe pneumothorax
d. Right-sided pleural effusion
e. Right lower lobe atelectasis

112. A 34-year-old nursing student is referred to your office because of the onset of a recent cough productive of dark-colored sputum. She is febrile but does not appear ill. She has been able to continue working with her symptoms. Examination of the posterior thorax is normal, but there is dullness at the anterior right hemithorax below the fifth rib. Crackles, as well as localized pectoriloquy, are audible over the same area. Which of the following is the most likely diagnosis?

a. Right lower lobe pneumonia
b. Left lower lobe pneumonia
c. Right lower lobe atelectasis
d. Right middle lobe pneumonia
e. Right upper lobe pneumonia

113. A 14-year-old boy presents with a history of chronic sinusitis and frequent pneumonias. On physical examination, the patient has normal vital signs and is afebrile. He has mild frontal and maxillary sinus tenderness with palpation. Transillumination of the sinuses is normal. Heart sounds are best heard on the right side of the chest. The boy is coughing copious amounts of yellowish sputum. Which of the following is the most likely diagnosis?

a. Cystic fibrosis
b. Kartagener's syndrome
c. Pulmonary dysplasia
d. Tuberculosis
e. Pulmonary hypertension

114. A 30-year-old woman presents with the chief complaint of shortness of breath with minimal activity. In retrospect, she feels she has been dyspneic for at least one year but has now progressed to the point where she has difficulty climbing stairs and walking short distances. She denies fever, cough, or chest pain. On physical examination, the patient has jugular venous distension (JVD) and a palpable right ventricular lift. On heart auscultation, there is a loud S_2 and a systolic murmur that increases with inspiration. Lungs are clear. There is no clubbing. Which of the following is the most likely diagnosis?

a. Sarcoidosis
b. Coronary heart disease
c. Idiopathic pulmonary fibrosis
d. Primary pulmonary hypertension
e. Systemic lupus erythematosus

115. A 54-year-old obese woman presents with the chief complaint of hemoptysis. She states that over the last day she has coughed up approximately 10 mL of blood-streaked sputum. She denies fever, chills, chest pain, or shortness of breath. She does admit to a recent upper respiratory tract infection with cough and a copious amount of sputum production. She remembers similar episodes of cough with bloody sputum occurring after colds for the last several years. She has smoked one pack of cigarettes per day since high school. Examinations of the pharynx and lungs are normal. Which of the following is the most likely diagnosis?

a. Chronic bronchitis
b. Tuberculosis
c. Adenocarcinoma of the lung
d. Congestive heart failure
e. Pulmonary infarction

116. A 70-year-old man with a history of chronic obstructive pulmonary disease (COPD) presents complaining of worsening shortness of breath for the last several days. He is coughing large amounts of yellow-colored sputum and is receiving no relief from his β_2 agonist and ipratropium aerosolized pumps. On physical examination, the patient's respiratory rate is 40 breaths per minute and his heart rate is 110 beats per minute. His blood pressure is 150/85 mmHg. The patient is afebrile. He is using his accessory muscles of respiration (sternocleidomastoids and intercostals) to assist in breathing. Lung examination reveals inspiratory and expiratory diffuse wheezing. Which of the following is the most likely diagnosis?

a. Acute exacerbation of COPD
b. α_1 antitrypsin deficiency
c. Chronic bronchitis
d. Exacerbation of asthma
e. Pneumonia

117. A 53-year-old woman presents with a four-month history of cough productive of bloody sputum. She denies fever, chills, and night sweats but has occasional flushing that she feels is secondary to menopause. She has had two pneumonias over the last three years that required short-term hospitalization. Physical examination reveals wheezing localized to the left midlung field. Chest radiograph is normal. Which of the following is the most appropriate next diagnostic step?

a. Pulmonary function tests
b. Pulmonary angiography
c. Fiberoptic bronchoscopy
d. Ventilation-perfusion scan
e. Video-assisted thorocoscopy

118. A man is stabbed and arrives at the emergency room within 30 minutes. You notice that the trachea is deviated away from the side of the chest with the puncture. The most likely lung finding on physical examination of the traumatized side is which of the following?

a. Increased fremitus
b. Increased breath sounds
c. Dullness to percussion
d. Hyperresonant percussion
e. Wheezing
f. Stridor

119. A 16-year-old high school student presents with the sudden onset of sharp right-sided chest pain associated with shortness of breath. He denies any history of trauma. On physical examination, the patient is afebrile with a respiratory rate of 28 breaths per minute. His blood pressure is 100/70 mmHg and his heart rate is 120 beats per minute. Neck examination reveals no tracheal deviation. On lung auscultation, the patient has decreased fremitus, hyperresonance, and diminished breath sounds over the right posterior hemithorax. Which of the following is the most likely diagnosis?

a. Tension pneumothorax
b. Secondary pneumothorax
c. Pulmonary embolus
d. Spontaneous pneumothorax
e. Pneumonia

120. A 41-year-old woman with a past medical history significant for rheumatoid arthritis presents with shortness of breath and dyspnea on exertion. She has right-sided chest pain that worsens with cough and deep breath. Her cough is nonproductive; she denies fever, chills, and night sweats. Physical examination reveals diminished breath sounds halfway down the right posterior hemithorax with an audible pleural rub. Chest radiograph reveals a right-sided pleural effusion. Which of the following is most likely to be seen on thoracentesis?

a. High amylase level
b. High glucose level
c. Bloody fluid
d. High complement levels
e. Cholesterol crystals

121. A 66-year-old man presents with a scanty cough and pleuritic chest pain. He also complains of fever and watery diarrhea. He smokes one pack of cigarettes per day and lives in an apartment building that is undergoing renovation. He has no past medical history and takes no medications. Physical examination reveals a toxic-appearing man with a temperature of 39.5°C (103.2°F). His heart rate is 60 beats per minute. Chest auscultation reveals bilateral scattered crackles. Abdominal examination reveals diffuse tenderness. Laboratory results reveal hyponatremia, hypophosphatemia, elevated liver function tests, and thrombocytopenia. A chest radiograph reveals bilateral infiltrates. Which of the following is the most likely diagnosis in this patient?

a. Pontiac fever
b. Legionnaires' disease
c. Influenza
d. Tuberculosis
e. Psittacosis

122. A 37-year-old woman was recently extubated after requiring a ventilator for 10 days for an exacerbation of her asthma. After the uncomplicated extubation, the patient complains of hoarseness and dyspnea. On physical examination, her lungs are clear, with normal fremitus and dullness. There is no tracheal deviation, and heart examination is normal. The patient's chest radiograph is normal. Which of the following is the most likely diagnosis?

a. Oxygen toxicity
b. Premature extubation
c. Pneumonia
d. Tracheal stenosis
e. Aspiration pneumonia

123. A 41-year-old woman presents to the emergency room after being given naloxone by paramedics for a probable heroin overdose. The paramedics state that the patient began to vomit excessively, and they fear she may have aspirated gastric contents. Physical examination reveals a respiratory rate of 32 breaths per minute, and pulse oximetry reveals a saturation of 82%. The patient appears cyanotic. Lung examination is significant for bilateral crackles. There is no S_3 gallop. Chest radiograph reveals bilateral basilar alveolar infiltrates. The patient is immediately intubated and stabilized. Which of the following is the most appropriate next step in management?

a. High-dose steroids
b. Broad-spectrum antibiotics
c. β agonist therapy
d. Intravenous theophylline
e. No other therapy is needed

124. A 23-year-old college student presents to the emergency room unresponsive. He has been depressed at school and may have ingested 20 phenobarbitol pills his roommate had for a seizure disorder. Paramedics report that the patient was found in the supine position. Vital signs reveal a blood pressure of 90/50 mmHg, a heart rate of 54 beats per minute, and a respiratory rate of 10 breaths per minute. Pupils are equally dilated and constrict to light. Lung examination reveals right-sided crackles. Neurologic examination is significant for decreased muscle tone and hyporeflexia. Gag reflex is not tested. You suspect that the patient has aspirated. Which of the following is the most likely lung segment to be affected?

a. Medial segment of the right middle lobe
b. Lateral segment of the right middle lobe
c. Posterior segment of the right upper lobe
d. Apical segment of the right upper lobe
e. Anterior segment of the right upper lobe

125. A 65-year-old man presents with severe right-sided chest pain over several months. He has been a lifelong smoker and worked most of his life as a shipbuilder. On physical examination, the patient appears to be dyspneic at rest. Lung auscultation reveals scattered rhonchi anteriorly and posteriorly. The patient has clubbing. Chest radiograph reveals the lungs to have a ground-glass appearance, and bilateral pleural plaques with some areas of calcification and pleural thickening are evident. Which of the following is the most likely diagnosis?

a. Byssinosis
b. Berylliosis
c. Silicosis
d. Asbestosis
e. Farmer's lung

126. A newborn has an Apgar score of 0 at one minute and an Apgar score of 10 at five minutes. Which of the following statements is true regarding the Apgar score?

a. It has good predictive value regarding the newborn's long-term outcome
b. It has no predictive value regarding the newborn's long-term outcome
c. It should be repeated a third time at 10 minutes
d. It tells you very little about the infant's respiratory efforts

127. A 21-year-old man presents with a two-month history of anterior and posterior cervical lymphadenopathy. He denies recent illness, weight loss, and fever. His physical examination reveals scattered nontender 1-cm cervical nodes bilaterally. Lung, heart, and abdominal examinations are normal. Chest radiograph reveals bilateral hilar adenopathy. Which of the following is the most likely diagnosis?

a. Pneumonia
b. Sarcoidosis
c. Bagassosis
d. Löffler's syndrome
e. Hamman-Rich syndrome

128. A 45-year-old woman presents with a two-year history of nonproductive cough. The cough is not associated with time of day or year, and the patient denies any occupational or environmental exposures. She has never smoked cigarettes. She finds herself clearing her throat frequently during the day and night. She has no nasal discharge, heartburn, or cardiac symptoms. She denies fever, chest pain, or shortness of breath. She takes no medications. On physical examination, her nasopharynx reveals mucopurulent secretions and a cobblestone-appearing mucosa. Lung examination is normal. Chest radiograph is normal. Which of the following is the most likely diagnosis?

a. Reflux disease
b. Asthma
c. Bronchitis
d. Postnasal drip
e. Use of angiotensin converting enzyme (ACE) inhibitors
f. Congestive heart failure

129. A 20-year-old college student presents with a three-month history of left-sided pleuritic chest pain, shortness of breath with exertion, and night sweats. He admits to a 10-lb weight loss over the last several months. He is a nonsmoker and does not use illicit drugs. He is heterosexual. He recalls a negative purified protein derivative (PPD) when he started college two years ago. On physical examination, his temperature is 38.3°C (100.9°F) and his respiratory rate is 24 breaths per minute. Lung examination reveals decreased fremitus, dullness to percussion, and diminished breath sounds over the left posterior lung. A pleural friction rub is audible at the left lung base. Which of the following is the most likely diagnosis?

a. Pneumonia
b. Pneumothorax
c. Pleural effusion
d. Lung abscess
e. Pulmonary nodule

130. A 26-year-old sexually promiscuous intravenous drug abuser presents with fever and shortness of breath. He complains of dyspnea on exertion and some bilateral pleuritic chest pain. He admits to a recent 30-lb weight loss. On physical examination, heart rate is 124 beats per minute, respiratory rate is 28 breaths per minute, blood pressure is 100/70 mmHg, and temperature is 39.1°C (102.4°F). Pulse oximetry reveals a saturation of 85% on room air. Lung auscultation reveals scattered bilateral crackles posteriorly. Chest radiograph reveals bilateral interstitial infiltrates and no cardiomegaly. Which of the following is the most likely diagnosis?

a. Pulmonary edema
b. *Pneumocystis carinii* pneumonia
c. Cytomegalovirus pneumonia
d. Kaposi's sarcoma
e. Varicella zoster pneumonia

131. A 22-year-old graduate student presents with a two-week history of a dry cough. Her symptoms include sore throat at the start of the illness, low-grade fever, and generalized malaise. She is otherwise healthy and does not drink alcohol or smoke cigarettes. Several of her colleagues at school are ill with a similar illness. Physical examination reveals normal vital signs, and lung examination reveals some crackles at the right midaxillary line. Which of the following is the most likely diagnosis?

a. Pneumococcal pneumonia
b. *Mycoplasma* pneumonia
c. Aspiration pneumonia
d. Primary pulmonary hypertension
e. *Legionella* pneumonia

132. A 55-year-old man with emphysema will have which pattern of breathing?

a. Biot respiration
b. Apneustic breathing
c. Cheyne-Stokes respiration
d. Rapid and shallow breathing
e. Kussmaul breathing

133. A 22-year-old man is brought to the emergency room after being found unconscious in a swimming pool. The patient is mildly cyanotic. Blood pressure is 80/50 mmHg, heart rate is 60 beats per minute, and respiratory rate is 26 breaths per minute. His core body temperature is 31.7°C (89°F). Pupils are 4 mm bilaterally and reactive. The patient is moving all extremities and responds appropriately to questions. Crackles are heard bilaterally on lung auscultation. Pulse oximetry reveals a saturation of 94% on 50% oxygen. Chest radiograph reveals bilateral perihilar infiltrates with a normal-sized heart. Which of the following is the most likely diagnosis?

a. Partial fracture of the C5 vertebral body
b. Subdural frontal hematoma
c. Congestive heart failure
d. Noncardiogenic pulmonary edema
e. Drowning

134. Forty-eight hours after a motor vehicle accident, a 47-year-old man develops restlessness and hypoxemia. He has retinal and conjunctival hemorrhages, and fat is seen in the retinal vessels. A petechial rash is visible in the upper chest and supraclavicular areas. Lung examination reveals bilateral crackles, and chest radiograph shows interstitial bilateral infiltrates. Fat globules are present in the urine. The patient requires immediate endotracheal intubation. Which of the following is the most likely diagnosis?

a. Fat embolism
b. Hospital-acquired pneumonia
c. Mendelson's syndrome
d. Cardiac pulmonary edema
e. *Pneumocystis carinii* pneumonia

135. A 60-year-old man presents to your office with an 80-pack-per-year history of cigarette smoking. He complains of some dyspnea on exertion. He has an asthenic body habitus and pursed-lip breathing. He has an increased anteroposterior thickness of the thorax. Lung examination reveals decreased fremitus, hyperresonance on percussion, and diminished breath sounds. Which of the following is the most likely diagnosis?

a. Bronchiectasis
b. Asthma
c. Emphysema
d. Pleural effusion
e. Pneumonia

136. A 45-year-old alcoholic man with a history of blackouts when intoxicated presents with fever, chills, and cough productive of putrid, foul-smelling sputum. On physical examination the patient appears inebriated. He is febrile with a temperature of 39.5°C (103.2°F). Mouth examination reveals numerous dental caries and poor dental hygiene. Lung examination reveals normal fremitus, dullness, and auscultation. Which of the following is the most likely diagnosis?

a. Spontaneous pneumothorax
b. Bronchogenic carcinoma
c. Lung abscess
d. Pleural effusion
e. Empyema

137. A patient arrives at the emergency room cyanotic with severe shortness of breath. The patient was found unconscious and face down in a swimming pool, and was intubated and then resuscitated by paramedics using advanced cardiac life support measures. On arrival, the patient has a blood pressure of 90/60 mmHg, a heart rate of 120 beats per minute, and a respiratory rate of 28 breaths per minute. There is no tracheal deviation. Lung auscultation reveals crackles anteriorly and posteriorly. Arterial blood gas reveals a P_{O_2} of 50 mmHg on 100% oxygen. The chest radiograph reveals bilateral whiteout of the lungs consistent with interstitial and alveolar infiltrates. There is no cardiomegaly. Which of the following is the most likely diagnosis?

a. Acute respiratory distress syndrome
b. Pulmonary contusion
c. Pneumothorax
d. Cardiogenic pulmonary edema
e. Pulmonary infarction

138. A 42-year-old man with a history of Osler-Weber-Rendu disease presents with platypnea. He states that he has difficulty breathing in the upright position, which is relieved promptly by recumbency. Pulse oximetry in the sitting position confirms the desaturation (orthodeoxia). Which of the following best explains the likely cause of these results?

a. Upright posture increases venous return to the heart, thereby causing desaturation
b. Upright posture increases perfusion to the upper lobes, thereby causing desaturation
c. Upright position increases perfusion to the lower lobes, thereby causing desaturation
d. Upright position causes abdominal paradox, thereby causing desaturation
e. Upright position causes respiratory alternans, thereby causing desaturation

139. A 6-year-old boy who had a mild respiratory tract infection for two days awakens in the middle of the night with shortness of breath and difficulty breathing, and his parents bring him to the emergency room. His respiratory rate is 36 breaths per minute and his heart rate is 150 beats per minute. He has a prolonged expiratory phase when breathing. He is afebrile. Lung auscultation reveals high-pitched, squeaky, musical breath sounds in all lung fields during inspiration and expiration. Which of the following is the most likely diagnosis?

a. Epiglottitis
b. Asthma
c. Croup
d. Tonsillitis
e. Pneumonia

140. A 19-year-old college student develops a positive PPD skin test. The area of induration is 15 cm in diameter at 48 hours. A PPD skin test done four years earlier was negative. The patient has no past medical history and does not know anyone with tuberculosis. She has not received the BCG (extract of *Mycobacterium bovis*) vaccine. She has no fever, chills, night sweats, weight loss, or respiratory symptoms. Which of the following statements best explains the PPD skin test results?

a. The patient does not have tuberculosis
b. The patient has never had tuberculosis in the past
c. The positive reaction may be a false positive due to nontuberculosis mycobacteria
d. The patient is not a candidate for isoniazid chemoprophylaxis
e. The first positive test requires a booster PPD

141. A 36-year-old woman complains of frequent headaches accompanied by abdominal pain, nausea, weakness, and palpitations. A mass located in the posterior mediastinum is seen on chest radiograph. Which of the following masses is most likely to be found in this compartment of the mediastinum?

a. Thymoma
b. Teratoma
c. Thyroid adenoma
d. Parathyroid adenoma
e. Bronchogenic cyst
f. Pericardial cyst
g. Pheochromocytoma

DIRECTIONS: Each group of questions below consists of lettered options followed by a set of numbered items. For each numbered item, select the **one** lettered option with which it is **most** closely associated. Each lettered option may be used once, more than once, or not at all.

Questions 142–143

For each chest description, select the appropriate skeletal deformity.

a. Pectus excavatum
b. Kyphosis
c. Barrel chest
d. Pectus carinatum
e. Lordosis

142. A 4-year-old boy has a marked depression of the sternum below the clavicular-manubrial junction.

143. A 9-year-old girl has a chest deformity in which the sternum protrudes from the thorax.

Questions 144–145

For each patient with a sleep disturbance, select the most appropriate disorder.

a. Narcolepsy
b. Depression
c. Obstructive sleep apnea syndrome
d. Obesity hypoventilation syndrome
e. Cataplexy
f. Somnambulism

144. A 35-year-old man complains of daytime sleepiness and disruptive snoring. He admits to falling asleep several times a day while at work. He does not smoke. He is 72 in. tall and weighs approximately 210 lb.

145. A morbidly obese woman is admitted to the intensive care unit after being found in bed with lethargy, cyanosis, and hypoxemia.

Respiratory System

Answers

105. The answer is e. *(Goldman, pp 519–522.)* **Bronchiectasis** is an acquired disease that causes abnormal dilatation of the bronchi leading to pooling of secretions in the airways and recurrent infections. Patients typically present with cough and production of purulent sputum. Lung auscultation may be normal or remarkable for wheezes, rhonchi, or crackles. Chest radiograph may be normal, but occasionally the damaged, dilated airways will appear as **tram tracks** or **ring shadows.** Bronchiectasis may be a sequela of foreign body aspiration, cystic fibrosis, rheumatic diseases (rheumatoid arthritis, Sjögren's disease), pulmonary infections (tuberculosis, pertussis, *Mycoplasma*), AIDS, or allergic bronchopulmonary aspergillosis (ABPA).

106. The answer is a. *(Tierney, pp 250–252.)* The patient has been in the hospital for 48 hours and has developed a **hospital-acquired pneumonia.** Patients develop fever, leukocytosis, cough productive of purulent sputum, and a new or progressive infiltrate on chest radiograph. The most likely organisms are *P. aeruginosa, Staphylococcus aureus, Enterobacter, Klebsiella pneumoniae,* and *Escherichia coli.*

107. The answer is b. *(Tierney, p 218.)* The rule for recumbent position in lung disease is **good side down.** Gravity will increase perfusion to the good lung. This patient with right-sided lung disease should be lying in the left lateral decubitus position to maximize gas exchange in the dependent (good) lung, allowing for improved oxygenation, ventilation/perfusion (V/Q) matching, and more comfortable respiration. **However, with unilateral lung diseases in which there is a chance that pus or blood could spill from the bad lung to the good lung, lying with the good lung down would be detrimental.**

108. The answer is a. *(Tierney, pp 243–244.)* **Idiopathic bronchiolitis obliterans with organizing pneumonia** (**BOOP**) is also called **cryptogenic organizing pneumonia.** It is a disorder of granulation tissue proliferation within the small ducts and airways. Usually, patients present with an acute illness followed by exertional dyspnea. Patients with **allergic bronchopulmonary aspergillosis (ABPA)** have a history of asthma and have peripheral eosinophilia, elevated IgE levels, skin reactivity to *Aspergillus* antigen, precipitating antibodies to *Aspergillus* antigen, a chest radiograph showing transient or fixed infiltrates, and central bronchiectasis. The presence of six or seven criteria makes the diagnosis almost certain. **Wegener's granulomatosis** typically involves the upper airways (i.e., nasal ulcers, sinus infections), lungs, joints, and kidneys, and antineutrophil cytoplasmic antibodies (c-ANCA) is positive. **Goodpasture's syndrome** causes glomerulonephritis and pulmonary hemorrhage, and patients have antibodies to renal and lung alveolar basement membranes.

109. The answer is e. (*Seidel, pp 337–339.*) The tongue may fall posteriorly to obstruct the oropharynx and is the major cause of airway obstruction. This may occur in patients with a decreased level of consciousness and may be corrected by utilizing the **head tilt–chin lift maneuver.**

110. The answer is d. (*Tierney, pp 276–282.*) The most frequent presenting clinical sign of **pulmonary embolus (PE)** is shortness of breath. Patients may also present with pleuritic chest pain, hemoptysis, and tachycardia. An excellent clue to the diagnosis of PE is deep venous thrombosis (DVT), but absence of signs of DVT does not exclude the diagnosis of PE. Embolus from a thrombus in the lower extremities (DVT) is the most common cause of PE. Common settings for PE include prolonged immobilization, sedentary lifestyle, use of oral contraceptives, obesity, recent surgery, burns, severe trauma, congestive heart failure, malignancy, pregnancy, sickle cell anemia, polycythemias, inherited deficiencies of the anticoagulating proteins (protein C, protein S, antithrombin III), and the Leiden factor V mutation. Chest radiograph in PE may be normal but may demonstrate a peripheral wedge-shaped density above the diaphragm (**Hampton's hump**), focal oligemia (**Westermark's sign**), or abrupt occlusion of a vessel (**cutoff sign**). A **loud** S_2 is often heard in disorders that cause pulmonary hypertension, such as pulmonary embolism. The best next step in making the diagnosis would be to order a ventilation-perfusion (V/Q) scan. If the V/Q scan results are of low or indeterminate probability, the patient may need further studies, such as pulmonary arteriogram or venous ultrasonography of the lower extremity. The absence of D-dimer is strong evidence against thromboembolism. **Helical (spiral) CT scans** are comparable to V/Q scans and are becoming the emerging first step in diagnosing pulmonary embolus.

111. The answer is b. (*Tierney, pp 244–250.*) The patient described most likely has **community-acquired pneumonia** (**CAP**) due to *Streptococcus pneumoniae.* Other pathogens responsible for CAP include *Mycoplasma pneumoniae,* viruses, and *Chlamydia pneumoniae.* In smokers, even without documented chronic lung disease, *Haemophilus influenzae* must be considered. **Fremitus** refers to vibrations that are perceived in a tactile manner; these are increased in patients with consolidation from pneumonia. **Vocal fremitus (bronchophony, egophony, bronchial breath sounds,** and **pectoriloquy)**, **increased dullness to percussion,** and fine crackles may be evident in patients with pneumonia. Areas of **atelectasis** have decreased fremitus, decreased breath sounds, and dullness to percussion. The **trachea is shifted** to the side of the atelectasis. A limited area of egophony is heard above the area of atelectasis.

112. The answer is d. (*Seidel, p 369.*) The best areas to listen for **right middle lobe** findings would be: (1) the right anterior midclavicular line between the fifth and sixth ribs and (2) the right midaxillary line between the fourth and sixth ribs. The right middle lobe is not heard posteriorly, and the lung examination is incomplete if the physician does not listen anteriorly or medially.

113. The answer is b. (*Goldman, p 382.*) **Kartagener's syndrome** is the inheritable disorder of **dextrocardia,** chronic sinusitis (with the formation of nasal polyps), and bronchiectasis. Patients may also present with **situs inversus.** The disorder is due to a defect that causes the cilia within the respiratory tract epithelium to become immotile, thereby predisposing patients to frequent pneumonias. Cilia of the sperm are also affected.

114. The answer is d. (*Tierney, pp 286–288.*) **Primary pulmonary hypertension** (**PPH**) is of unknown etiology and primarily affects women in their thirties or forties. The underlying problem in the disorder is a fixed increased resistance to pulmonary blood flow. Pulmonary function in PPH is usually normal, but the elevation in pulmonary artery pressure causes a decrease in cardiac output and eventually right ventricular failure. Patients become dyspneic and hypoxemic due to the mismatch of pulmonary ventilation and perfusion and the reduced cardiac output. Physical examination reveals signs of right ventricular hypertrophy, right- and left-sided heart failure, and tricuspid and pulmonic regurgitation. The mean survival for this disease is two to three years from the time of diagnosis.

115. The answer is a. *(Tierney, p 217.)* Massive **life-threatening hemoptysis** is more than 100 mL of blood in 24 hours. The most common cause for nonmassive hemoptysis (<30 mL/day) in smokers and nonsmoking patients with a normal chest radiograph is **bronchitis.** Chronic bronchitis is characterized by excessive secretions manifested by a productive cough, often purulent or bloody, for three months or more for two consecutive years in the absence of any other disease to explain the symptoms. Patients are often obese and cyanotic (**blue bloater**). The mnemonic is **BBB = Bronchitis/Blue Bloater.**

116. The answer is a. *(Tierney, pp 235–240.)* COPD is defined as a condition in which there is chronic obstruction to airflow due to chronic bronchitis or emphysema. An exacerbation of COPD occurs when the patient develops the acute onset of marked dyspnea and tachypnea requiring the use of accessory muscles that is unresponsive to medications. α_1 **antitrypsin deficiency** should be suspected in nonsmokers who present with COPD of the lung **bases** in their fifties without any predisposing history, such as occupational exposure, to support the diagnosis. α_1 antitrypsin deficiency is rare in African Americans and Asian–Pacific Islanders.

117. The answer is c. *(Tierney, p 269.)* Carcinoid and bronchial gland tumors are called bronchial adenomas but are actually low-grade malignant neoplasms. They are resistant to radiation and chemotherapy. Patients are usually below the age of 60; common symptoms include hemoptysis, chronic cough, focal wheezing, and recurrent pneumonia (due to obstruction and atelectasis). The chest radiograph may be normal. The classic presentation of flushing, diarrhea, wheezing, and hypotension (**carcinoid syndrome**) is rare. These tumors are centrally located, and bronchoscopy will often reveal a tumor in a central airway. CT scanning and octreotide scintigraphy also may help to localize the lesion.

118. The answer is d. *(Tierney, p 299.)* The patient has a **tension pneumothorax,** as evidenced by the trachea deviating away from the side of the traumatized lung. This occurs secondary to trauma or during mechanical ventilation. Breath sounds will be faint or distant, percussion will be hyperresonant, and fremitus will be decreased. The increased air on the affected side is in the pleural space, not in the lung. As an attempt is made to inflate the lung, air moves into the pleural space from the puncture site, resulting in a collapsed lung with a large pleural space. The contralateral lung is also at risk for collapse. Anytime the trachea is deviated from the involved side, it is considered a medical emergency and the tension pneumothorax must be relieved or the patient will die from hypoxemia or inadequate cardiac output.

119. The answer is d. *(Tierney, p 299.)* The patient most likely has a **spontaneous pneumothorax.** This disorder affects tall, thin men and may be recurrent. It is thought to be due to the rupture of subpleural blebs in response to high negative intrapleural pressures. Physical examination often reveals unilateral chest expansion, decreased fremitus, hyperresonance, and diminished breath sounds. Patients with COPD, cystic fibrosis, *Pneumocystis carinii* pneumonia (PCP), and tuberculosis may have blebs and are at risk for secondary pneumothoraxes.

120. The answer is e. *(Tierney, pp 296–299.)* The pleural effusion of **rheumatoid arthritis** typically has a high LDH, low complement level, **low glucose level,** high rheumatoid factor, and characteristic **cholesterol crystals.** The fluid is usually **greenish-yellow** in color, not grossly bloody (this is seen with pulmonary infarction and with malignancy). Pancreatitis and esophageal rupture produce pleural effusions that have elevated amylase levels; these effusions are typically left-sided. Patients with pleural effusions often have bronchial breath sounds (increased fremitus) immediately above the pleural effusion. There is dullness to percussion, and the trachea may be shifted to the opposite side of the effusion.

121. The answer is b. *(Tierney, p 1373.)* The clinical presentation is most consistent with Legionnaires' disease. Patients are usually elderly or immunocompromised or have chronic lung disease. Air conditioners, whirlpools, water-using machinery, and cooling towers have been linked to outbreaks of the disease. Clinical signs of the disease include fever, relative bradycardia, abdominal complaints, scanty cough, and laboratory abnormalities. **Pontiac fever** is an acute, self-limited, flulike illness due to *Legionella,* but it does not cause pneumonia. **Psittacosis** (*Chlamydia*) is pneumonia associated with the handling of birds.

122. The answer is d. *(Tierney, p 308.)* **Tracheal stenosis** may occur days after intubation and is a sequela of the balloon cuff of the tracheal tube pressing against the tracheal wall, causing necrosis and scar tissue formation. Patients are typically hoarse and dyspneic.

123. The answer is e. *(Tierney, p 291.)* The patient most likely has **Mendelson's syndrome** (acute aspiration of gastric contents). The more acidic the gastric contents, the greater the degree of chemical pneumonitis and the more extensive the desquamation of the bronchial epithelium and the subsequent pulmonary edema. There is no evidence to support the use of antibiotics or high-dose steroids. Treatment consists of supplemental oxygen and other supportive measures.

124. The answer is c. *(Tierney, p 252.)* The right main stem bronchus is wider, shorter, and vertically placed, and therefore, if the patient aspirates while supine, the **posterior segment of the right upper lobe** is anatomically susceptible to aspiration. The **superior segments of the right lower and left lower lobes** are also susceptible to aspiration pneumonia if the patient is supine. These three segments are often referred to as the **aspiration segments of the lung.** The **basilar segments of both lungs are susceptible to aspiration if the patient aspirates while erect or sitting up.**

125. The answer is d. *(Tierney, pp 292–295.)* Persons in certain occupations, such as asbestos mining, shipbuilding, construction, insulation, automobile brake repair, pipe fitting, plumbing, electrical repair, and railroad engine repair are at risk for **asbestos** exposure. Even persons handling the clothes of the person exposed to asbestos are at risk for asbestosis (bystander exposure). Asbestosis means that the patient has developed pulmonary fibrosis, scarring (plaques), and calcification. Asbestosis is a bilateral disease that starts from the bottom of the thorax and works upward, so it is not uncommon for the diaphragm to be involved early on in the disease process. Patients with asbestosis are at risk not only for lung cancer and mesothelioma but also for pharyngeal, gastric, and colon cancers. This patient has clubbing, and malignancy must be considered. **Farmer's lung** results from exposure to moldy hay containing spores. **Berylliosis** causes bilateral hilar adenopathy; patients have a history of occupational exposure to nuclear weapons, fluorescent lights, and ceramics. Patients who work as miners, sandblasters, stonecutters, or foundry or quarry workers are at risk for exposure to **silica.** The chest x-ray typically reveals eggshell calcification of the hilar nodes. **Byssinosis** occurs with exposure to cotton, flax, or hemp.

126. The answer is b. *(Seidel, p 391.)* The **Apgar score** has no predictive value regarding long-term outcome but tells you a great deal about the newborn's respiratory efforts. It is repeated a third time at 10 minutes only if the score is poor at 5 minutes. The Apgar scoring system (a score of 0 to 10 is possible) is based on **APGAR = A**ppearance, **P**ulse, **G**rimace, **A**ctivity, and **R**espirations:

	0	1	2
Heart rate	Absent	<100/min	>100/min
Respiratory effort	Absent	Slow or irregular	Good
Muscle tone	Limp	Some flexion	Active motion
Response to catheter in nostril	None	Grimace	Cough/sneeze
Color	Blue/pale	Body pink/ extremities blue	All pink

127. The answer is b. *(Tierney, pp 273–276.)* **Sarcoidosis** is a multisystemic disease of unknown cause. The histologic hallmark of the disease is noncaseating granulomas, and the most common chest radiograph finding is bilateral hilar adenopathy. Lymphadenopathy is found in 70 to 90% of all patients with sarcoidosis. **Hamman-Rich syndrome** is also called **idiopathic pulmonary fibrosis (IPF)**. It is as common as sarcoidosis but is found more in males than females; the usual age of onset is the fifth or sixth decade of life. Chest radiograph usually reveals fibrosis. **Bagassosis** is a hypersensitivity pneumonitis (HP) due to exposure to sugar cane. **Löffler's syndrome** is a disorder of unknown etiology that causes an acute pneumonia with peripheral blood eosinophilia.

128. The answer is d. *(Tierney, p 216.)* The most common cause of chronic cough in adults is **postnasal drip** due to sinusitis or rhinitis (allergic, vasomotor, irritant, perennial nonallergic). Patients typically complain of having to clear the throat or a feeling of something dripping in the back of the throat. Physical examination reveals mucopurulent secretions and a **cobblestone** appearance of the mucosa. **Asthma** is more of an episodic disease with wheezing, but occasionally patients complain of only cough. **Gastroesophageal reflux disease (GERD)** must be considered in patients who complain of heartburn or regurgitation. Other causes of chronic cough include bronchitis, congestive heart failure, and use of ACE inhibitors.

129. The answer is c. *(Seidel, p 397.)* This patient has a **pleural effusion** most likely due to tuberculosis. Chest examination of a pleural effusion reveals distant or absent breath sounds, a **pleural friction rub,** decreased fremitus, and flatness to percussion. A pleural friction rub is a raspy, grating sound heard in both inspiration and expiration due to inflamed surfaces rubbing against each other. Occasionally, exaggerated bronchial breath sounds are audible at the area of the effusion.

130. The answer is b. *(Tierney, pp 1489–1491.)* Based on the patient's risk factors for human immunodeficiency virus (HIV), **Pneumocystis carinii pneumonia (PCP)** is the most likely diagnosis in this patient, but PCP rarely presents with any physical examination findings that distinguish it from other pneumonias. The chest radiograph may reveal bilateral interstitial infiltrates, and patients are often hypoxemic. Congestive heart failure may present with a similar chest radiograph, but patients will have jugular venous distension (JVD) and an S_3 gallop. Cytomegalovirus (CMV), varicella zoster, and Kaposi's sarcoma (due to herpesvirus type 8) are opportunistic infections seen in immunocompromised patients.

131. The answer is b. *(Tierney, pp 244–247.)* **Pneumococcal pneumonia** is abrupt in onset, with fever, pleuritic chest pain, and purulent sputum production. In young, otherwise healthy patients who present with a localized pneumonia (in this case, right middle lobe) of gradual onset accompanied by dry cough and a predominance of extrapulmonary symptoms (i.e., malaise, headache, diarrhea), the most likely diagnosis is atypical pneumonia due to **Chlamydia pneumoniae** or **Mycoplasma pneumoniae.** Patients often complain of a sore throat at the beginning of the illness and a protracted course of symptoms. Physical examination is often unimpressive compared to radiograph findings. **Legionella pneumoniae** is an atypical organism, but patients usually have renal and hepatic abnormalities, hypo-natremia, and mental status changes.

132. The answer is d. *(Seidel, p 372.)* In emphysema, there is destruction of alveolar septa and reduced elastic recoil. This causes collapse of the small airways and prolongs the expiratory phase of respiration. During the prolonged expiration, patients will **purse their lips** to avoid collapse of the small airways [**this causes auto–positive end-expiratory pressure (auto-PEEP)**]. The respiratory rate is increased by having a markedly shortened inspiratory interval. **Kussmaul respirations** are fast and deep respirations to increase the tidal volume and combat the metabolic acidosis seen in patients with diabetic ketoacidosis. **Biot respirations,** seen in patients with increased intracranial pressure, are irregular, unpredictable periods of apnea alternating with periods of noisy hyperventilation. **Cheyne-Stokes respiration** is a rhythmic, gradually changing pattern of apnea and hyperpnea that is cardiac or neurologic in origin. **Apneustic breathing** is characterized by a long period of inspiration or gasping with almost no expiratory phase.

133. The answer is d. *(Tierney, pp 1552–1554.)* The definition of **drowning** is death from suffocation after submersion. Freshwater drowning in swimming pools is actually more common than saltwater drowning. The patient described has noncardiogenic pulmonary edema, which is a complication of **near drowning** (survival after suffocation from submersion). This is a result of direct pulmonary injury, loss of surfactant, and contaminants in the water. Respiratory failure, severe hypothermia, and neurologic injury are the three most common threats to life after submersion.

134. The answer is a. *(Goldman, p 567.)* Patients with severe long bone injuries are at risk for developing widespread **fat embolism syndrome.** Several days after the trauma, patients develop restlessness, hypoxemia, delirium, seizures, retinal and conjunctival hemorrhages, visible fat in the retinal vessels, a petechial chest rash, bilateral interstitial infiltrates, fat globules in the urine, and renal failure. There is no treatment for fat embolism other than supportive care and early diagnosis.

135. The answer is c. *(Tierney, p 235.)* The increased anteroposterior thickness of the thorax indicates the presence of a **barrel chest,** which in association with a smoking history and exertional dyspnea is a typical presentation of emphysema. **Pursed-lip breathing** is often a learned behavior that occurs with emphysema to prolong the expiratory phase of respiration and prevent sudden collapse of the small airways. Patients have an **asthenic body habitus,** since energy expenditure is in excess of calorie intake. There is often **hypertrophy of the accessory muscles** of respiration. Breath sounds in emphysema are usually diminished, and there is hyperresonance with percussion. Emphysema begins as a centriacinar process but eventually becomes panacinar, involving both the central and the peripheral tissues.

136. The answer is c. *(Tierney, p 252.)* The signs and symptoms of lung abscess include a history of loss of consciousness due to seizure, alcoholism, or illicit drug use. Patients complain of several days or weeks of malaise and fever while the abscess develops. Patients eventually complain of chills, cough, pleuritic chest pain, and cough productive of putrid sputum. Due to position at the time of loss of consciousness and to the anatomy of the lung, the lung segments most often involved in lung abscesses include the **posterior segment of the right upper lobe** (wide, short, and vertically placed) and the **superior segments of both lower lobes.** Patients with poor dental hygiene are prone to developing anaerobic infections if aspiration occurs.

137. The answer is a. *(Tierney, pp 305–307.)* **Acute respiratory distress syndrome** (**ARDS**) can occur due to conditions unrelated to pulmonary disease, such as burns, transfusion, or trauma, but may also be due to sepsis and shock. ARDS is due to severe and widespread increased alveolar capillary permeability secondary to injury of the alveolar and capillary epithelium. This leads to the accumulation of protein-rich edematous fluid within the septal walls, followed by escape of the fluid into the alveolar spaces, where it coagulates to form hyaline membranes lining the alveoli. There is marked impairment of gas exchange that causes severe dyspnea, diffuse crackles, tachypnea, hypoxemia, and cyanosis. The cyanosis may be refractory to oxygen therapy. Chest radiograph reveals bilateral infiltrates.

138. The answer is c. *(Tierney, p 215.)* **Platypnea** (supine respiration) is often associated with **orthodeoxia** (hemoglobin oxygen desaturation in the upright position). **Orthopnea** may be due to either cardiac or pulmonary disease; the upright position decreases venous return to the heart and effectively reduces lung congestion. Platypnea is due to bilateral lower lobe lung disease, not cardiac disease. An upright position increases perfusion to the lower lobes and worsens V/Q matching. Platypnea has been described in patients with pulmonary emboli, bibasilar pneumonia, and diseases with bibasilar arteriovenous shunting, such as cirrhosis and **Osler-Weber-Rendu disease. Abdominal paradox** is when the abdomen collapses in inspiration instead of rising; this is a sign of respiratory muscle weakness and fatigue.

139. The answer is b. (*Tierney, p 223.*) **Asthma** is an airway disease characterized by a hyperreactive tracheobronchial tree that manifests physiologically as narrowing of the airway passages. The classic triad of symptoms is dyspnea, cough, and wheezing. Attacks are usually episodic and nocturnal and often follow exposure to specific allergens, exertion, viral infection, or emotional excitement. Wheezing is described as whistling and is typically heard in both inspiration and expiration. The expiratory phase becomes prolonged, and the patient develops tachypnea, tachycardia, and mild systolic hypertension. Accessory muscles of respiration (sternocleidomastoid and intercostals) may be used to improve breathing. If the asthma attack is severe, the patient will develop a **pulsus paradoxus** (an inspiratory drop in systolic blood pressure of more than 10 mmHg). Patients with **epiglottitis** present with fever, drooling, and dysphagia; lung examination will be normal. Children with **croup** or **laryngotracheobronchitis** present with labored breathing and stridor and use accessory muscles to assist breathing.

140. The answer is c. (*Tierney, p 256.*) Patients with a **positive PPD** require isoniazid chemoprophylaxis. A positive PPD may mean that the patient currently has tuberculosis or may have had tuberculosis in the past. A positive PPD may be a false positive due to nontuberculosis mycobacterium. A booster PPD is placed in patients (typically over the age of 55) one week after a negative PPD to boost a response. A negative boost implies the patient is anergic or uninfected. A PPD skin test is classified as positive by the American Thoracic Society and the Centers for Disease Control and Prevention (1995) according to the reaction size and patient population:

$\geq$5 mm: HIV patients or HIV at-risk patients; close contacts of patients with active TB; persons with CXR showing healed TB
$\geq$10 mm: immigrants; intravenous drug abusers; medically underserved; residents of nursing homes, prisons, and mental institutions; persons with underlying disease
$\geq$15 mm: all other persons

141. The answer is g. (*Tierney, p 271.*) The area between the pleural sacs—the mediastinum—is divided anatomically into the anterior mediastinum, middle mediastinum, and posterior mediastinum. The most common masses found in the **anterior mediastinum** are the **four T's =** **T**hymomas, **T**eratomas, **T**hyroid masses, and para**T**hyroid masses. Lymphomas may also be found in the anterior mediastinum. Masses in the

middle mediastinum include enlarged lymph nodes, lymphomas, vascular masses, pleuropericardial cysts, and bronchogenic cysts. The **posterior mediastinum** is the likely area for neurogenic tumors, lymphomas, pheochromocytomas, myelomas, meningoceles, meningomyeloceles, gastroenteric cysts, and diverticula.

142–143. The answers are 142-a, 143-d. (*Seidel, p 371.*) **Pectus excavatum,** or **funnel breast,** is a congenital, hereditary malformation characterized by depression of the sternum below the clavicular-manubrial junction with symmetric inward bending of the costal cartilages. This may affect pulmonary and heart function. **Pectus carinatum,** or **pigeon breast,** is a deformity where the sternum protrudes from the narrowed thorax. **Kyphosis** is posterior deviation of the spine. **Scoliosis** is lateral deviation of the spine. **Lordosis** is an exaggerated convex curvature of the lumbar spine.

144–145. The answers are 144-c, 145-d. (*Tierney, pp 300–302.*) The patient with **obstructive sleep apnea syndrome** (**OSAS**) presents complaining of disruptive snoring and daytime hypersomnolence. Obesity is a risk factor for OSAS, but many patients with OSAS are not obese. Patients have upper airway narrowing from enlarged soft tissues, and good respiratory effort occurs against the airway obstruction. Diagnosis is best made by overnight polysomnography to document the apneic periods (10 to 15 events per hour of sleep, each event more than 10 seconds in duration). Obesity represents a mechanical load to the respiratory system, since excess weight reduces chest wall compliance. Patients with **obesity hypoventilation syndrome** demonstrate a decrease in central respiratory drive (no respiratory effort), especially during sleep (sleep-induced hypoventilation), since vital capacity is further reduced in the recumbent position. **Narcolepsy** is excessive daytime sleepiness associated with abnormalities in REM sleep. Narcoleptic sleep attacks are brief and may occur during sedentary periods or when the patient is driving, eating, or conversing. Cataplexy occurs when strong emotion (i.e., laughing or crying) precipitates sudden loss of muscle tone. Somnambulism is sleepwalking.

Cardiovascular System

Questions

DIRECTIONS: Each item below contains a question followed by suggested responses. Select the **one best** response to each question.

146. A 47-year-old woman presents with chest pain that worsens with inspiration and improves when she bends forward. Pain is relieved when the patient holds her breath. Blood pressure is 140/90 mmHg. Heart examination reveals coarse, scratchy sounds heard throughout the cardiac cycle. Electrocardiogram (ECG) reveals T wave inversions. Which of the following is the most appropriate next step in management?

a. Intravenous heparin
b. Oral prednisone
c. Fibrinolytics
d. Oral aspirin
e. Primary angioplasty
f. Chest radiograph
g. Echocardiogram

147. A 47-year-old perimenopausal woman presents for her annual checkup. She denies chest pain, shortness of breath, and palpitations. She has no family history of heart disease and does not smoke cigarettes. She has no past medical history of hypertension or diabetes mellitus. She takes no medications, and she exercises in a fitness center three times a week. Her blood pressure is 110/75 mmHg and her heart rate is 66 beats per minute and regular. Physical examination reveals no jugular venous distention. Lung examination is normal. A split S_1 best heard over the tricuspid area is now audible but was not present one year ago. There is no peripheral edema. Which of the following is the most appropriate next step in diagnosis?

a. Transthoracic echocardiogram
b. Transesophageal echocardiogram
c. Cardiac isoenzymes
d. Cardiac catheterization
e. Electrocardiogram
f. Cardiac stress test
g. Holter monitor

148. A 16-year-old boy is found to have an unexpected sound audible in the right side of the neck. The sound is loudest in diastole and with the patient in the sitting position. The sound disappears when the patient is lying down or with the Valsalva maneuver. He has no complaints and is very athletic in school. He has no clubbing or cyanosis. Blood pressure and heart rate are normal. The rest of the physical examination is normal. Which of the following is the most likely diagnosis?

a. Thyroid bruit
b. Venous hum
c. Carotid bruit
d. AV malformation
e. Transmitted murmur

149. A 31-year-old woman presents with a two-year history of palpitations. She denies chest pain and dizziness. Past medical history is significant for pectus excavatum. Blood pressure and heart rate are normal. Physical examination reveals a late systolic murmur preceded by a midsystolic click that increases with standing. Transthoracic echocardiogram confirms your suspicion of mitral valve prolapse. Which of the following is the most likely complication of mitral valve prolapse?

a. Severe mitral regurgitation
b. Myocardial infarction
c. Pulmonary embolism
d. Ventricular arrhythmia
e. Congestive heart failure
f. Cerebrovascular accident

150. You are called to evaluate a 57-year-old man with pressure-like chest pain that occurred while he was shoveling snow. The pain radiates to the jaw and medial aspect of the left arm. The patient denies dizziness, nausea, vomiting, or palpitations. He has a past medical history of hypertension and he smokes two packs of cigarettes per day. He has a brother who had a myocardial infarction that required balloon angioplasty when he was in his forties. The patient has recently been told to modify his diet because of high glucose and cholesterol levels. On physical examination the patient appears pale and diaphoretic. Blood pressure is 160/100 mmHg and pulse is 108 beats per minute. His extremities are cool. Heart examination reveals an S_4 gallop. Lungs are normal. Peripheral pulses are palpable and bilaterally equal. He has no peripheral edema. Which of the following is the most likely diagnosis?

a. Right ventricular infarction
b. Cardiogenic shock
c. Acute myocardial infarction
d. Congestive heart failure (CHF)
e. Prinzmetal's angina

151. A 41-year-old intravenous drug abuser presents with shortness of breath and pleuritic chest pain. He is febrile with a temperature of 39.7°C (103.5°F). He has no skin lesions, and funduscopic exam is negative. He has jugular venous distension that increases with compression of the liver. The liver is pulsatile. The jugular venous pulse shows a prominent v wave. The patient has splenomegaly. Heart auscultation reveals a holosystolic murmur heard best at the left lower sternal border. The murmur increases with inspiration (Müller maneuver). Which of the following is the most likely diagnosis?

a. Bacterial endocarditis
b. Pericarditis
c. Rheumatic fever
d. Mitral valve prolapse
e. Pericardial effusion

152. A 58-year-old man presents to the emergency room with shortness of breath for two days. He has three-pillow orthopnea but no paroxysmal nocturnal dyspnea. He denies chest pain, palpitations, dizziness, and cough. His blood pressure is 170/90 mmHg and his heart rate is 130 beats per minute. He has jugular venous distension. Heart examination reveals a high-pitched extra heart sound that appears to be louder than an isolated S_3 or S_4 gallop. It occurs in diastole, is best heard with the bell of the stethoscope, and is palpable. Lung examination reveals crackles at the bases; the patient has 1+ bilateral peripheral edema. Which of the following is the most likely cause of his abnormal heart sound?

a. It is a ventricular gallop
b. It is an atrial gallop
c. It is quadruple rhythm
d. It is a summation gallop
e. It is a diastolic murmur

153. An 18-year-old woman presents with arthritis that is asymmetrical and involves more than three joints. The arthritis is migratory, affecting one joint for several days and improving, then affecting another joint. On physical examination, the patient has several subcutaneous nodules and her cardiac exam reveals an S_3 gallop. Which of the following is the most likely diagnosis?

a. Lyme disease
b. Endocarditis
c. Rheumatoid arthritis
d. Gout
e. Rheumatic fever

154. A 37-year-old man presents to the emergency room after three days of feeling weak. He drinks alcohol daily but denies illicit drug use. He called the paramedics when he began to experience palpitations and light-headedness with exertion. On physical examination, his blood pressure is 120/80 mmHg and his pulse is irregularly irregular at a rate of 126 beats per minute. Electrocardiogram for this patient would most likely demonstrate which of the following?

a. Sinus tachycardia
b. Ventricular premature beats (VPCs)
c. Atrial fibrillation (AF)
d. Premature atrial contractions (PACs)
e. Sinus arrhythmia

155. A 23-year-old student presents to your office for health clearance to play collegiate sports. He is asymptomatic and exercises daily. On physical examination, his blood pressure is 160/50 mmHg and his pulse rate is 60 beats per minute. There is pulsus bisferiens. Heart examination reveals an early diastolic rumble at the apex and a blowing diastolic murmur at the left sternal border. Nail beds reveal a Quincke pulse. Which of the following is the most likely diagnosis?

a. Cardiac tamponade
b. Aortic insufficiency (AI)
c. Mitral stenosis (MS)
d. Atrial septal defect (ASD)
e. Tetralogy of Fallot

156. While palpating the pulse of a patient, you note that the pulse wave has two peaks. You auscultate the heart and are certain that there is only one heartbeat for each two pulse waves. Which of the following best describes this finding?

a. Pulsus alternans
b. Dicrotic pulse
c. Pulsus parvus et tardus
d. Pulsus bigeminus
e. Pulsus bisferiens

157. A 68-year-old woman with a history of hypertension and diabetes mellitus presents with shortness of breath. She denies chest pain and palpitations. Physical examination reveals a blood pressure of 130/60 mmHg and a heart rate of 72 beats per minute. The patient's lungs are normal, and heart auscultation reveals an S_4 gallop. She has no jugular venous distention (JVD) and no peripheral edema. Chest radiograph shows a normal-size heart, and ECG shows left ventricular hypertrophy. Echocardiogram reveals concentric left ventricular hypertrophy (LVH) with a hyperdynamic left ventricle. Which of the following is the most likely diagnosis?

a. Systolic dysfunction
b. Diastolic dysfunction
c. Left heart failure
d. Right heart failure
e. Normal heart

158. A 50-year-old woman presents with malaise and weight loss. She denies chest pain, shortness of breath, dizziness, and palpitations. Her temperature is 38.3°C (100.9°F), and her heart rate is 80 beats per minute. There is a diastolic murmur that is variable from cycle to cycle. Splinter hemorrhages are visible in the fingernails of both hands. Which of the following is the most likely diagnosis?

a. Mitral stenosis
b. Endocarditis
c. Aortic insufficiency
d. Atrial myxoma
e. Tricuspid stenosis

159. A 30-year-old woman presents for a routine checkup. She has no complaints and denies previous medical problems. On heart examination, the patient has a loud S_1. She has a grade 2 low-pitched mid-to-late diastolic murmur that is heard best at the apex. Immediately preceding the murmur is a loud extra sound. Which of the following is the most likely diagnosis?

a. Mitral valve prolapse (MVP)
b. Mitral stenosis
c. Ventricular septal defect
d. Aortic insufficiency
e. Atrial septal defect

160. A 16-year-old boy is referred to your practice for leg claudication. His right arm blood pressure is 150/110 mmHg, while his left leg blood pressure is 80/60 mmHg. On auscultation, a systolic murmur best heard over the middle of the upper back is detected. You also find that the patient's femoral pulses are diminished when compared to his brachial pulses. Which of the following is the most likely diagnosis?

a. Patent ductus arteriosus
b. Ventricular septal defect
c. Coarctation of the aorta
d. Atrial septal defect
e. Tetralogy of Fallot

161. A 66-year-old man presents with worsening shortness of breath and dyspnea on exertion. His blood pressure and heart rate are normal. Physical examination is positive for jugular venous distension, ascites, and peripheral edema. A loud and high-pitched extra sound is heard in early diastole corresponding to early ventricular filling. Which of the following is the most likely diagnosis?

a. Pericardial effusion
b. Pericardial tamponade
c. Pericarditis
d. Constrictive pericarditis
e. Restrictive cardiomyopathy

162. A 57-year-old man presents with midsternal pressure-like chest pain that radiates to the left arm accompanied by diaphoresis and nausea. He has a blood pressure of 80/50 mmHg and neck vein distention with inspiration. The rest of the physical examination is normal. Electrocardiogram reveals ST elevations in leads 2, 3, and AVF. Which of the following is the most likely diagnosis?

a. Congestive heart failure
b. Pericardial tamponade
c. Right ventricular infarction
d. Rupture of the chordae tendinae
e. Rupture of the papillary muscle

163. A mother brings her 11-year-old son to your office because he easily becomes short of breath while running. She states that he does not seem to be able to play for as long a period of time as his friends. The patient's blood pressure is 140/60 mmHg, and he has bounding peripheral pulses. On auscultation of the heart, you detect a harsh, loud continuous murmur heard best below the left clavicle. Which of the following is the most likely diagnosis?

a. Cervical venous hum
b. Hepatic venous hum
c. Coarctation of the aorta
d. Patent ductus arteriosus
e. Mammary soufflé

164. A 54-year-old man with a 20-year history of chronic obstructive lung disease has a heave that is palpable at the lower left sternal border at the third, fourth, and fifth intercostal spaces. He has no palpable thrill. Which of the following best explains the etiology of the heave?

a. It is probably a displaced point of maximum impulse (PMI)
b. It means the patient has congestive heart failure
c. It means the patient has aortic stenosis
d. It means the patient has right ventricular hypertrophy
e. It means the patient has a pericardial effusion

165. A 64-year-old man with a history of hypertension presents with sharp midsternal chest pain that is intermittent and radiates to his back between his shoulder blades. Blood pressure is 170/110 mmHg in his right arm and 90/60 mmHg in his left arm. Heart auscultation reveals a diastolic murmur. He has a tracheal tug sign. ECG is normal. Chest radiograph reveals a widened mediastinum. Which of the following is the most likely diagnosis?

a. Myocardial infarction
b. Pulmonary embolus
c. Aortic dissection
d. Coarctation of the aorta
e. Aortic stenosis

166. An 81-year-old woman presents with syncope. Blood pressure is 120/80 mmHg; heart rate is 40 beats per minute. There is no jugular venous distension, but cannon *a* waves are visible. Lung and heart examinations are otherwise normal. Which of the following is the most likely cause of her syncope?

a. Ventricular tachycardia
b. Complete heart block
c. Atrial flutter
d. Atrial fibrillation
e. Cardiac tamponade
f. Myocardial infarction

167. A 16-year-old boy is referred to your office for a blood pressure of 140/55 mmHg. He has a well-healed surgical scar about 12 cm long over the medial aspect of his left thigh. On questioning, he states that he acquired the scar four years ago by impaling his thigh on a large nail after falling. Auscultation of the scar reveals a bruit, and there is a palpable thrill. Which of the following is the most likely diagnosis?

a. Premature atherosclerosis
b. Arteriovenous fistula
c. Scar tissue compressing the femoral artery
d. Congenital femoral artery bruit
e. Patent ductus arteriosus

168. A 16-year-old boy presents with the chief complaint of palpitations while in gym class. The palpitations occur with moderate exertion and are relieved with rest. He denies shortness of breath, dizziness, and chest pain. Heart examination reveals a systolic murmur that increases with standing. Which of the following is the most likely diagnosis?

a. Mitral regurgitation (MR)
b. Aortic insufficiency (AI)
c. Tricuspid regurgitation (TR)
d. Hypertrophic cardiomyopathy (HCM)
e. Mitral stenosis (MS)

169. A 51-year-old man is involved in a motor vehicle accident. He was not wearing a seat belt and remembers striking the steering wheel during the collision. On arrival at the emergency room, the patient is complaining of chest pain and shortness of breath. His blood pressure is 120/80 mmHg but decreases to 90/50 mmHg at the end of inspiration. He has JVD with distant heart sounds. Lung examination reveals normal breath sounds bilaterally. Which of the following is the most likely diagnosis?

a. Aortic dissection
b. Ruptured aorta
c. Pneumothorax
d. Congestive heart failure
e. Cardiac tamponade

170. A 71-year-old man complains of occasional lower back pain. His blood pressure is 150/85 mmHg and his pulse is 80 beats per minute. Cardiac examination reveals an S_4 gallop. Abdominal examination reveals a pulsatile mass approximately 5.0 cm in diameter palpable in the epigastric area. Peripheral pulses are normal. Which of the following is the most likely diagnosis?

a. Abdominal aortic aneurysm
b. Cancer of the proximal colon
c. Peptic ulcer disease
d. Chronic pancreatitis
e. Lipoma of the abdominal wall

171. A 47-year-old man has been at home recovering from an anterior myocardial infarction that occurred 10 days ago. He presents to your office complaining of persistent chest pain that is worse on inspiration and that is different from his heart attack pain. The pain radiates to both clavicles. The pain is worse when the patient is lying down and improves with sitting up and leaning forward. The patient has a temperature of 38.4°C (101.2°F) and a normal blood pressure. Heart auscultation reveals a pericardial rub. Lung examination is positive for dullness and diminished breath sounds at the right base. Chest radiograph reveals a small right-sided pleural effusion. Laboratory data reveal that the patient has a mild leukocytosis and an increased erythrocyte sedimentation rate (ESR). Which of the following is the most likely diagnosis?

a. Extension of the myocardial infarction
b. Unstable angina
c. Prinzmetal's angina
d. Pulmonary embolus
e. Post–myocardial infarction syndrome

172. A 41-year-old woman has a split second heart sound on physical examination. The split S_2 is audible with deep inspiration and disappears with expiration. Which of the following is the most likely cause of these physical examination findings?

a. Delayed aortic valve closure
b. Shortened right ventricular ejection time
c. Decreased pulmonary vasculature compliance
d. Decreased thoracic pressure
e. Decreased stroke volume

173. An 82-year-old woman presents for her annual physical examination. She has a history of hypertension, for which she takes a calcium channel blocker. She does not smoke cigarettes. Physical examination reveals a blood pressure of 135/85 mmHg. Heart examination is remarkable for a short systolic murmur that peaks early in systole. The second heart sound is normal in intensity. Which of the following is the most likely diagnosis?

a. Aortic sclerosis
b. Aortic stenosis
c. Mitral regurgitation
d. Tricuspid regurgitation
e. Mitral valve prolapse

174. A 10-year-old boy is brought to the emergency room because of chest pain. He has had a fever for the last five days. Physical examination is remarkable for conjunctival injection, strawberry tongue, cervical lymphadenopathy, a diffuse polymorphous rash, and edema of the hands and feet. Electrocardiogram is consistent with a myocardial infarction. Which of the following is the most appropriate next step in management?

a. Intravenous fibrinolytics
b. Percutaneous angioplasty
c. Intravenous steroids
d. Intravenous gamma globulin
e. Coronary artery bypass surgery

175. You are asked to provide a consult on a 13-year-old boy who wishes to join his high school track team. The patient is asymptomatic but carries a diagnosis of having a functional heart murmur. Heart examination reveals a nonradiating systolic ejection murmur heard best at the left sternal border. The murmur does not increase with Valsalva maneuver, hand grip, or inspiration. Which of the following is the most appropriate next step in management?

a. No further management is necessary
b. Transthoracic echocardiogram
c. Transesophageal echocardiogram
d. Electrocardiogram
e. Holter monitor
f. Stress test

176. A 73-year-old man with a history of hypertension presents for a blood pressure check. He is compliant with his four antihypertensive medications. He does not drink alcohol or smoke cigarettes. He walks several miles each day and follows a low-salt diet. His blood pressure in your office is 170/90 mmHg. The brachial artery is palpable when the sphygmomanometer cuff is inflated above systolic blood pressure. Which of the following is the most appropriate next step in management?

a. Add a fifth antihypertensive medication
b. Maximize present antihypertensive medication
c. Measure intraarterial pressure directly
d. Stress the importance of compliance with medications
e. No further management is indicated

177. A 14-year-old boy experiences shortness of breath while in gym class. Heart exam reveals fixed splitting of S_2. Which of the following is the most likely etiology?

a. Right bundle branch block
b. Left bundle branch block
c. Aortic stenosis
d. Atrial septal defect
e. Pulmonic stenosis
f. Mitral insufficiency
g. Mitral stenosis

178. A 25-year-old woman presents with a blood pressure of 125/50 mmHg. She complains of palpitations. Which of the following is the most likely cause of her abnormal blood pressure reading?

a. Aortic stenosis
b. Pregnancy
c. Mitral regurgitation
d. Pericardial tamponade
e. Tricuspid regurgitation
f. Constrictive pericarditis

DIRECTIONS: Each group of questions below consists of lettered options followed by a set of numbered items. For each numbered item, select the **one** lettered option with which it is **most** closely associated. Each lettered option may be used once, more than once, or not at all.

Questions 179–182

For each patient with a heart murmur, select the heart lesion most likely responsible for the murmur.

a. Aortic stenosis
b. Mitral stenosis
c. Aortic insufficiency
d. Mitral regurgitation
e. Pulmonic stenosis
f. Pulmonic insufficiency
g. Tricuspid regurgitation
h. Tricuspid stenosis
i. Hypertrophic cardiomyopathy
j. Mitral valve prolapse
k. Ventricular septal defect
l. Atrial septal defect
m. Idiopathic calcific aortic stenosis

179. A 50-year-old man presents with syncope that occurred while he was dancing at his high school reunion party. His blood pressure is normal but his pulse pressure is narrow. Heart examination reveals a crescendo-decrescendo systolic murmur heard best at the second left intercostal space that radiates to the carotid artery. The patient has a soft S_2 heart sound.

180. A 19-year-old man presents after having a syncopal episode while playing in a college intramural basketball game. His father died suddenly at the age of 30. Physical examination reveals a rapid, brisk carotid upstroke. Heart examination reveals a holosystolic murmur heard best in the left sternal border. The murmur increases with Valsalva maneuver.

181. A 31-year-old woman with a long history of a heart murmur diagnosed by her pediatrician over 20 years ago wishes reassurance that the murmur is normal. On heart examination, S_2 is widely split and does not change with respiration. There is a crescendo-decrescendo systolic murmur heard best in the left second intercostal space.

182. A 56-year-old man is four days post–myocardial infarction. On heart auscultation, a new holosystolic murmur is heard that radiates to the right of the sternum. A thrill is palpable.

Cardiovascular System

Answers

146. The answer is d. (*Tierney, pp 394–396.*) The pericardium is a double-walled sac that protects the heart; inflammation and roughening of the sac may result in the formation of a pericardial rub. The sounds represent heart movement against the inflamed pericardium and are best heard with the diaphragm of the stethoscope placed at the left lower sternal border with the patient leaning forward. The scratchy nature of the **triphasic sound** represents systole and diastole of the ventricle and atrial systole. The ECG in pericarditis often reveals ST elevation and PR depression early and T wave inversion later. The treatment for benign pericarditis is anti-inflammatory agents.

147. The answer is e. (*Goldman, pp 246–248.*) S_1 consists of mitral valve closure followed by tricuspid closure. **Splitting of S_1** is seldom heard. In most cases, the valves close together and make a single sound, but if right ventricular contraction is delayed—as in the case of right bundle branch block (RBBB)—closure of the tricuspid valve occurs long after the mitral valve has closed, and a split S_1 is heard.

148. The answer is b. (*Seidel, pp 474–475.*) **Venous hums** are innocent murmurs (occur in 25% of young adults) caused by flow through the internal jugular vein. They are heard best in the sitting position and disappear on lying down, with Valsalva maneuver, or with compression of the ipsilateral jugular vein. Venous hums are often confused with carotid bruits; in adults, they are seen with anemia, pregnancy, and hyperthyroidism. Systolic heart murmurs that transmit to the neck are usually accompanied by a precordial murmur. **Carotid bruits** are usually heard in systole.

149. The answer is a. (*Tierney, p 323.*) The diagnosis of **mitral valve prolapse** (**MVP**) is clinical but can be confirmed by echocardiography. It is diagnosed in 10% of all healthy women. Many are thin, and some have minor chest wall abnormalities. Most patients with MVP have a benign course, and complications are rare. Patients with thickened leaflets may develop severe mitral regurgitation often due to rupture of the chordae tendinae. Other complications include endocarditis (patients require prophylactic antibiotics), supraventricular arrhythmias, and sudden death due to ventricular arrhythmias (rare). Association between MVP and cerebrovascular accident has been reported but not confirmed in subsequent studies.

150. The answer is c. *(Tierney, pp 344–345.)* **Myocardial infarction** occurs when an atherosclerotic plaque ruptures or ulcerates. Patients having a myocardial infarction are typically anxious, restless, and uncomfortable secondary to the extreme pain. They may be demonstrating **Levine's sign** (clenching of the fist over the sternum to demonstrate the severity of the pain). Risk factors for this patient include male gender, positive family history, hypertension, diabetes mellitus, tobacco use, and hyperlipidemia. ECG will show ST elevations, and cardiac isoenzymes (troponin, CPK-MB fraction, and LDH) will be elevated. Patients with **Prinzmetal's angina** have recurrent attacks of chest pain at rest or while asleep (unstable angina) due to a focal spasm of an **epicardial** coronary artery. The diagnosis is confirmed by detecting the spasm after provocation during coronary arteriography. **Cardiogenic shock** is a form of severe left ventricular heart failure; patients are typically hypotensive. **Right ventricular infarction** is a complication of inferoposterior myocardial infarction; patients present with jugular venous distension (JVD), Kussmaul's sign, and hypotension. Diagnosis is made by a right-sided electrocardiogram in which the leads are placed to the right of the sternum instead of the left.

151. The answer is a. *(Tierney, p 327.)* The increased venous return of inspiration (the **Müller maneuver** is sucking in with the nares held closed) increases murmurs of the right side of the heart, and expiration increases murmurs of the left side of the heart. The murmur of **tricuspid regurgitation** is a holosystolic murmur heard best at the left lower sternal border that increases with inspiration. Other findings in tricuspid regurgitation include distended neck veins, prominent *v* waves, hepatomegaly, pulsatile liver, edema, and a positive **Pasteur-Rondot sign** or hepatojugular reflex (pressure applied over the liver causes increased distension of the neck veins). Intravenous drug abusers are at risk for developing acute endocarditis of the tricuspid valve due to *Staphylococcus aureus* bacteria. Other signs of bacterial endocarditis include splinter hemorrhages (subungual streaks), **Roth spots** (oval retinal hemorrhages with a pale center), **Osler nodes** (tender nodules on finger or toe pads), **Janeway lesions**

(small hemorrhages on the palms and soles), clubbing, and splenomegaly. Rheumatic heart disease predisposes patients to endocarditis; the organism is often *Streptococcus viridans,* and the mitral valve is most commonly involved. Mitral valve prolapse also predisposes patients to endocarditis.

152. The answer is d. *(Seidel, p 441.)* A **summation gallop** is often referred to as an S_7; it is due to tachycardia reducing diastole, thus leading to a fusion of S_3 and S_4 into a loud S_7. Summation gallops may be heard in fluid overload states. A **quadruple rhythm** is characterized by the presence of both an S_3 and an S_4, each separately audible.

153. The answer is e. *(Tierney, pp 392–393.)* **Subcutaneous nodules** may be seen in rheumatic fever, gout, rheumatoid arthritis, and syphilis. Rheumatic fever is due to group A streptococci and often presents with a migratory polyarthritis. Patients have a history of sore throat two weeks prior to presentation. Rheumatic fever is often diagnosed using the **Jones minor = FEAR** (**F**ever, prolonged **P**R interval on **E**lectrocardiogram, **A**rthralgia, blood results indicating an elevated acute-phase **R**eactant) and **Jones major = CASES** (**C**arditis, migratory poly**A**rthritis, **S**ydenham's chorea, **E**rythema marginatum, and **S**ubcutaneous nodules) criteria (**FEAR CASES**). The diagnosis of rheumatic fever requires demonstration of previous streptococcal infection and either **two major or one major and two minor criteria** with evidence of previous group A streptococci. **Aschoff bodies** (histiocytes) are found histologically in rheumatic fever. The characteristic rash of Lyme disease is erythema migrans. A chronic arthritis may develop in up to 10% of untreated patients infected with *Borrelia burgdorferi,* but this arthritis is usually monoarticular or oligoarticular, affecting the knees, ankles, hips, elbows, and wrists (large joints).

154. The answer is c. *(Tierney, pp 364–366.)* **Atrial fibrillation** is a common dysrhythmia that can occur in normal people, especially during emotional stress, after surgery or exercise, in patients who have hyperthyroidism, in patients with underlying heart disease, or following an alcoholic binge (**holiday heart syndrome**). It may also be seen in patients with hypoxemia, hypercapnea, or some metabolic or hemodynamic disturbance. Chronic AF occurs in patients with cardiovascular disease, rheumatic heart disease, mitral valve disease, cardiomyopathy, atrial septal defect (ASD), thyroid disease, pulmonary embolus, or chronic lung disease. Whenever the pulse is found to be **irregularly irregular,** AF is almost always the diagnosis. A major complication of AF is formation of mural thrombi, which may embolize to cerebral vessels, causing stroke or transient ischemic attacks (TIAs).

155. The answer is b. (*Tierney, pp 326–327.*) The patient has physical findings consistent with **aortic insufficiency (AI)**. Etiologies may include dissecting aorta, Marfan's syndrome, bicuspid aortic valve, rheumatic heart disease, ankylosing spondylitis, endocarditis, and syphilis. Associated signs of AI (all due to the large stroke volume) include pulsus bisferiens (double wave pulse), **deMusset's sign** (head bobbing with the heartbeat), **water-hammer pulse** (rapidly rising pulse), **Corrigan pulse** (collapsing pulse that follows rising pulse), **Hill's sign** (an increase of >20 mmHg in femoral artery systolic BP compared to brachial artery BP), **Quincke pulse** (blanching of the root of the nail when pressure is applied to the tip), **capillary pulsations, pistol shots** (booming sound heard over the femoral arteries), and **Duroziez's sign** (bruit auscultated over the femoral artery when compressed). Patients with AI have a **wide pulse pressure** (due to increased stroke volume) and a rumbling bruit (from the aortic regurgitant flow displacing the mitral valve, often called the **Austin Flint murmur**).

156. The answer is e. (*Seidel, pp 472–473.*) **Pulsus bisferiens (bisferious pulse)** is seen in AI and in hypertrophic cardiomyopathy (HCM). In the latter, the first wave or percussion wave is due to the rapid flow rate of initial contraction, and the second wave or tidal wave is due to the slower rate of continued contraction. The **dicrotic pulse** has two palpable pulses, but one is in systole and the other is in diastole. **Pulsus bigeminus** is an alteration in pulse amplitude that follows a ventricular premature beat. **Pulsus alternans** is a regular alternating pulse amplitude due to alternating left ventricular contractile force; it is usually seen with severe left ventricular decompensation and cardiac tamponade. **Pulsus parvus et tardus** (small and slow rising) represents a delayed systolic peak due to obstruction to left ventricular ejection. It is seen in aortic stenosis (AS).

157. The answer is b. (*Goldman, pp 293–295.*) **Systolic dysfunction** is an inability of the ventricle to contract normally (hypodynamic). Patients (especially older patients) with hypertension and diabetes mellitus are predisposed to **diastolic dysfunction** (inability of the ventricle to relax for filling) and typically have an S$_4$ gallop, elevated filling pressures, and a hyperdynamic (ejection fraction > 50%) ventricle. Patients with left heart failure present with pulmonary congestion (i.e., crackles); patients with right heart failure present with JVD, an S$_3$ gallop, hepatomegaly, ascites, and peripheral edema.

158. The answer is d. *(Tierney, p 398.)* **Atrial myxomas** are benign tumors of the heart that may embolize systemically. Patients present with fever, malaise, weight loss, leukocytosis, and emboli. If the tumor is large, signs of low cardiac output may result. A **tumor plop** is the hallmark sound of atrial myxoma; it is a diastolic sound that is variable from cycle to cycle (related to the motion of the tumor). The plop represents the diastolic prolapse of the myxoma through an opened mitral or tricuspid valve.

159. The answer is b. *(Seidel, pp 447–451.)* **Mitral stenosis (MS)** is characterized by an opening snap just prior to a low-pitched, rumbling diastolic murmur. **Aortic regurgitation** is characterized by a high-pitched diastolic murmur. **MVP** consists of a midsystolic click with a late systolic murmur. **ASD** is characterized by a systolic murmur. Murmurs are caused by turbulent blood flow and are graded (since 1933, using the **Levine scale**) based on intensity from grades 1 to 6:

Grade 1 murmurs are faint and just audible.
Grade 2 murmurs are quiet but audible with a stethoscope.
Grade 3 murmurs are not loud but are easily heard and should not be missed.
Grade 4 murmurs are loud with a palpable thrill.
Grade 5 murmurs are very loud and can be heard with the chest piece tilted.
Grade 6 murmurs are heard with the stethoscope off the chest.

160. The answer is c. *(Seidel, pp 457–458, 493.)* **Coarctation of the aorta** is narrowing of the aorta usually just distal to the origin of the ductus arteriosus and subclavian artery. Patients may complain of epistaxis, headache, cold peripheral extremities, and claudication. Absent, delayed, or markedly diminished femoral pulses may also be found. The low arterial pressure in the legs in the face of hypertension in the arm is also a clue toward the diagnosis. Chest radiograph in coarctation shows **rib notching**

secondary to the dilated collateral arteries. **Patent ductus arteriosus (PDA)** is associated with a loud, continuous murmur. **Tetralogy of Fallot** consists of ventricular septal defect (VSD), pulmonary stenosis (PS), dextroposition of the aorta, and right ventricular hypertrophy (RVH).

161. The answer is d. *(Tierney, pp 391, 396.)* A **pericardial knock** is an early mid-diastolic sound and is due to constrictive pericarditis. The diagnosis is confirmed by showing a thickened pericardium on CT scan or MRI. The treatment is pericardiectomy. **Constrictive pericarditis** may be idiopathic (60% of cases) or due to tuberculosis, mediastinal irradiation, or cardiac surgery. **Restrictive cardiomyopathy** is the least common form of cardiomyopathy; potential etiologies include sarcoidosis, amyloidosis, and hemochromatosis. Often, the patient with restrictive cardiomyopathy presents with other signs of the systemic illness.

162. The answer is c. *(Tierney, p 396.)* **Kussmaul's sign** (inspiratory distension of the neck veins) is seen in right ventricular infarction, right heart failure, constrictive pericarditis, superior vena cava syndrome, and tricuspid stenosis. Inspiration normally generates a negative intrapleural pressure, which sucks blood into the heart. With certain diseases, there is impairment of right heart filling and blood cannot enter the heart, causing venous pressure to rise. In these patients, inspiration will cause a paradoxical rise in venous pressure (Kussmaul's sign). *Kussmaul's sign is never seen in uncomplicated pure cardiac tamponade.* Right ventricular infarction is seen in up to 30% of inferior wall infarctions; patients usually present with hypotension and raised venous pressure (Kussmaul's sign).

163. The answer is d. *(Tierney, p 317.)* The ductus arteriosus, which is patent in the fetal circulation, may fail to close at birth. Patients with **PDA** may be asymptomatic or may complain of dyspnea, palpitations, and exercise intolerance. The pulse pressure is usually widened and pulses are bounding due to the runoff of blood through the ductus. The **continuous machinery murmur** of PDA is best heard in the first and second intercostal spaces below the left clavicle. Other **continuous murmurs** include the **cervical venous hum** (due to increased blood flow in the internal jugular vein; disappears with compression of the vein), the **hepatic venous hum** (disappears with compression of epigastrium), and the **mammary soufflé** (heard over the breast, due to increased blood flow in pregnancy).

164. The answer is d. (*Seidel, p 430*.) The left parasternal border at the third, fourth, and fifth intercostal spaces should be palpated for a **right ventricular tap,** which is also called a **lift** or **heave.** It is a nondiagnostic finding and results from any etiology of right ventricular hypertrophy. A **heave** that is palpable at the apex is consistent with LVH. A **precordial thrill** is a palpable murmur that may accompany heart disease. It is always considered pathologic and may be felt during systole (i.e., AS, VSD, MR, PDA, tetralogy of Fallot) or diastole (i.e., AI, MS). The presence of a thrill characterizes a murmur as at least grade 4 in intensity.

165. The answer is c. (*Tierney, pp 435–436*.) **Dissection of the aorta** occurs when the intima is interrupted so that blood enters the wall of the aorta and separates its layers, forming a second lumen. It is almost always fatal if left undiagnosed, but with prompt treatment most patients survive. Anything that weakens the media can lead to dissection, but hypertension is the most common risk factor. Aortic dissection is a major cause of morbidity and mortality in Marfan's syndrome. Other etiologies of dissection include cystic medial necrosis (described in patients with bicuspid aortic valves), syphilis, Ehlers-Danlos syndrome, trauma, and bacterial infections. Patients often have murmurs due to aortic insufficiency. The treatment for dissection is to control the blood pressure and heart rate to prevent extension of the dissection. A **tracheal tug** is considered positive if the pulsating aorta is felt when the trachea is pulled upward, a sign that the expanding aorta is contacting the left mainstem bronchus.

166. The answer is b. (*Seidel, p 467*.) Exaggerated *a* waves are called **cannon waves** and are due to the right atrium contracting against increased resistance [i.e., PS, tricuspid stenosis (TS), complete heart block]. The activity of the right side of the heart is transmitted normally through the jugular veins as a visualized pulse. The *a* **wave** is due to venous distension caused by atrial contraction. It is the most dominant wave, especially during inspiration. The *a* wave is not present during atrial fibrillation. The **c** **wave** of the venous pressure curve occurs as a result of ventricular contraction, which forces the tricuspid valve (TV) back toward the atrium. For that reason, it is simultaneous with the carotid pulse. If the TV is incompetent, the *c* wave will be increased. The *v* wave is the result of atrial filling while the AV valves are closed. The **v wave** becomes large with TR. The downward **x slope** is caused by atrial filling, and the **y slope** is caused by the open TV and the rapid filling of the ventricle. The y descent is abolished in cardiac tamponade.

167. The answer is b. (*Seidel, p 490.*) An acquired **arteriovenous fistula** may be diagnosed by the presence of a continuous murmur and a palpable thrill over an area of previous trauma. The large pulse pressure is an indication that a large portion of the cardiac output is bypassing the systemic vascular resistance through the fistula.

168. The answer is d. (*Tierney, pp 390–391.*) Squatting to standing and the Valsalva maneuver both decrease right ventricular filling and decrease venous return, thereby increasing the murmurs of HCM and MVP. **Standing decreases venous return because of pooling of the blood in the lower extremities caused by gravity.** The Valsalva maneuver decreases cardiac output and increases heart rate. Standing decreases all other murmurs. **MR murmurs are increased by hand grip or squatting** (**increases systemic vascular resistance**), and right-sided heart murmurs are increased by inspiration.

169. The answer is e. (*Tierney, p 395.*) **Cardiac tamponade** is the accumulation of fluid in the pericardial sac in amounts sufficient to cause obstruction of blood flow back to the heart. Cardiac tamponade may follow trauma or surgery. It may be a complication of malignancy (i.e., lung, breast, lymphoma), chronic renal failure, or hypothyroidism. The patient has the classic signs of cardiac tamponade, including **pulsus alternans, pulsus paradoxus,** JVD, and distant heart sounds. Patients may also present with hypotension. ECG may show low voltage and pulsus alternans. Chest radiograph may show enlargement of the cardiac shadow (globular-shaped). **Pulsus paradoxus** is an inspiratory drop (from expiration) in systolic blood pressure of more than 10 mmHg (normal <10 mmHg). Pulsus paradoxus may also be seen in severe asthma and constrictive pericarditis.

170. The answer is a. (*Tierney, pp 430–432.*) **Abdominal aortic aneurysms** (**AAAs**) are usually due to atherosclerosis, and more than 90% originate below the renal arteries. The aneurysms are typically asymptomatic until they rupture, but patients may complain of lower back or hypogastric pain. The aneurysms may be associated with emboli to the feet and kidneys. Normal diameter of the aorta is less than 2 cm. When the diameter of the AAA is more than 4.5 cm, repair is generally suggested. Risk of rupture is 1 to 2% over five years when the AAA is less than 5 cm, but 20 to 40% when the AAA reaches 6 cm in diameter. The best method of evaluating the AAA is by ultrasound or CT scan.

171. The answer is e. (*Tierney, p 395.*) **Post–myocardial infarction syndrome,** or **Dressler's syndrome,** is an autoimmune complication of myocardial infarction. It occurs from three days to six weeks after the infarction and usually responds quickly to salicylates. The fever, pericarditis, leukocytosis, elevated ESR, and pleural effusion are all part of the autoimmune process.

172. The answer is d. (*Seidel, p 437.*) A normal S_2 consists of closure of the aortic valve (A_2) followed by closure of the pulmonic valve (P_2). It is best heard at the base of the heart, where it is louder than S_1. **Inspiration** (increases venous return and decreases thoracic pressure) **normally** increases the split of S_2 by two mechanisms. First, there is delayed pulmonic valve closure, which is due to prolonged right ventricular ejection time from increased stroke volume. Second, inspiration increases the compliance of the pulmonary vasculature and thereby decreases the return of blood to the left heart and shortens its ejection time by the same mechanism.

173. The answer is a. (*Tierney, pp 324–325.*) **Aortic sclerosis** is found in 65% of patients over the age of 65. Approximately 20% of these will progress to significant aortic stenosis. Degenerative valve disease is more common in men, in smokers, and in patients with hypertension. The murmur of aortic sclerosis is more likely to be short and to occur earlier in systole than the murmur of aortic stenosis; the intensity of the second heart sound is preserved (loud S_2 in aortic stenosis) in patients with aortic sclerosis.

174. The answer is d. (*Seidel, p 494.*) The patient has **Kawasaki's disease** (mucocutaneous lymph node syndrome), an acute illness of uncertain etiology that affects young males more than females; Asian children are at higher risk. Patients present with fever, conjunctival injection, cervical lymphadenopathy, rash, and edema. Cardiac involvement may include myocardial infarction, coronary artery aneurysms, or generalized vasculitis of the small vessels of the heart. The treatment is gamma globulin. Steroids may worsen aneurysmal dilatation.

175. The answer is a. *(Tierney, p 310.)* The patient has a **functional or innocent heart murmur.** These are nonpathologic murmurs generated by flow abnormalities (systolic ejection), not structural heart abnormalities. Functional murmurs are extremely common in children (>50% of children) and may be found in 50% of patients over 50 years old (aortic sclerosis). Functional murmurs are the most common kinds of murmurs encountered by physicians.

176. The answer is c. *(Tierney, p 410.)* The patient has a positive **Osler's sign** (a palpable brachial or radial artery when the cuff is inflated above systolic pressure). Older patients may have noncompressible vessels and falsely elevated blood pressure readings by sphygmomanometry. It may be necessary to measure intraarterial pressure before increasing or adding blood pressure medication.

177. The answer is d. *(Seidel, p 437.)* Normally, S_2 is split during inspiration. **Wide splitting of S_2** occurs in both inspiration and expiration. Delayed closure of the pulmonic valve due to a right bundle branch block, pulmonic stenosis, or mitral regurgitation causes a wide splitting of S_2. **Fixed splitting of S_2** is unaffected by respiration. It is due to ASD or a VSD with left-to-right shunting. **Paradoxical splitting of S_2** is caused by anything that delays A_2 or speeds up P_2 to the point where P_2 occurs prior to A_2. For this reason, expiration, not inspiration, separates a paradoxical split by prolonging left ventricular ejection and shortening right ventricular ejection. The causes of a paradoxical split S_2 are left bundle branch block and aortic stenosis, both of which prolong left ventricular outflow.

178. The answer is b. *(Tierney, p 326.)* A **widened pulse pressure** is due to conditions associated with a high stroke volume, such as AI, PDA, fever, pregnancy, hyperthyroidism, beriberi, anemia, and Paget's disease. A **narrowed pulse pressure** suggests a low stroke volume and is seen in pericardial tamponade, constrictive pericarditis, AS, and tachycardia.

179–182. The answers are 179-a, 180-i, 181-l, 182-k. *(Tierney, pp 314–324.)* Patients with AS may present with symptoms of angina, syncope, dyspnea, or congestive heart failure. The etiologies of AS include rheumatic fever and congenital bicuspid valve. **Idiopathic calcific AS** is a common disorder in the elderly and may produce the murmur of AS, but it is usually a mild disorder and of no significance. **Hypertrophic obstruc-**

tive cardiomyopathy (HOCM or HCM) is the most common cause of sudden cardiac death in young adults. Patients may be asymptomatic, and over half have a positive family history of sudden death. **ASD** is a common anomaly in adults; **VSD** may be a congenital anomaly or a complication of myocardial infarction. Both defects may cause a left-to-right shunt, which may lead to pulmonary hypertension (loud S_2) and pulmonary obstruction (**Eisenmenger's syndrome**).

Gastrointestinal System

Questions

DIRECTIONS: Each item below contains a question followed by suggested responses. Select the **one best** response to each question.

183. A 42-year-old woman presents to the emergency room complaining of the sudden onset of right upper abdominal pain. Her pain started after she ate a hamburger for lunch. She is nauseated and vomited twice at home. She denies diarrhea. Her temperature is 39°C (102.2°F), blood pressure is 140/90 mmHg, and pulse is 110 beats per minute. She appears anxious and distressed. She is not jaundiced. Abdominal examination reveals normal bowel sounds. While you are palpating under her right costal margin, the patient abruptly arrests her inspiration and pulls away because of sharp pain. Which of the following is the most appropriate next step in management?

a. Abdominal radiograph
b. Ultrasound of the abdomen
c. Dimethyl iminodiacetic acid (HIDA) scan
d. MRI of the abdomen
e. Upper endoscopy

184. A 16-year-old boy presents to the emergency room with a history of a football injury to the left flank earlier that day while at practice. He reports that at the time of the injury he only had the wind knocked out of him and he recovered in a few minutes. About one hour later he began to experience pain in the left upper quadrant and left shoulder. He also feels dizzy and lightheaded on standing. Physical examination demonstrates orthostatic changes in blood pressure and heart rate. Heart and lung examinations are normal. Abdominal auscultation reveals normal bowel sounds, but the patient complains of tenderness when palpating the left upper quadrant. Rectal exam is normal. Which of the following is the most likely diagnosis?

a. Dislocation of the left shoulder
b. Left rib fracture
c. Left pneumothorax
d. Ruptured spleen
e. Contusion of the left kidney

185. A 71-year-old man presents to your office with the chief complaint of a 40-lb weight loss over the last four months. He has anorexia and generalized weakness. Abdominal examination is positive for a scaphoid abdomen and a palpable nodule found in the area of the umbilicus. The nodule is irregular and appears to replace part of the umbilicus. Which of the following is the most likely cause of the physical examination findings?

a. Pancreatic cancer
b. Esophageal cancer
c. Hepatocellular cancer
d. Renal cell carcinoma
e. Hodgkin's lymphoma
f. Tuberculosis
g. Lung cancer

186. A 40-year-old man presents to the emergency room complaining of severe abdominal pain that radiates to his back, accompanied by several episodes of vomiting. He drinks alcohol daily. On physical examination, the patient is found on the stretcher lying in the fetal position. He is febrile and appears ill. The skin of his abdomen has an area of bluish periumbilical discoloration. There is no flank discoloration. Abdominal examination reveals decreased bowel sounds. The patient has severe midepigastric tenderness on palpation and complains of exquisite pain when your hands are abruptly withdrawn from his abdomen. Rectal examination is normal. Which of the following is the most likely diagnosis?

a. Acute cholecystitis
b. Pyelonephritis
c. Necrotizing pancreatitis
d. Chronic pancreatitis
e. Diverticulitis
f. Appendicitis

187. A 60-year-old man with a history of appendectomy 30 years ago presents to the emergency room complaining of abdominal pain. He describes the pain as colicky and crampy and feels it builds up, then it improves on its own. He has vomited at least 10 times since the pain started this morning. He states that he has not had a bowel movement for two days and cannot recall the last time he passed flatus. The abdomen is slightly distended. Abdominal auscultation reveals high-pitched bowel sounds and peristaltic rushes. Percussion reveals a tympanic abdomen. The patient is diffusely tender with palpation but has no rebound tenderness. Rectal examination reveals the absence of stool. Which of the following is the most likely diagnosis?

a. Cholecystitis
b. Diverticulitis
c. Pancreatitis
d. Gastroenteritis
e. Intestinal obstruction

188. A 51-year-old woman presents with a history of increasing abdominal girth over the last several weeks. She has no past medical history and takes no medications. She does not drink alcohol or smoke cigarettes. Abdominal examination reveals the presence of engorged veins on the lateral abdominal wall, which seem to drain upward. Which of the following is the most likely cause of the physical examination findings?

a. Obstruction of the portal system
b. Obstruction of the superior vena cava
c. Obstruction of the inferior vena cava
d. Obstruction of the abdominal aorta
e. Obstruction of the mesenteric artery

189. A 51-year-old woman presents to the emergency room complaining of right upper quadrant pain for five hours. She has nausea and vomiting. She denies jaundice, hematemesis, and melena. She is febrile. Abdominal examination reveals a positive Boas's sign and an audible rub over the gallbladder. Which of the following is the most likely diagnosis?

a. Cancer of the biliary tract
b. Cancer of the pancreas
c. Cirrhosis of the liver
d. Acute cholecystitis
e. Acute viral hepatitis

190. A 32-year-old man presents with severe abdominal pain, which he describes as sharp and diffuse. He does not drink alcohol or take any medications. He has a medical history significant for peptic ulcer disease over five years ago. He has stable vital signs and has no orthostatic changes. You observe that the patient is lying very still on the emergency room stretcher. On physical examination, he has a rigid abdomen and decreased bowel sounds. He has localized left upper quadrant guarding and rebound tenderness. He has referred rebound tenderness on palpation of the right upper quadrant. Rectal examination is fecal occult blood test (FOBT) negative. Which of the following is the best method of confirming the diagnosis in this patient?

a. Barium swallow
b. Leukocytosis
c. Upper endoscopy
d. Abdominal radiograph
e. Colonoscopy

191. A 74-year-old man presents with the abrupt onset of pain in the left lower abdomen, which has been progressively worsening over the last two days. He states that the pain is unremitting. He has some diarrhea but no nausea or vomiting. He has no dysuria or hematuria. His temperature is 38.9°C (102°F). Bowel sounds are decreased. The patient has involuntary guarding. There is tenderness and rebound tenderness when the left lower quadrant is palpated. The referred rebound test is positive. A fixed sausage-like mass is palpable in the area of tenderness. There is no costovertebral angle (CVA) tenderness. Rectal examination reveals brown stool, which is fecal occult blood test (FOBT) positive. Bloodwork demonstrates a leukocytosis. Which of the following is the most likely diagnosis?

a. Colon cancer
b. Diverticulitis
c. Pancreatitis
d. Pyelonephritis
e. Appendicitis

192. A 32-year-old man presents with fever and diffuse abdominal pain. On physical examination, his temperature is 39.4°C (103°F) and his heart rate is 120 beats per minute. He has abdominal pain on vibration and severe pain when palpating one-third of the way along a line drawn from the right anterior superior iliac spine to the umbilicus. He has a positive Rovsing's sign. Which of the following is the most appropriate next step in diagnosis?

a. CT of the abdomen
b. Ultrasound of the abdomen
c. Surgical intervention
d. Electrocardiogram
e. Plain film of the abdomen
f. Paracentesis

193. A 71-year-old woman with a history of chronic congestive heart failure presents to her family physician for a routine checkup. The physician notices that she has lost 20 lb since her last visit six months ago. When questioned, the patient gives a history of intermittent periumbilical pain that begins 30 minutes after eating and lasts two to three hours. She claims the pain is worse after large meals, so she has begun to eat less out of fear of precipitating the pain. Which of the following is the most likely diagnosis?

a. Pancreatitis
b. Intestinal ischemia
c. Cholecystitis
d. Small-bowel obstruction
e. Peptic ulcer disease

194. A patient with a long history of cirrhosis presents with asterixis. He is alert and oriented to person, place, and time. His breath is positive for fetor hepaticus. His abdomen is significant for caput medusae and a positive fluid wave. He has no focal neurologic deficit. His wife states that the patient is very functional at home but is moderately confused and drowsy. Which is the most likely stage of hepatic encephalopathy in this patient?

a. Stage 1 hepatic encephalopathy
b. Stage 2 hepatic encephalopathy
c. Stage 3 hepatic encephalopathy
d. Stage 4 hepatic encephalopathy

195. A 38-year-old man arrives at the emergency room with the chief complaint of hematemesis for three hours. He does not drink alcohol and has no previous medical history. He spent the previous night vomiting approximately 10 to 12 times after eating some "bad chicken." The patient is squirming on the stretcher and is retching. He is afebrile, with a heart rate of 120 beats per minute and a blood pressure of 90/60 mmHg. Abdominal exam is positive for diffuse tenderness, but the patient has no rigidity, guarding, or rebound tenderness. There is no hepatosplenomegaly. Rectal exam is negative for occult blood. A nasogastric tube is inserted and reveals bright red blood. Which of the following is the most likely diagnosis?

a. Esophageal varices
b. Mallory-Weiss tear
c. Gastritis
d. Peptic ulcer disease
e. Boerhaave's syndrome
f. Dieulafoy's lesion

196. A 24-year-old HIV-positive patient who has had AIDS for three years presents with painful swallowing and dysphagia to solids and liquids. He has no previous history of heartburn or reflux disease. His CD4 count is 41/μL, and he recently required three weeks of antibiotics for *Pneumocystis carinii* pneumonia. Examination of the pharynx reveals no oral thrush. Barium swallow demonstrates multiple nodular filling defects of various sizes that resemble a cluster of grapes. Which of the following is the most likely diagnosis?

a. *Candida* esophagitis
b. Reflux disease
c. Barrett's esophagus
d. *Pneumocystis* esophagitis
e. Achalasia
f. Plummer-Vinson syndrome
g. Schatzki's ring

197. A 47-year-old woman is admitted to the hospital with new onset of jaundice and ascites. Physical examination is positive for caput medusae and shifting dullness. Liver size is 12 cm in the midclavicular line (MCL); nodules less than 1 mm are palpable throughout the liver. Liver edge is firm but nontender. Which of the following is the most likely etiology of the patient's liver disease?

a. Hepatitis B
b. Hepatitis C
c. Alcoholism
d. Hemachromatosis
e. Hepatocellular carcinoma

198. A 70-year-old woman with a 25-year history of diabetes mellitus presents with early satiety, bloating, and nausea after meals. She has had previous surgery for gallbladder stones and appendicitis. Her diabetes is complicated by retinopathy and peripheral neuropathy. On physical examination, bowel sounds are normal. A succussion splash is audible. The abdomen is tympanic, and there is no hepatosplenomegaly. There is no tenderness. Rectal examination is normal. Serum glucose is 310 mg/dL. Which of the following is the most likely diagnosis?

a. Celiac sprue
b. Whipple's disease
c. Gastroparesis
d. Gluten-sensitive enteropathy
e. Tropical sprue

199. A 49-year-old man with a four-year history of peptic ulcer disease requires hospital admission for blood transfusions because of symptoms relating to anemia. His primary care physician has been doing annual fecal occult blood testing, and results have been negative. The patient does not drink alcohol or smoke cigarettes. He denies medication use. He has no nausea, vomiting, melena, hematochezia, or abdominal pain. Endoscopy reveals several duodenal ulcers; colonoscopy is normal. Which of the following factors may have caused a false-negative FOBT result in this patient?

a. Vitamin C
b. Turnips
c. NSAIDs
d. Red meat
e. Aspirin
f. Horseradish
g. Poultry
h. Fish

200. A 42-year-old morbidly obese woman complains of a nonproductive cough for eight months. She denies abdominal discomfort after eating and has never suffered from heartburn. Rarely, she has regurgitation, and when she does, it has a sour taste. Abdominal examination is normal. Rectal examination is FOBT negative. Which of the following is the most likely diagnosis?

a. Carcinoma of the lung
b. Gastroesophageal reflux disease
c. Chronic obstructive lung disease
d. Lactose deficiency
e. Chronic cholestasis

201. A 16-year-old boy has had lifelong constipation. He requires suppositories and, often, enemas to initiate bowel movements. His abdomen is distended. Palpation reveals a tubular mass in the left lower quadrant. Rectal exam reveals no stool in the vault. Barium enema reveals a dilated colon above a normal-appearing rectum. Which of the following is the most likely diagnosis?

a. Colon carcinoma
b. Gardner's syndrome
c. Peutz-Jeghers syndrome
d. Hirschsprung's disease
e. Volvulus

202. A 45-year-old patient presents with altered mental status. His wife states that over the last week her husband has been taking acetaminophen for some abdominal discomfort. He uses no illicit drugs but drinks four to five beers daily. Over the last 24 hours, the patient has become progressively lethargic. Vital signs reveal a temperature of 36.1°C (97°F), blood pressure of 100/70 mmHg, heart rate of 120 beats per minute, and respiratory rate of 26 breaths per minute. The patient is jaundiced with right upper quadrant (RUQ) abdominal tenderness on palpation. He has no rebound tenderness or splenomegaly but has an enlarged liver. There is no ascites or peripheral edema. Heart and lung examinations are normal. The patient responds to painful stimuli and has asterixis. He has no focal neurologic deficit. Which of the following is the most likely diagnosis?

a. Alcohol intoxication
b. Alcohol withdrawal
c. Delirium tremens
d. Acetaminophen toxicity
e. Wilson's disease

203. A 19-year-old girl attending school in Massachusetts presents with the chief complaint of bloody diarrhea for two months. She has abdominal discomfort and feels she has lost some weight. She also complains of tenesmus. Abdominal examination is normal. Rectal exam reveals stool containing blood and pus. Which of the following is the most likely diagnosis?

a. Irritable bowel syndrome
b. Ulcerative colitis
c. Giardiasis
d. Hemorrhoids
e. Diverticulosis

204. A 50-year-old man has a 10-year history of chronic active hepatitis from the hepatitis C virus. He is brought to the emergency room because of cachexia and disturbed mental status. On physical examination, the patient has palmar erythema and clubbing. He is jaundiced with massive ascites. He has asterixis. Laboratory data reveal severe hypoalbuminemia and hyperbilirubinemia. Which of the following is the most likely diagnosis?

a. Child's class A cirrhosis
b. Child's class B cirrhosis
c. Child's class C cirrhosis
d. Child's class D cirrhosis
e. Child's class E cirrhosis

205. A 44-year-old man with a history of peptic ulcer surgery presents with palpitations, tachycardia, lightheadedness, and diaphoresis after eating a meal. The symptoms typically begin 30 minutes after eating. Which of the following is the most likely diagnosis?

a. Malabsorption
b. Peptic ulcer recurrence
c. Gastric carcinoma
d. Gastritis
e. Dumping syndrome
f. Esophagitis

206. A 21-year-old woman presents with jaundice and hepatomegaly. She has nausea, vomiting, and diarrhea. She recalls eating raw oysters one to two months ago. She has not traveled recently and denies drug use or unprotected sexual intercourse. She has no history of blood transfusion. Which of the following is the most likely viral etiology?

a. Hepatitis A
b. Hepatitis B
c. Hepatitis C
d. Hepatitis D
e. Hepatitis E
f. Hepatitis G

DIRECTIONS: Each group of questions below consists of lettered options followed by a set of numbered items. For each numbered item, select the **one** lettered option with which it is **most** closely associated. Each lettered option may be used once, more than once, or not at all.

Questions 207–208

For each patient with a gastrointestinal bleed, select the most likely diagnosis.

a. Gastric ulcer
b. Erosive gastritis
c. Dieulafoy's lesion
d. Mallory-Weiss syndrome
e. Duodenal ulcer
f. Esophageal varices

207. A 44-year-old man presents to the emergency room with the acute onset of hematemesis after drinking heavily for the last several days. He appears jaundiced and has some mild ascites.

208. A 51-year-old man has massive hematemesis and melena. He had no antecedent symptoms. Endoscopy fails to identify a bleeding source.

Questions 209–210

For each description for detection of ascites, select the appropriate named sign.

a. Shifting dullness
b. Fluid wave
c. Puddle sign
d. Bulging flanks

209. The patient is on all fours, and the umbilicus is percussed for dullness.

210. The border of dullness moves to the dependent side and tympany moves toward the top when the patient turns to the side from the supine position.

Questions 211–216

For each patient with liver disease, select the most likely disorder.

a. Hemochromatosis
b. Primary biliary cirrhosis
c. Sclerosing cholangitis
d. Hepatocellular carcinoma
e. Zollinger-Ellison syndrome
f. Alcoholic hepatitis
g. Wilson's disease
h. α_1 antitrypsin deficiency
i. Metastatic carcinoma of the liver
j. Budd-Chiari syndrome

211. A 54-year-old woman presents with generalized pruritus that keeps her awake at night. Liver size by percussion in the MCL is 17 cm. There is no splenomegaly. Serum alkaline phosphatase level is three times the normal value.

212. A 44-year-old man with a 20-year history of ulcerative colitis presents with fever and right upper quadrant pain. Physical examination reveals jaundice and RUQ tenderness with palpation. Endoscopic retrograde cholangiopancreatography (ERCP) shows multifocal strictures of the extrahepatic biliary tree.

213. A 41-year-old woman has a history of recurrent duodenal ulcer disease. She takes no medications and has no evidence of *Helicobacter pylori* infection. Her serum gastrin level is 800 pg/mL.

214. A 53-year-old alcoholic presents with mild RUQ tenderness and jaundice. Liver function tests reveal an elevated aspartate aminotransferase (AST) and alanine aminotransferase (ALT) level, but the AST is two times greater than the ALT.

215. A 39-year-old man presents with jaundice and ascites. He has a history of diabetes mellitus and was recently diagnosed as having heart disease. On physical examination, he has a bronze appearance to his skin, arthritic changes of the fingers, and testicular atrophy.

216. A 43-year-old man presents with cirrhosis. Slit-lamp examination reveals a yellow-brown ring in the limbus of the cornea. The patient has recently developed an unsteady gait, tremors, and involuntary chorea-like movements.

Questions 217–218

For each patient with jaundice, choose the most likely liver disorder.
a. Dubin-Johnson syndrome
b. Rotor's syndrome
c. Crigler-Najjar type 1 syndrome
d. Crigler-Najjar type 2 syndrome
e. Gilbert's syndrome

217. A 23-year-old man presents with mild, persistent jaundice. His serum bilirubin is always less than 5 mg/dL and is primarily unconjugated bilirubin. The jaundice is exacerbated by fasting, surgery, fever, infection, and alcohol ingestion.

218. A 17-year-old woman presents with moderate jaundice, which is primarily conjugated bilirubin. She develops jaundice during pregnancy and in times of illness. She has mild hepatomegaly. Liver biopsy reveals black pigment in the hepatocytes.

Gastrointestinal System

Answers

183. The answer is c. (*Tierney, pp 664–665.*) The finding of abruptly arresting inspiration with palpation of the right upper quadrant (RUQ) is called **Murphy's sign,** and it is consistent with a diagnosis of cholecystitis. The liver and gallbladder (GB) move inferiorly as the diaphragm contracts on deep inspiration. The inferior movement of the diaphragm causes the inflamed gallbladder to become compressed against the inverted wall; the patient experiences sharp pain and abruptly halts inspiration. Cholecystitis risk factors are the **four F's** (**F**at, **F**orty, **F**emale, and **F**ertile). Other risk factors include diabetes, a positive family history, and medications such as oral contraceptives. The most sensitive test for detecting gallstones is the **HIDA scan** (98% sensitive and 81% specific for cholecystitis). It shows obstruction of the cystic duct (the primary cause of cholecystitis). Plain films detect gallstones in 15% of cases. Abdominal ultrasound has a sensitivity of 67% and a specificity of 82% for detection of gallstones.

184. The answer is d. (*Goldman, p 645.*) The clinical picture is most consistent with a **ruptured spleen.** Intense pain in the left upper quadrant that radiates to the top of the left shoulder (**Kehr's sign**) is due to diaphragmatic irritation by blood from the ruptured spleen. The spinal levels supplying most of the sensory fibers of the diaphragm (**C3 to C5 and the phrenic nerve**) are the same levels as for some of the sensory supply to the shoulder. Therefore, diaphragmatic irritation is sometimes perceived as shoulder pain. The blood loss from the spleen causes signs of shock, including hypotension and orthostatic changes.

185. The answer is a. (*Seidel, p 540.*) The patient has a metastatic nodule of the umbilicus often referred to as a **Sister Mary Joseph nodule.** Because of its vascular and embryologic connections, the umbilicus is a susceptible site for metastatic disease. The primary sites for umbilical metastases are the stomach, ovary, colon, rectum, and pancreas (in descending order). A **scaphoid abdomen** in this patient implies malnourishment; the abdomen appears hollow or concave. *Scaphoid* may also refer to the normal boatlike appearance of the abdomen seen in thin patients.

The costal margins, anterior iliac spines, and pubis represent the sides of the boat, while the bottom of the boat is represented by the abdominal wall, which appears sunken in the supine patient in response to gravity.

186. The answer is c. *(Tierney, pp 671–674.)* The patient most likely has **necrotizing pancreatitis,** which is a complication of acute pancreatitis. Other complications of pancreatitis include pseudocyst, abscess, and phlegmon. The periumbilical discoloration (**Cullen's sign**) suggests a hemoperitoneum. Discoloration of the flanks would be a positive **Turner's sign.** When the patient experiences pain as the hands of the examiner are abruptly withdrawn from the abdomen, he or she is said to have **rebound tenderness** (a sign of peritonitis). Decreased bowel sounds are another sign of peritonitis. Risk factors for acute pancreatitis include alcohol use, trauma, hyperlipidemia, gallstones, and medications. An abdominal radiograph in acute pancreatitis might show a **sentinel loop** (air-filled small intestine in the LUQ) and **colon cutoff sign** (air in the transverse colon). Patients with **chronic pancreatitis** present with bouts of abdominal pain and signs of pancreatic insufficiency (weight loss, steatorrhea, and diabetes). The abdominal radiograph in patients with chronic pancreatitis demonstrates calcifications in the pancreas (pathognomonic).

187. The answer is e. *(Tierney, p 589.)* The patient has a past medical history of appendectomy, which predisposes him to adhesions and **small-bowel obstruction** (**SBO**). Other etiologies for SBO include incarcerated hernia, stricture, and malignancy. The high-pitched bowel sounds, **peristaltic rushes,** and tympany with percussion are physical findings when air is under pressure in viscera and intestinal fluid is present (i.e., obstruction). The hallmarks of intestinal obstruction are abdominal pain, distension, vomiting, and obstipation. Abdominal radiographs may reveal dilated loops of bowel in a ladder-like pattern and **air-fluid levels. Large-bowel obstruction** (**LBO**) is due to malignancy, diverticulitis, and volvulus. A mnemonic for **abdominal distension** is the **six F's:** Fat, Fluid, Food, Fetus, Feces, and Flatus.

188. The answer is c. *(Seidel, p 537.)* There are **three collateral venous circulations** that may be seen on the abdominal wall. The patient described (veins that drain upward) has **obstruction of the inferior vena cava. Obstruction of the superior vena cava** is characterized by veins with flow directed downward. **Obstruction of the portal system** causes the development of periumbilical veins that drain both upward (located in the upper abdomen) and downward (located in the lower abdomen). The flow of collateral veins can be demonstrated by placing the two index fingers over the engorged vein, then sliding the fingers apart, leaving a stretch of empty vein between the fingers. Refilling direction can be identified by releasing first the caudal end and then the cephalad end.

189. The answer is d. (*Seidel, p 550.*) **Boas's sign** (a positive area of hyperesthesia over the right costophrenic angle) and **an audible rub over the edge of the gallbladder** are signs of acute cholecystitis. Patients with cholecystitis also may have a palpable tender gallbladder. **Courvoisier's gallbladder** is an enlarged nontender gallbladder in a patient with painless jaundice; it is not due to cholecystitis but to cancer of the biliary tract or head of the pancreas.

190. The answer is d. (*Seidel, p 557.*) Guarding, rigidity, absent or diminished bowel sounds, rebound and referred rebound tenderness, and lying perfectly still are all signs of **peritonitis.** A plain film of the abdomen in this patient with a probable perforated ulcer might show **free intraperitoneal air under the diaphragm** (in up to 75% of patients). The free air establishes the diagnosis, and no further studies are needed. Barium studies are contraindicated in perforation.

191. The answer is b. (*Tierney, pp 612–614.*) Complications of diverticular disease include diverticulitis and gastrointestinal bleeding. **Diverticulitis** is an acute inflammatory process caused by bacteria in a diverticulum (outpouching of the mucosa or submucosa). It may occur in up to 50% of patients with diverticulosis. The patient most likely has diverticulitis, which is usually left-sided, since the diameter of the sigmoid colon is the smallest of the colon (higher wall tension and intraluminal pressure in this area are probably responsible for the diverticular formation). The palpable mass reflects adherent loops of bowel. Peritonitis often results in **involuntary guarding** (abdominal rigidity due to reflex muscle spasm from the peritoneal irritation). Decreased bowel sounds may be heard in peritonitis or in any condition that causes an ileus (absence of peristalsis). Tenderness upon abrupt withdrawal of the hand (rebound tenderness or **Blumberg's**

sign) occurs because when the abdominal wall passively springs back into place, it carries with it the inflamed peritoneum. The **referred rebound test** is conducted in the same way but in a location away from the area of tenderness. The patient will experience pain in the area of stated tenderness rather than the site where the test is performed.

192. The answer is c. *(Seidel, p 558.)* There are many signs pertaining to the abdominal examination. **Rovsing's sign** occurs when palpation of the left lower quadrant (LLQ) causes pain in the right lower quadrant (RLQ). **Markle's sign** (a maneuver to detect peritoneal irritation) is tested by the **heel jar test;** the patient stands on his or her toes, then allows his or her heels to hit the floor, thus jarring the body and causing abdominal pain in peritonitis. The **obturator sign** is pain occurring when the bent leg is rotated laterally and medially. The **iliopsoas** sign occurs when the patient tries to raise the leg up against the hand of the examiner pushing down against the leg above the knee. Markle's sign, the obturator sign, the iliopsoas sign, and Rovsing's sign are seen in appendicitis. A patient with appendicitis may also have pain on rectal examination if the posterior appendix is involved. **Courvoisier's sign** is a palpable, nontender gallbladder, which suggests neoplasm. **Dance's sign** is the absence of bowel sounds in the RLQ due to intussusception. **McBurney's point** is the point on the abdomen that overlies the anatomic position of the appendix and is the site of maximum tenderness in a patient with appendicitis. It is located 1.5 to 2 in. from the anterior spinous process of the ileum on a straight line drawn from the process to the umbilicus. The next best step for the patient who presents with appendicitis is surgical intervention.

193. The answer is b. *(Tierney, pp 442–443.)* **Intestinal ischemia** is the result of reduction of the blood supply to the intestine; clinical manifestations range from mild chronic symptoms to an acute catastrophic event causing rectal bleeding, peritonitis, and shock. This patient has mild intestinal ischemia characterized by the triad of **postprandial pain,** anorexia from fear of eating, and weight loss. The pain is typically intermittent; it occurs 30 minutes after eating and persists for up to three hours. This is often referred to as **abdominal angina.** The diagnosis may be confirmed by angiography; embolectomy or surgery is required in selected cases. Patients with cardiac disease are at risk for intestinal ischemia.

194. The answer is b. (*Tierney, p 648.*) **Asterixis** is also referred to as liver flap or flapping tremor. It is a nonrhythmic, asymmetric lapse in a sustained position of an extremity. It is nonspecific for cirrhosis and may be seen in other metabolic derangements (i.e., renal disease and metabolic acidosis). **Fetor hepaticus** (due to mercaptans) is a musty odor of the breath and urine and is part of the encephalopathy. **Caput medusae** is the dilated abdominal veins (i.e., **reopened umbilical veins**) seen in patients with portal hypertension. It is often helpful to stage the hepatic encephalopathy to follow the course of the illness:

Stage 1: euphoria/depression, mild confusion, slurred speech, disordered
    sleep, +/–asterixis
Stage 2: lethargy, moderate confusion, +asterixis
Stage 3: marked confusion, incoherent speech, sleeping but arousable,
    +asterixis
Stage 4: comatose, –asterixis

195. The answer is b. (*Tierney, pp 533–534.*) **Mallory-Weiss tears** are longitudinal tears in the mucosa of the gastroesophageal junction due to prolonged and violent retching or vomiting. A bleeding **peptic ulcer** or **gastritis** can cause hematemesis, but usually, if the blood has been retained in the stomach, the digestive processes change the hemoglobin to a brown or black pigment commonly referred to as **coffee ground emesis.** **Esophageal varices** may cause gastrointestinal bleeding, but this patient has no history of alcoholism and no past history of liver disease. **Boerhaave's syndrome** is a transmural tear of the esophagus that causes gastric contents to escape into the mediastinum, leading to severe mediastinal complications. **Dieulafoy's lesion** is a large submucosal artery, which may rupture and cause massive bleeding.

196. The answer is a. (*Tierney, pp 546–554.*) **Odynophagia** (painful swallowing) is the most common presenting symptom of infectious esophagitis. In an HIV-positive patient, *Candida albicans* (even without oral thrush) is the most common organism. Other organisms include cytomegalovirus and herpes simplex virus. Reflux disease may cause a noninfectious esophagitis, but it is less likely in this patient. **Barrett's esophagus** (premalignant lesion for adenocarcinoma of the esophagus) is replacement of the squamous epithelium by columnar epithelium and may also result in esophagitis. **Achalasia** is failure of the lower esophageal sphincter to relax (motor disorder of smooth muscle); patients complain of dysphagia (difficulty swallowing) to liquids and solids. Patients with cancer typically present with dysphagia to solids, which progresses to liquids, accompanied by weight loss. Middle-aged women develop **Plummer-Vinson syndrome (hypopharyngeal web)**; they present with dysphagia to solids and iron-deficiency anemia. **Schatzki's ring** is a weblike constriction near the lower esophageal sphincter (LES) that produces dysphagia to solids. The first step in the workup of dysphagia is a barium swallow.

197. The answer is c. *(Tierney, pp 647–649.)* Normal liver span is 6 to 12 cm in the MCL and 4 to 8 cm in the midsternal line (MSL). **Micronodular cirrhosis (Laennec's cirrhosis)** is typically uniform throughout the liver, and the nodules are **less than 1 mm** in size. It is due to a metabolic insult such as alcohol use. The nodules of **macronodular cirrhosis,** which are less uniform, are **more than 1 mm** in size and are due to drugs or infection.

198. The answer is c. *(Tierney, pp 583–586.)* Diabetic patients, especially those with poor control, may develop delayed gastric emptying (autonomic dysfunction). Often, patients will have a **succussion splash** (a splash is heard with the stethoscope when shaking the patient, due to air-fluid level). Diagnosis is made by a gastric emptying study. Patients with **celiac sprue** (also called **gluten-sensitive enteropathy**) present with bloating, diarrhea, and excessive flatus. They typically have signs of malabsorption, such as hypoalbuminemia, iron-deficiency anemia, hypocholesterolemia, and decreased carotene level. The diagnosis is made by small-bowel biopsy, and the treatment is a wheat-free diet. **Whipple's disease** is a multisystemic disorder characterized by arthralgias, abdominal pain, fever, weight loss, lymphadenopathy, heart disease, and neurologic disease. Finding **periodic acid–Schiff (PAS) positive-staining foamy macrophages** in tissues makes the diagnosis, and treatment for this previously fatal disease is antibiotics (for *Tropheryma whippelii*). **Tropical sprue** often responds to antibiotics and may occur months or even years after a patient returns from the tropics.

199. The answer is a. *(Tierney, p 623.)* Vitamin C may cause a **false-negative fecal occult test.** The false-positive rate for FOBT is 1 to 5%, and patients must be told to abstain from acetylsalicylic acid (ASA), nonsteroidal anti-inflammatory drugs (NSAIDs), poultry, fish, red meat, and vegetables with peroxide activity (horseradish and turnips) for 72 hours before testing.

200. The answer is b. (*Tierney, pp 547–550.*) The risk factors for **gastroesophageal reflux disease** (**GERD**) include obesity, pregnancy, scleroderma, and diet (caffeine, alcohol, nicotine, chocolate, fatty foods). The most common etiology of GERD is transient LES relaxation, but it may also be due to hiatal hernia and acidic gastric contents. The sour taste of GERD is often referred to as **water brash.** A complication of GERD is Barrett's esophagus. Atypical symptoms of GERD may include asthma, chronic cough, chronic laryngitis, sore throat, and chest pain. Peptic ulcer disease (PUD) produces epigastric pain that typically improves with eating. Patients with **lactose intolerance** present with bloating, cramps, and diarrhea after ingesting a milk product.

201. The answer is d. (*Tierney, pp 616–618.*) **Hirschsprung's disease** (aganglionic megacolon) is a disorder characterized by the absence of enteric neurons in the submucosal and myenteric plexuses. The contracted segment of bowel is unable to relax, and a mass may become palpable. Hirschsprung's disease may lead to **megacolon,** but resection of the affected bowel is curative. **Peutz-Jeghers syndrome** is autosomal dominant (AD) and is characterized by hamartomatous polyps in the small intestine and perioral melanin deposits. **Gardner's syndrome** (also AD) is familial adenomatous polyposis syndrome. Gardner's syndrome and Peutz-Jeghers syndrome are risk factors for colon cancer. **Volvulus** (malrotation that leads to gangrene) is usually seen in the first year of life; infants present with bilious vomiting, bloody stools, rigid and discolored abdomen, and shock.

202. The answer is d. (*Tierney, pp 1566–1567.*) This patient with underlying liver disease probably has **fulminant hepatitis** from acetaminophen toxicity. Because of his alcohol use, he has insufficient glutathione stores and induced P450 enzymatic activity and is at greater risk for developing toxicity. Patients who survive the complication of fulminant hepatic failure will begin to recover over the following week, but some require liver transplantation. A serum acetaminophen level should be obtained, and immediate treatment with **N-acetylcysteine** (**NAC**), which provides cysteine for glutathione synthesis, is indicated. Signs of **alcohol intoxication** include euphoria, dysarthria, ataxia, labile mood, lethargy, coma, respiratory depression, and death. Patients experiencing **alcohol withdrawal** present with a hyperexcitable state (i.e., hypertension, tachycardia, flushing, sweating, and mydriasis) and have tremors, disordered perceptions, seizures, and delirium tremens (DTs). **Delirium tremens** occurs two to four days after alcohol abstinence and is characterized by hallucinations that may lead to dangerous, combative, and destructive behavior.

203. The answer is b. *(Tierney, pp 602–609.)* It is often difficult to distinguish clinically between **ulcerative colitis** (**UC**) and **Crohn's disease** (**CD**). Patients with CD usually have less rectal bleeding and rarely have tenesmus. Barium enema showing involvement of the colon supports UC. Typically, patients with CD have skip lesions and rectal sparing. Patients with **irritable bowel syndrome** complain of abdominal pain with altered frequency or consistency of stool but have no weight loss or bleeding. More than half of patients with irritable bowel syndrome have psychiatric disorders. Patients with **diverticulosis** (saclike protrusions of the mucosa through the muscularis) are usually older and asymptomatic; hemorrhage occurs in a small percentage of patients. **Giardiasis** may be found in immunocompromised patients, day care workers, male homosexuals, individuals who drink untreated water (hikers and campers), and international travelers (especially to Russia).

204. The answer is c. *(Tierney, p 648.)* Patients with **cirrhosis** may have erythema of the palms, spider angiomas, decreased body hair, gynecomastia, testicular atrophy or menstrual irregularities, and parotid and lacrimal gland enlargement. Many of these changes are due to hormonal disturbances (production of estrogen). Patients with cirrhosis may also have clubbing of the fingers. Portal hypertension may cause **caput medusae** (prominent abdominal vasculature), splenomegaly, and ascites. Patients may have jaundice and signs of hepatic encephalopathy (asterixis). Child's classification is a factor that determines survival in patients with end-stage liver disease; the patient described most likely has Child's class C cirrhosis (six-month survival of 50%).

Child's Classification			
	A	**B**	**C**
Bilirubin	<2.0	2.0–3.0	>3.0
Albumin	>3.5	3.0–3.5	<3.0
Ascites	None	Easily controlled	Not controlled
Neurologic	None	Minimal	Advanced (coma)
Nutrition	Excellent	Good	Wasting

205. The answer is e. (*Goldman, p 804.*) Some patients with a history of ulcer surgery experience the **dumping syndrome** 30 minutes after eating. They present with palpitations, tachycardia, lightheadedness, and diaphoresis after eating a meal, due to the rapid emptying of hyperosmolar gastric contents into the small intestine.

206. The answer is a. (*Seidel, p 577.*) Hepatitis A, C, D, E, and G are all RNA viruses, while hepatitis B is a DNA virus. **Hepatitis A (HAV)** is almost exclusively transmitted via the fecal-oral route and is spread from person to person. Outbreaks have been traced to contaminated food, water, milk, and shellfish. **Hepatitis B (HBV)** is transmitted sexually, perinatally, and through blood products. **Hepatitis C (HCV)** is transmitted primarily via blood products. Perinatal transmission and sexual transmission of HCV is less than 5%. HCV is the most common cause of chronic hepatitis in the United States. **Hepatitis D (HDV)** is endemic in patients with HBV in the Mediterranean countries, but in the United States it is confined to blood products. HDV was probably introduced into the United States by intravenous drug abusers. **Hepatitis E (HEV)** resembles HAV (fecal-oral route) but is found primarily in India, Africa, Asia, and Central America. **Hepatitis G (HGV)** is bloodborne, and its mode of transmission parallels that of HCV.

207–208. The answers are 207-f, 208-c. (*Tierney, p 534.*) A **Dieulafoy's lesion** is the rupture of an aberrantly large artery in the submucosa of either the stomach or the duodenum. It is a rare lesion that is often missed at endoscopy; multiple endoscopies may be required to make the diagnosis. The cause of the bleeding may be related to pressure necrosis of the epithelium overlying the lesion. **Esophageal varices** are dilated submucosal veins that develop in patients with portal hypertension. Bleeding varices have the highest morbidity and mortality rate of all causes of gastrointestinal bleeding.

209–210. The answers are 209-c, 210-a. (*Seidel, p 554.*) **Shifting dullness** and a **positive fluid wave** are the best physical examination findings for diagnosing ascites. In patients with ascites, the border of dullness shifts (shifting dullness) to the dependent side (approaches the midline) as the fluid resettles with gravity when the patient rolls to the side. A **shock wave** (fluid wave) occurs when a sharp tap at one end of the abdomen is felt on the other side. The patient places his or her hand in the middle of the abdomen to stop the transmission through adipose tissue. Asking the patient to go into the uncomfortable position of being on all fours and percussing the umbilicus for dullness is the **puddle sign** (low sensitivity and specificity). **Bulging flanks** (flanks are pushed outward) are seen in obese patients as well as in patients with ascites.

211–216. The answers are 211-b, 212-c, 213-e, 214-f, 215-a, 216-g. (*Tierney, pp 668–669.*) **Sclerosing cholangitis** is a complication of ulcerative colitis; patients have fibrosing inflammation of the intrahepatic and extrahepatic bile ducts that is best diagnosed by ERCP. Patients present with the **Charcot triad** of fever, jaundice, and RUQ pain. The Charcot triad occurs in 70% of cases of acute cholangitis. The **Reynolds pentad** is the Charcot triad with shock and altered mental status. Sclerosing cholangitis is a life-threatening illness requiring emergency bile duct decompression. Patients with **primary biliary cirrhosis** (**PBC**) often present with generalized pruritus, asymptomatic cholestasis, or an isolated alkaline phosphatase level. It occurs most frequently in women, and antimitochondrial antibodies (AMAs) are present in over 90% of affected patients. **Wilson's disease** is diagnosed by a low ceruloplasmin level, and hemochromatosis is diagnosed by an elevated serum iron level, an elevated ferritin level, and an elevated transferrin saturation (>55%). Patients with Wilson's disease have **Kayser-Fleischer rings** (yellow-brown) in the Descemet membrane and neurologic involvement. Patients with **hemochromatosis** present with suntan-like pigmentation ("**bronze diabetes**"), degenerative arthritis of the hands and fingers (PIPs), impotence, amenorrhea, testicular atrophy, cardiac disease, liver disease, and glucose intolerance. **Zollinger-Ellison syndrome** should be considered in patients with a history of recurrent duodenal ulcer disease. Serum gastrin levels are typically elevated (>150 pg/mL). Gastrinomas may be single or multiple, and up to two-thirds are malignant. Twenty-five percent are associated with multiple endocrine neoplasia (MEN) type 1 and may be found in the pancreas or duodenum.

α_1 **antitrypsin deficiency** is characterized by liver disease and emphysema. AST is elevated by twice as much as ALT in alcoholic hepatitis because alcohol inhibits ALT synthesis more than AST synthesis. **Budd-Chiari syndrome** is occlusion of the inferior vena cava or hepatic veins. The most common malignancy of the liver is metastatic (in order of decreasing frequency: colon, pancreas, breast, and lung).

217–218. The answers are 217-e, 218-a. *(Tierney, p 630.)* **Gilbert's disease** is the most common cause of mild unconjugated hyperbilirubinemia. It is found in up to **10%** of the population and is due to a **partial deficiency of glucuronosyltransferase.** Patients with **Dubin-Johnson syndrome** develop jaundice with stress, but it is primarily conjugated bilirubin. **Rotor's syndrome** is similar to Dubin-Johnson syndrome, but in Dubin-Johnson syndrome there is black pigment in the hepatocytes whereas in Rotor's syndrome there is no pigment. **Crigler-Najjar type 1 syndrome** (predominance of unconjugated bilirubin) is severe (absence of glucuronosyltransferase), and patients typically have bilirubin levels of more than 20 mg/dL. **Crigler-Najjar type 2 syndrome** is a relatively benign disorder due to partial deficiency of glucuronosyltransferase; patients present as adolescents with bilirubin levels of 6 to 20 mg/dL.

Genitourinary System

Questions

DIRECTIONS: Each item below contains a question followed by suggested responses. Select the **one best** response to each question.

219. A 24-year-old man presents with a painless testicular mass. He denies any past medical history and has no family history of cancer. He does not smoke, drink alcohol, or use illicit drugs. He recalls being kicked in the groin during karate practice 10 days ago. Physical examination reveals a 3-cm mass in the right scrotum that is hard and tender. The mass cannot be transilluminated. There is no lymphadenopathy. The serum α-fetoprotein level is elevated. Which of the following is the most likely diagnosis?

a. Seminoma
b. Nonseminoma
c. Hematoma
d. Leydig cell tumor
e. Sertoli cell tumor
f. Penile carcinoma
g. Testicular lymphoma

220. An 18-year-old man presents with a mass in the right inguinal area. When the examining finger is inserted into the lower part of the scrotum and carried along the vas deferens into the inguinal canal to inspect for herniation, the mass (viscus) strikes the lateral aspect of the examining finger when the patient is asked to cough. When the right inguinal area over the internal ring is compressed, and the patient is asked to cough again, the examining finger does not sense any mass striking it. Which of the following statements is true?

a. This type of hernia almost always resolves spontaneously before puberty
b. If the hernial sac extends into the scrotum, then this is a true surgical emergency
c. Inguinal hernias are more common in women than men
d. The appendix may be found in the hernial sac
e. This type of hernia is frequently present in elderly women

221. A 19-year-old student presents for a precollege screening visit. On physical examination, the patient has a scant beard (he states that he needs to shave only every other month) and gynecomastia. His testes are firm and measure less than 2 cm each. The patient states that he functions as a normal man sexually, although he feels his libido is diminished compared to that of his friends. Which of the following is the most likely diagnosis?

a. Turner's syndrome
b. Klinefelter's syndrome
c. Ambiguous genitalia
d. Late puberty
e. Normal male

222. A 22-year-old man presents one day after having been a restrained passenger in a moderate-speed motor vehicle accident (MVA). He states that his scrotum became discolored blue after the accident. He denies any trauma to the scrotum. On examination, the scrotum is bluish but the discoloration is gravity dependent. Which of the following is the most likely diagnosis?

a. Fournier's gangrene
b. Testicular torsion
c. Inguinal hernia
d. Hematocele
e. Hydrocele

223. A 48-year-old man presents with peripheral edema. He has been healthy and physically active all of his life. His family history is unremarkable. His blood pressure is normal. On physical examination, the patient is noted to have anasarca. Kidneys are not palpable. Urinalysis reveals a moderate amount of proteinuria, and "grape clusters" are seen under light microscopy. Which of the following is the most likely diagnosis?

a. Glomerulonephritis
b. Rhabdomyolysis
c. Nephrotic syndrome
d. Acute interstitial nephritis
e. Acute tubular necrosis

224. While examining the genitalia of an uncircumcised patient, you are unable to retract the foreskin. There is no evidence of erythema. Which of the following is the most likely diagnosis?

a. Balanitis
b. Phimosis
c. Escutcheon
d. Smegma
e. Priapism

225. A 34-year-old man complains of lumps in his scrotal skin. On physical examination, the lesions are small and mobile. An oily material can be extruded from the lesions. Which of the following is the most likely diagnosis?

a. Scrotal rings
b. Scrotal carcinoma
c. Epidermoid cysts
d. Molluscum contagiosum
e. Condyloma acuminatum

226. A 41-year-old man complains of soft, raised, flesh-colored growths or projections on his glans penis, prepuce, and penile shaft. Several excisional biopsies are done to look for malignancy. Which of the following is the most likely diagnosis?

a. Genital herpes
b. Condyloma acuminatum
c. Molluscum contagiosum
d. Condylomata lata
e. Peyronie's disease

227. A 21-year-old man who recently recovered from the mumps presents to the emergency room complaining of a swollen and painful left testicle. Physical examination reveals testicular tenderness. Which of the following is the most likely diagnosis?

a. Orchitis
b. Epididymitis
c. Testicular tumor
d. Varicocele
e. Spermatocele

228. A 32-year-old woman is referred to the emergency room for renal failure that was discovered in a preemployment screening examination. The patient has a blood urea nitrogen (BUN) of 100 mg/dL and a serum creatinine of 8.4 mg/dL. Her only complaint is bilateral flank pain. Family history reveals that her mother and one sibling have renal failure and receive hemodialysis. Her mother has had a recent stroke. The patient's blood pressure is 170/100 mmHg. Heart examination reveals a midsystolic click and murmur that increases with Valsalva maneuver. Kidneys are palpated bilaterally and are each 20 cm. Which of the following is the most likely diagnosis?

a. Horseshoe kidney
b. Polycystic kidney disease
c. Bilateral hydronephrosis
d. Kidney carcinoma
e. Medullary sponge kidney

229. A 34-year-old man presents to the emergency room complaining of protracted penile erection. The erection is not associated with sexual desire but is associated with severe pain. He denies any recent illicit drug or medication use. He has a past medical history significant for sickle cell disease. Which of the following is the appropriate next step in management?

a. Narcotics
b. Hydroxy urea
c. Folic acid
d. Exchange transfusion
e. Oxygen by nasal cannula

230. A 34-year-old firefighter presents to the emergency room complaining of the sudden onset of severe right-sided flank pain that radiates to the right groin and genitalia. He is unable to lie still on the stretcher. He denies any history of trauma. He denies any dysuria, frequency, nocturia, or fever. Examination of the genitalia is normal. Abdominal and rectal examinations are normal. There is positive right costovertebral angle (CVA) tenderness. Urinalysis reveals blood. Which of the following is the most likely diagnosis?

a. Pyelonephritis
b. Renal calculi
c. Testicular torsion
d. Strangulated hernia
e. Acute prostatitis

231. A 68-year-old man presents for his annual checkup. He has no complaints. He has no past medical history and takes no medications. He does not smoke cigarettes or drink alcohol. Physical examination is normal except for the rectal examination, which is positive for a 3-mm prostatic nodule. Which of the following is the appropriate next step in management?

a. Urology consult
b. Prostate-specific antigen (PSA) level
c. Transrectal ultrasound
d. Prostate biopsy
e. Blood urea nitrogen
f. Creatinine level

232. A 10-year-old boy with no history of trauma presents to the emergency room with a 14-hour history of a painful scrotum. Elevation of the scrotum does not relieve the pain. He also complains of nausea and vomiting. Examination reveals an enlarged, tender, erythematous scrotum that does not transilluminate. The testicle is in a transverse (horizontal) position. Cremasteric reflex is absent on the side of the swelling. Which of the following is the most likely diagnosis?

a. Spermatocele
b. Hydrocele
c. Epididymitis
d. Varicocele
e. Testicular torsion

233. A 16-year-old uncircumcised male presents to the emergency room with severe penile pain. On physical examination, the foreskin is retracted to reveal an enlarged and bluish-colored glans penis. The patient complains of severe pain on attempting to reposition the foreskin. Which of the following is the most likely diagnosis?

a. Hypospadias
b. Balanitis
c. Priapism
d. Paraphimosis
e. Phimosis
f. Epispadias

234. A 49-year-old man with multiple myeloma presents with glucosuria, hypophosphatemia, hypokalemia, hypouricemia, aminoaciduria, and proteinuria. Further analysis of the electrolytes reveals the patient has a metabolic acidosis. The urine pH is less than 5.5. Which of the following is the most likely diagnosis?

a. Fanconi's syndrome
b. Type 1 renal tubular acidosis
c. Distal renal tubular acidosis
d. Type 4 renal tubular acidosis
e. Kimmelstiel-Wilson disease

235. A 14-year-old boy complains of gradually worsening scrotal pain and swelling. He also complains of dysuria. On physical examination, the scrotum is edematous and erythematous. There is exquisite tenderness when palpating posterolaterally to the testicle. When you elevate the testicle, the scrotal pain is relieved. Which of the following is the most likely diagnosis?

a. Orchitis
b. Epididymitis
c. Testicular torsion
d. Varicocele
e. Hydrocele

236. A 19-year-old woman presents with severe right-sided flank pain accompanied by fever, shaking, chills, dysuria, and frequency. She is sexually active with one partner and always uses condoms. Her last menstrual period was five days ago. On physical examination, her temperature is 39.9°C (103.8°F) and her heart rate is 120 beats per minute. Blood pressure and respirations are normal. Abdominal examination reveals suprapubic tenderness with palpation. The patient complains of pain when percussion is performed with the ulnar surface of the fist over the right costovertebral angle (CVA). Pelvic examination is normal. Which of the following is the most likely diagnosis?

a. Diverticulitis
b. Acute cystitis
c. Renal calculi
d. Pyelonephritis
e. Appendicitis

237. A 15-year-old boy complains of worsening scrotal pain. On palpation of the scrotum, you find a pea-sized, tender mass at the upper pole of the testis. With transillumination, the mass appears as a blue dot. Which of the following is the most likely diagnosis?

a. Testicular torsion
b. Epididymitis
c. Hernia with hydrocele
d. Appendix testis torsion
e. Orchitis with hydrocele

238. A 13-year-old boy is complaining of heaviness in his scrotum and some vague pain in the area that worsens with exertion. Palpation of the scrotum reveals a freely moveable, nontender, tubular mass ("bag of worms") above the left testis. Which of the following is the most likely diagnosis?

a. Orchitis
b. Testicular torsion
c. Epididymitis
d. Varicocele
e. Hematocele

239. A 71-year-old man presents with a history of nocturia, frequency, and urgency about half the time. He states that for the last month he has had difficulty starting and maintaining his urine stream (has to push or strain) more than half of the time. He always feels like his bladder is not empty after urinating. On physical examination, the prostate gland is enlarged, nodular, and nontender. The PSA level is 2.7 ng/mL. Which of the following is the most likely diagnosis?

a. Mild BPH
b. Moderate BPH
c. Severe BPH
d. Prostate cancer
e. Prostatitis

240. A 23-year-old man presents complaining of hematuria for one day. He has no other symptoms but states that the hematuria started after he played in a fast-paced basketball game. He takes no medications and does not drink alcohol or use illicit drugs. He recalls having a sore throat yesterday but denies cough or fever. He takes no medications and has no family history of renal disease. Physical examination is normal. Rapid streptococcal antigen test is negative. Urinalysis reveals erythrocytes and erythrocyte casts. Which of the following is the most likely diagnosis?

a. Bladder carcinoma
b. IgA nephropathy
c. Poststreptococcal glomerulonephritis
d. Alport's syndrome
e. Minimal change disease

241. A 63-year-old woman with a history of end-stage renal disease presents after having missed two dialysis sessions. She complains of shortness of breath and fatigue. Her blood pressure is 150/105 mmHg and her heart rate is 115 beats per minute. Her point of maximum impulse (PMI) is displaced laterally. She has jugular venous distension and an S_4 gallop. She has some crackles at the lung bases posteriorly but no peripheral edema. Laboratory data reveal elevation of the BUN and creatinine levels. Her serum potassium level is 6.0 mg/dL (normal range is 3.5 to 5.5 mg/dL). Electrocardiogram is normal. After 80 mg of furosemide, the patient is no longer short of breath. Which of the following is an indication for emergency dialysis in this patient?

a. Heart rate of 115 beats per minute
b. Blood pressure of 150/105 mmHg
c. Fluid overload
d. Elevated potassium level
e. Elevated BUN
f. Elevated creatinine level
g. No need for emergency dialysis

242. An 18-year-old woman presents to your office for a blood pressure check. The patient has a history of hypertension diagnosed by a previous physician who recently retired. The patient takes three antihypertensives and is compliant. Except for an occasional headache, she has no complaints. There is no family history of hypertension. Blood pressure is 145/90 mmHg in both arms. Funduscopic examination reveals exudates and hemorrhages. Heart and lungs are normal. Abdominal examination reveals a systolic and diastolic bruit heard in the right midabdomen and through to the back. The remainder of the examination is normal. Which of the following is the most likely diagnosis?

a. Pheochromocytoma
b. Coarctation of the aorta
c. Renal artery stenosis
d. Hyperaldosteronism
e. Cushing's disease

243. A 24-year-old man has a lifelong history of voiding difficulty. He usually experiences hesitancy and interruption of flow when voiding. He has no past history of sexually transmitted disease, urinary tract infection, or kidney stones. Physical examination and urinalysis are normal. Examination of expressed prostatic secretions is normal. Which of the following is the most likely diagnosis?

a. Acute bacterial prostatitis
b. Prostatodynia
c. Tuberculous prostatitis
d. Chronic bacterial prostatitis
e. Nonbacterial prostatitis

244. A 41-year-old patient with a long history of schizophrenia presents with confusion and disorientation. His wife states that he drinks several liters of water daily. His blood pressure is 110/70 mmHg, pulse is 104 beats per minute, respirations are 20 breaths per minute, and temperature is 37°C (98.6°F). The patient has no orthostatic changes in blood pressure or pulse. Heart and lung examinations are normal. The neurologic exam reveals a dysarthric man who is oriented only to person. He has no focal neurologic deficits. Laboratory data reveal a serum sodium concentration of 105 meq/L and the diagnosis of primary polydipsia is made. The patient is admitted and the sodium is corrected to normal (135 meq/L) within 12 hours. While awaiting a psychiatry consult, the patient develops flaccid quadriplegia, then becomes comatose. Which of the following is the most likely diagnosis?

a. Relapse into hyponatremia
b. Acute schizophrenia
c. New stroke
d. Myocardial infarction
e. Central pontine myelinolysis

245. Which of the following is most likely to cause hematuria?

a. Femoral hernia
b. Hydrocele
c. Nephrotic syndrome
d. Renal artery stenosis
e. Cryoglobulinemia
f. Renal tubular acidosis

DIRECTIONS: Each group of questions below consists of lettered options followed by a set of numbered items. For each numbered item, select the **one** lettered option with which it is **most** closely associated. Each lettered option may be used once, more than once, or not at all.

Questions 246–247

For each patient with hematuria, select the most likely diagnosis.

a. Prostate cancer
b. Renal cell carcinoma
c. Bladder cancer
d. Carcinoma of the ureter

246. A 55-year-old man presents with hematuria, flank pain, and fever. Physical examination reveals the presence of an abdominal mass.

247. A 57-year-old man with a history of smoking presents with hematuria. He has owned and operated a chain of dry cleaners for over 30 years.

Genitourinary System

Answers

219. The answer is b. *(Tierney, pp 941–943.)* **Germ cell tumors** are the most common tumors in men between 20 and 35 years of age. A man who presents with a testicular mass and an **elevated serum α-fetoprotein (AFP) level** most likely has **nonseminomatous** testicular cancer. The elevated AFP implies yolk sac or nonseminomatous elements. Patients with **seminomas** (more common than nonseminomas) often have elevations in **human chorionic gonadotropin (hCG)**. All germ cell tumors, even if advanced, are curable with chemotherapy. **Leydig and Sertoli cell tumors** tend to produce estrogen, causing gynecomastia and impotence. Squamous cell carcinoma of the penis presents as a painful, nonhealing ulceration and is often found in uncircumcised men with poor hygiene. Testicular lymphoma is often bilateral. Swellings containing serous fluid transilluminate; those containing blood and tissue do not.

220. The answer is d. *(Seidel, pp 657–658.)* The digital examination described is consistent with an **indirect hernia** (a hernia that lies within the inguinal canal), which is the most common of all hernias. A **direct hernia** (a hernia through the posterior wall of the inguinal canal) is present if the viscus is felt medial to the external canal on digital examination. The appendix—or, for that matter, any visceral organ—may be found in a hernial sac. All hernias except femoral hernias are more common in males than in females. Hernias become surgical emergencies if they become incarcerated and irreducible. When the circulation is compromised due to the incarceration, the hernia is strangulated.

221. The answer is b. *(Seidel, p 673.)* **Klinefelter's syndrome,** the most common (1 in 500) disorder of sexual differentiation, is associated with XXY chromosomal inheritance and is characterized by tall stature, hypogonadism or small scrotum with pea-sized testes (normal testes are 5 cm long), a female distribution of pubic hair, and gynecomastia. Newborns require prompt chromosomal studies if born with ambiguous genitalia (small penis with hypospadias or enlarged clitoris). Patients with gonadal dysgenesis or **Turner's syndrome** are 45,X0; the syndrome is characterized by primary amenorrhea, short stature, webbed neck, and multiple congenital abnormalities.

222. The answer is d. *(Tierney, p 904.)* The presence of a patent processus vaginalis allows communication of intraperitoneal contents with the scrotum. Clear intraperitoneal fluid can form a **hydrocele**. Purulent material from a ruptured appendix can cause a hot scrotum. **Fournier's gangrene** is a polymicrobial infection of the subcutaneous tissues of the scrotum often seen in diabetic patients. Abdominal trauma, as from a car seat belt, can disrupt intraabdominal contents, and the blood can migrate through a patent processus vaginalis. The scrotal blood will not transilluminate and will be gravity dependent (**hematocele**). There have been unusual cases of scrotal swelling due to meconium in the newborn and due to migration of ventriculoperitoneal shunt tubing.

223. The answer is c. *(Tierney, p 890.)* **Anasarca** is generalized body edema that is often seen in the nephrotic syndrome. The "grape clusters" (lipid deposits or oval fat bodies in sloughed tubular epithelial cells) that appear under light microscopy appear as **Maltese crosses** under polarized light. One-third of patients with nephrotic syndrome have a systemic disease such as diabetes mellitus or systemic lupus erythematosus (SLE), and two-thirds have either (1) membranous nephropathy due to hepatitis C, SLE, syphilis, or medications; (2) minimal change disease; (3) focal glomerular sclerosis (HIV or heroin use); or (4) membranoproliferative glomerulonephritis. Patients with **glomerulonephritis** present with a nephritic syndrome (hypertension, hematuria, and edema). Patients with **acute interstitial nephritis** from drugs or infection usually present with rash, arthralgias, eosinophiluria, and eosinophilia. **Acute tubular necrosis** (**ATN**) typically occurs after an insult, such as ischemia or exposure to a nephrotoxin (i.e., contrast media, paraproteins in multiple myeloma, antibiotics). Myoglobinuria is a consequence of rhabdomyolysis that leads to ATN.

224. The answer is b. *(Seidel, p 655.)* **Phimosis** is the condition in which the foreskin in an uncircumcised patient cannot be retracted; this may occur normally in the first six years of life. Phimosis is usually congenital but may be due to recurrent infections or balanoposthitis (inflammation of the glans penis and prepuce). **Balanitis** is inflammation of the glans penis and occurs only in uncircumcised persons. **Escutcheon** is the hair pattern associated with genitalia. **Smegma** is a white, cheeselike material that collects around the glans penis in an uncircumcised man. **Priapism** is a painful, prolonged penile erection, which most often occurs in patients with sickle cell disease, sickle cell trait, or leukemia.

225. The answer is c. *(Seidel, pp 667–668.)* **Epidermoid** or sebaceous cysts appear as small lumps in the scrotal skin, which may enlarge and discharge oily material. **Molluscum contagiosum** appears as pearly white, umbilicated, dome-shaped papules caused by a poxvirus. **Condylomata acuminata** are warts caused by the human papillomavirus (HPV).

226. The answer is b. *(Seidel, pp 666–668.)* The lesions of **condyloma acuminatum,** or venereal warts, are soft, flesh-colored (may also be pink or red) growths or projections that are found on various parts of the penis. The etiologic agent is human papillomavirus (HPV), which is associated with dysplasia (i.e., squamous cell carcinoma of the cervix, penis, anus, vagina, and vulva). Warts are sexually transmitted with an incubation period of one to six months. **Condylomata lata** are the soft, flat-topped, moist, pale nodules and papules of secondary syphilis that appear two to six months after the primary chancre. These contagious lesions may be seen anywhere on the body, including the palms and soles. **Peyronie's disease** is unilateral deviation of the penis caused by a fibrous band in the corpus cavernosum. It results in deviation (and often pain) of the penis during erection. **Genital herpes** is a sexually transmitted disease characterized by a painful group of vesicles on an erythematous base.

227. The answer is a. *(Seidel, p 671.)* **Orchitis** is an uncommon occurrence except as a sequela of infection with mumps in young males. It is most often unilateral, and testicular atrophy occurs in 50% of cases. Testicular tumors are the most common neoplasms in men between the ages of 15 and 30 years. The tumors are nontender, are fixed to the testicle, and do not transilluminate.

228. The answer is b. *(Seidel, pp 551–552.)* The kidneys normally extend from T12 to L3 (11 cm long). The right kidney is lower than the left kidney due to the liver above it. The left kidney is usually not palpable. Bilateral large kidneys suggest polycystic kidney disease or bilateral hydronephrosis. **Polycystic kidney disease** **(PKD)** is the most common inherited disorder in the

United States and may be autosomal dominant (ADPKD) due to a defect on the short arm of chromosome 16. Patients develop hypertension and renal cysts and often require dialysis or transplantation by the age of 40. Extrarenal manifestations of ADPKD include mitral valve prolapse, berry aneurysms of the circle of Willis, diverticulosis, diverticulitis, and liver cysts. **Medullary sponge kidney** is a benign condition seen in older patients (40 to 50) that almost never leads to renal failure. **Horseshoe kidney** is a kidney that can be palpated crossing the midline. **Renal carcinoma** often presents as a hard mass. Patients with **bilateral hydronephrosis** typically have signs of infection, such as fever, hematuria, and dysuria.

229. The answer is d. *(Tierney, p 902.)* **Priapism** is protracted erection associated with pain but not associated with sexual desire. Local abnormalities such as malignancy or inflammatory diseases of the shaft may cause priapism. Priapism may also be secondary to systemic illness, such as leukemia and sickle cell disease. The patient with sickle cell disease who presents with priapism may benefit from exchange transfusion.

230. The answer is b. *(Tierney, pp 914–916.)* **Renal colic** is severe episodic pain localized to the flank that often radiates to the groin and genitalia. It is often accompanied by nausea and vomiting. Patients often move about (in contrast to an acute abdomen from peritonitis, where patients stay very still) in an effort to find a more comfortable position. The most common composition of stones is **calcium oxalate** (radiopaque on abdominal film). Patients with **acute bacterial prostatitis** present with fever, dysuria, urgency, frequency, and pain (suprapubic, perineal, and sacral). Rectal examination reveals a warm and exquisitely tender prostate gland. Pyelonephritis is unlikely without fever or urinary symptoms. The normal genitalia examination makes the other choices unlikely.

231. The answer is b. *(Tierney, pp 934.)* Serum **PSA,** although widely used as a screening test for adenocarcinoma of the prostate, is not specific for cancer. The PSA measurement, however, is more reliable than digital rectal exam (DRE) for detection of prostate cancer. The combined use of PSA and DRE affords a more complete evaluation for detecting prostate cancer. PSA levels of more than 10 ng/mL are considered high, results lower than 4 ng/mL are considered normal, and results between 4 and 10 ng/mL are considered borderline. The higher the PSA level, the more likely the presence of prostate cancer, but PSA should not be considered specific for cancer. Twenty percent of patients with prostate cancer will have a normal PSA level. Patients with suspicious DRE/PSA results should have transrectal ultrasound (TRUS) of the prostate with biopsies.

232. The answer is e. *(Seidel, p 672.)* The tunica vaginalis normally attaches the posterolateral surfaces of the testicle to the scrotum, thereby anchoring it and preventing rotation. When these attachments are missing, the testicle is free to rotate around the spermatic cord and the critical vascular pedicle. This is known as intravaginal **torsion** and is most common in patients between 10 and 20 years of age. Classically, the testicle will have a transverse lie within the scrotum, known as the **bell-clapper relationship.** The onset of pain is sudden, and there are no urinary complaints. The pain may be accompanied by nausea and vomiting. Many feel that the initiating factor may be contraction of the cremaster muscle, since loss of the cremasteric reflex (normally the testicle and scrotum rise on the side where the inner thigh is stroked with a blunt instrument or finger) is almost invariably found in torsion.

233. The answer is d. *(Seidel, p 665.)* **Paraphimosis** occurs when the foreskin cannot be returned to the extended position. It may lead to gangrene of the glans penis. **Phimosis** is the inability to retract the foreskin. **Hypospadias** is a congenital abnormality in which the urethra is situated on the ventral surface of the shaft of the penis. **Epispadias** is a congenital defect in which the urethral meatus appears on the dorsum of the penis.

234. The answer is a. *(Tierney, p 853.)* **Fanconi's syndrome** is a generalized defect in proximal tubule transport involving amino acids, glucose, uric acid, potassium, phosphate, sodium, and bicarbonate. It may be secondary to multiple myeloma, amyloidosis, or heavy metal toxicity. Fanconi's syndrome is a **type 2 (proximal) renal tubular acidosis (RTA). Type 1 RTA (distal)** causes a metabolic acidosis with an alkaline (>5.5) urine pH. **RTA type 4** causes hyperkalemia and is due to inadequate aldosterone production from diabetes mellitus, sickle cell disease, obstructive uropathy, or medication use (heparin, nonsteroidal anti-inflammatory drugs, ACE inhibitors). Diabetic patients may develop a specific kind of nephropathy (glomerulosclerosis) in which **Kimmelstiel-Wilson** lesions are found histologically (nodules that stain periodic acid–Schiff positive and are deposited in the periphery of the glomerulus).

235. The answer is b. *(Seidel, p 670.)* The epididymis is located on the posterolateral surface of the testis and should be smooth, discrete, nontender, and larger cephalad. **Epididymitis** in children usually occurs in the preteen years and is thought to be secondary to reflux of sterile urine that causes an inflammatory reaction in the epididymis. A urinary tract infection is occasionally seen. There is tenderness of the posterolaterally positioned epididymis with a normal testicle palpated anteriorly. **Prehn's sign** is positive when the patient experiences relief from pain on elevation of the testicle. This sign is not reliable, however, and testicular torsion must still be ruled out.

236. The answer is d. *(Tierney, pp 909–910.)* The patient presents with **pyelonephritis,** which is an infection of the kidney and renal pelvis. It is characterized by flank pain, fever, dysuria, and frequency. Patients often experience suprapubic and CVA tenderness. Patients with acute cystitis may present with dysuria, frequency, urgency, and suprapubic tenderness, but typically the patient is afebrile and the physical examination is normal. The organisms responsible for urinary tract infections are **SEEK PP =** **S**erratia marcescens, **E**scherichia coli, **E**nterobacter cloacae, **K**lebsiella pneumoniae, **P**roteus mirabilis, and **P**seudomonas aeruginosa.

237. The answer is d. *(Tierney, pp 904–905.)* The appendix testis and the appendix epididymis are embryonic ductal system remnants. The appendix epididymis is an irregularity on the cephalad surface of the epididymis. These two intrascrotal appendages may undergo torsion. The peak incidence of **torsion** occurs between the ages of 10 and 15 years. Onset of pain can be sudden or gradual, and the infarcted appendage can often be seen as a **blue dot** on the superior pole of the testis. Transillumination highlights the appearance.

238. The answer is d. *(Seidel, p 670.)* **Varicocele** is a collection of dilated veins of the pampiniform plexus. Compression of the left renal vein (varicocele is most common on the left side) at the level of the aorta causes venous stasis and reflux into the spermatic vein, causing the varicocele. Incidence is rare before the age of 8 years and is often seen during puberty.

The dilated veins are more easily seen and palpated with the patient standing. Varicocele is associated with reduced fertility.

239. The answer is b. *(Tierney, p 927.)* The patient has an **American Urologic Association (AUA) symptom index score** of 17/35 or moderate benign prostatic hyperplasia (BPH). This score is based on a patient's 0 to 5 response to seven questions (0 = not at all; 1 = less than one-fifth of the time; 2 = less than one-half of the time; 3 = one-half of the time; 4 = more than one-half of the time; 5 = almost always).

Over the last month, how often have you:

1. Had a sensation of not emptying your bladder after urinating?
2. Had to urinate again less than two hours after you finished urinating?
3. Stopped and started again several times when you urinated?
4. Found it difficult to postpone urination?
5. Had a weak urinary stream?
6. Had to push or strain to begin urination?
7. Had nocturia?

A score of 0 to 7 indicates mild BPH; 8 to 19, moderate BPH; and 20 to 35, severe BPH.

240. The answer is b. *(Tierney, pp 887–888.)* **IgA nephropathy (Berger's)** is the most commonly encountered form of focal glomerulonephritis worldwide, and patients will often have microhematuria. It may follow an upper respiratory tract infection or physical exertion. **Bladder cancer** is a common cause of asymptomatic microhematuria but is usually found in patients over the age of 50. Risk factors for bladder neoplasia include aniline, rubber, other organic solvents, industrial dyes, and tobacco use. **Minimal change disease** almost always presents with severe proteinuria, and erythrocyte casts are not seen in rhabdomyolysis. Patients with **Alport's syndrome** have the nephritic syndrome and hearing loss.

241. The answer is g. *(Tierney, p 882.)* Indications for dialysis are easily remembered with the vowel mnemonic of **A, E, I, O, U,** or **A**cidosis (pH < 7.20), **E**lectrolyte abnormality (hyperkalemia with EKG changes), fluid **O**verload unresponsive to diuretics, and **U**remic symptoms (pericarditis, encephalopathy, or coagulopathy). The **I** in the mnemonic is a reminder that ingestion of certain drugs (barbiturates, bromide, chloral hydrate, ethanol, ethylene glycol, isopropyl alcohol, lithium, methanol, procainamide, theophylline, salicylates, and heavy metals) is treatable with dialysis.

242. The answer is c. *(Tierney, p 884.)* **Renal artery stenosis (RAS)** accounts for less than 5% of hypertension (HTN). The most common cause is atherosclerosis, but in young women the etiology is often fibromuscular dysplasia. Patients may present with a high-pitched epigastric bruit. A positive captopril test (renin values increase greatly after a dose of the angiotensin converting enzyme is given, because the drug magnifies the impairment in blood flow and in the glomerular filtration rate caused by the RAS) is an excellent screening procedure. The diagnosis is then confirmed with a digital subtraction renal arteriogram, Doppler ultrasonography, or a magnetic resonance angiogram. Patients with **pheochromocytoma** often present with sudden episodes of hypertension, headache, profuse sweating, anxiety, and palpitations. The diagnosis is made by 24-hour urine collection for catecholamines or catecholamine metabolites. Patients with HTN due to **coarctation of the aorta** present with delayed or absent femoral pulses and complain of claudication. Patients with **primary hyperaldosteronism** (Conn's syndrome; etiology is usually bilateral adrenal hyperplasia) present with HTN, fatigue, polyuria, and muscle weakness due to potassium depletion. **Cushing's disease** is characterized by central deposition of adipose tissue, muscle weakness, amenorrhea, impotence, psychiatric abnormalities, and HTN.

243. The answer is b. *(Tierney, p 911.)* **Prostatodynia** is a noninflammatory disorder that affects young and middle-aged men. Patients present complaining of a lifelong history of difficulty voiding. The prostate is normal, and urinalysis is negative for bacteria and leukocytes. Prostatic secretions show a normal number of leukocytes. Treatment consists of alpha blocking agents. Patients with **nonbacterial prostatitis** (*Chlamydia, Mycoplasma, Ureaplasma,* and viruses) will have increased numbers of leukocytes in prostatic secretions with a negative culture. Patients with **chronic bacterial prostatitis** will have positive prostatic secretion leukocytes and a positive culture. **Expressing prostatic secretions in patients with acute bacterial prostatitis is contraindicated.**

244. The answer is e. *(Tierney, pp 839–842.)* The patient presents with euvolemic hyponatremia secondary to **primary polydipsia** (compulsive water consumption). Since the hyponatremia developed gradually in the absence of neurologic symptoms (i.e., seizures), it should not be corrected rapidly. The appropriate rate of correction should be 12 meq every 24 hours to prevent central pontine myelinolysis (CPM), which is an osmotically induced demyelination due to overly rapid correction of serum sodium. Patients develop paraplegia, quadriplegia, and coma.

245. The answer is e. *(Tierney, pp 906–908.)* An easy mnemonic to address hematuria is "If your doctor does not know how to work up hematuria, you should **SWITCH GPS.**"

S = stones, sickle cell disease, sickle cell trait, scleroderma, SLE, sulfonamides
W = Wegener's granulomatosis
I = infections, instrumentation, iatrogenic, interstitial nephritis
T = trauma, TB, tubulointerstitial disease, tumor, thrombocytopenic thrombotic purpura (TTP)
C = cryoglobulinemia, cyclophosphamide
H = hemolytic-uremic syndrome, hypercalciuria, hemophilia, Henoch-Schönlein purpura
G = Goodpasture's disease, glomerulonephritis
P = papillary necrosis, polycystic kidney disease, polyarteritis nodosa
S = schistosomiasis, sponge disease (medullary sponge disease)

246–247. The answers are 246-b, 247-c. *(Tierney, pp 937–941.)* Ninety-five percent of tumors of the kidney are **renal cell carcinomas.** Patients present with hematuria and the presence of an abdominal mass. Causal factors have been implicated in the development of renal cell carcinoma, but cigarette smoking and obesity are the strongest associations. **Bladder cancer** is strongly associated with cigarette smoking and chemical compounds (aromatic hydrocarbons). Chimney sweepers and dry cleaners are also at risk for bladder cancer (up to 25% of all bladder cancer is occupationally related). **Cancer of the ureter** (transitional cell like the bladder) is associated with chronic phenacetin use, cigarette smoking, and hydrocarbon chemical exposure.

Endocrinology

Questions

DIRECTIONS: Each item below contains a question followed by suggested responses. Select the **one best** response to each question.

248. A 41-year-old woman with no previous medical problems presents with the chief complaint of generalized weakness. The patient states that she has been irritable lately and finds it difficult to concentrate at work. She has been amenorrheic for 12 months and feels her symptoms might be related to early menopause. On physical examination, blood pressure is 160/90 mmHg. The patient has a "moon face" and a "buffalo hump." She is hirsute. Abdominal examination reveals purple striae. Her extremities appear to be atrophied. Her finger stick glucose is 210 mg/dL. Which of the following is the most likely diagnosis?

a. Cushing's syndrome
b. Cushing's disease
c. Pseudo-Cushing state
d. Polycystic ovary disease
e. Normal menopause

249. A 42-year-old man presents to your office for a checkup. He has been in excellent health except for a recent diagnosis of mild hypertension and bilateral carpal tunnel syndrome. On physical examination, the patient is tall, with large and doughy hands. His facial features are coarse, and he has a prominent mandible with wide-spaced teeth. His voice is deep, and he has macroglossia. Heart examination reveals the point of maximum impulse (PMI) to be displaced 2 cm laterally. Which of the following is the most likely diagnosis?

a. Acromegaly
b. Gigantism
c. Hypothyroidism
d. Familial prognathism
e. Amyloidosis

250. A 47-year-old woman presents complaining of redness and itchiness of the skin of her neck area. She has no other complaints. Physical examination is positive for redness of the skin overlying the thyroid gland (Marañón's sign). Which of the following is the most appropriate next step in the diagnosis?

a. Free thyroxine
b. Thyroid-stimulating hormone (TSH) level
c. Thyroid resin uptake
d. T_4
e. T_3

251. A 21-year-old woman presents to the emergency room with palpitations. Physical examination reveals an anxious and highly energetic patient. Her heart rate is 120 beats per minute. She has bilateral proptosis (exophthalmos), stare, and lid retraction. Thyroid examination reveals diffuse enlargement with an audible bruit. The thyroid gland is nontender. The patient has weakness of her quadriceps muscles (needs help to rise from a chair) and has fine tremors. Which of the following is the most likely diagnosis?

a. Graves' disease
b. Hashimoto's thyroiditis
c. Plummer's disease
d. Struma ovarii
e. Subacute thyroiditis

252. A 52-year-old woman presents to her private physician with the chief complaint of hoarseness. She sings in her church choir, and her friends have noticed a voice change. Her past medical history is significant for heart arrhythmias, which have been well controlled for three years with amiodarone. Physical examination reveals a woman with coarse hair and skin. Her fingernails are thick, and her eyes appear puffy. The thyroid gland is normal and nontender. Her muscle strength is excellent, but the relaxation phase of her ankle reflex is prolonged. Which of the following is the most likely diagnosis?

a. Cushing's disease
b. Acromegaly
c. de Quervain's disease
d. Amiodarone-induced hypothyroidism
e. Cretinism

253. You suspect that a 26-year-old woman presenting with galactorrhea and infertility has a large pituitary tumor. Which of the following is the most likely visual field defect on physical examination?

a. Bitemporal hemianopsia
b. Left homonymous hemianopsia
c. Right homonymous hemianopsia
d. Right homonymous inferior quadrantanopsia
e. Left homonymous inferior quadrantanopsia

254. A 51-year-old patient is seen in your office several weeks after a parathyroidectomy for a parathyroid adenoma. She is complaining of parethesias. Physical examination reveals contraction of the right facial muscles when you tap lightly over the right side of the patient's face. Which of the following is the most likely diagnosis?

a. Hypokalemia
b. Hypercalcemia
c. Hyperkalemia
d. Hypocalcemia
e. Hyponatremia

255. A 21-year-old woman presents with a 6-cm nontender mass located in the center of her neck. On physical examination the thyroid gland is normal in size and there are no bruits audible over the mass. She has no other symptoms or complaints. She does not smoke or drink alcohol. Which of the following is the most likely diagnosis?

a. Brachial cleft cyst
b. Thyroglossal ductal cyst
c. Lipoma
d. Carotid body tumor
e. Laryngocele

256. A 37-year-old woman who recently emigrated from Central America presents with a 20-lb weight loss over the last month. She also complains of generalized weakness and occasional nausea. She has no medical history and was in previous good health. On physical examination, the patient has increased skin pigmentation. She is afebrile. Her blood pressure is 90/60 mmHg supine and 70/50 mmHg standing. The rest of her physical examination is normal. Laboratory data reveal hyponatremia, hyperkalemia, and a metabolic acidosis. Which of the following is the most likely diagnosis?

a. Sheehan's syndrome
b. Craniopharyngioma
c. Addison's disease
d. Empty sella syndrome
e. Insulinoma
f. Schmidt's syndrome
g. Pituitary apoplexy

257. A 49-year-old man presents with a compression fracture of his sixth thoracic vertebra. He is a tobacco and alcohol user and takes diphenylhydantoin for a seizure disorder. Which of the following is the most likely diagnosis?

a. Osteomalacia
b. Premature osteoporosis
c. Scleromalacia
d. Paget's disease
e. Multiple myeloma

258. A 46-year-old man with lung cancer is brought to the emergency room with confusion. He is lethargic and oriented to person but not to place or time. An electrocardiogram reveals a shortened QT interval. Which of the following is the most appropriate initial step in management?

a. Intravenous corticosteroids
b. Intravenous mithramycin
c. Intravenous bisphosphonates
d. Hydrochlorothiazide
e. Subcutaneous calcitonin
f. Intravenous fluids

259. A 22-year-old woman presents with the chief complaint of hirsutism. She has had irregular periods since menarche at the age of 13. She has an ideal body weight and her facies is normal. Physical examination reveals excess back and chest hair. Pelvic examination is normal. The luteinizing hormone (LH) value is elevated. Serum 17-OH progesterone concentrations are highly elevated. Which of the following is the most likely diagnosis?

a. Cushing's syndrome
b. Congenital adrenal hyperplasia
c. Adrenal tumor
d. Idiopathic hirsutism
e. Polycystic ovary disease

260. A 13-year-old boy is worried that he is growing breasts and complains that the breasts are often painful, but he has no other complaints. He states that he has been growing taller this past year. On physical examination, you note some acne on the patient's face. His testes and phallus are appropriate for his age, and his scrotum is reddened, with some thinning of the skin. He has fine, sparse pubic hair. Which of the following is the most likely diagnosis?

a. Gonadal tumor
b. Pituitary tumor
c. Adrenal tumor
d. Normal puberty
e. Klinefelter's syndrome

261. A 19-year-old collegiate football player is sent to your office by the team's coach because of occasional outbursts of anger and hostility. The patient has no past medical history and denies using tobacco, alcohol, or illicit drugs. Physical examination reveals a blood pressure of 140/90 mmHg. The patient has gynecomastia and testicular atrophy. He states that his libido and sexual performance are adequate. Which of the following is the most likely diagnosis?

a. Prolactinoma
b. Kallman's syndrome
c. Anabolic steroid use
d. Chronic cocaine use
e. Diabetes mellitus

262. A 17-year-old woman presents with amenorrhea for three months. She states that she has had irregular periods since her menarche at the age of 12 years. Physical examination reveals a normal adolescent female. Breast examination reveals breast engorgement and tenderness. Pelvic examination is normal. The patient's prolactin level is elevated. Which of the following is the most likely diagnosis?

a. Hypothyroidism
b. Cushing's syndrome
c. Pregnancy
d. Prolactinoma
e. Premature menopause
f. Congenital adrenal hyperplasia

263. A 46-year-old woman complains of headache, sweating, and diaphoresis that occur on a daily basis or sometimes twice a day while she is at work. She has gone to the company nurse during these episodes and was told that her blood pressure was elevated. Aside from that, the nurse could not find any other problem. Physical examination is normal, including blood pressure, which is 130/80 mmHg. Which of the following is the most likely diagnosis?

a. Carcinoid syndrome
b. Thyroid storm
c. Pheochromocytoma
d. Syndrome X
e. CHAOS

264. A 63-year-old woman has a large retroclavicular goiter. Whenever she elevates her arms over her head, she experiences facial plethora and dizziness (Pemberton's sign). Which of the following is the most likely diagnosis?

a. Chronic obstructive lung disease
b. Bilateral vocal cord paralysis
c. Spinal cord compression
d. Superior vena cava syndrome
e. Congestive heart failure

265. A 47-year-old woman presents to your office complaining of bone pain. She has a past medical history significant for peptic ulcer disease and pancreatitis. Routine laboratory studies reveal a serum calcium of 12.0 mg/dL (normal is <10.5 mg/dL) and hypophosphatemia. Which of the following is the most likely diagnosis?

a. Underlying malignancy
b. Vitamin D intoxication
c. Familial hypocalciuric hypercalcemia
d. Osteitis fibrosa cystica
e. Primary hyperparathyroidism

266. A 15-year-old boy has noticed the descent of his scrotum. His penis has enlarged in length, and he has developed curly, pigmented hair around the base of the penis. Which of the following would best describe his Tanner stage of development?

a. Tanner stage 1
b. Tanner stage 2
c. Tanner stage 3
d. Tanner stage 4
e. Tanner stage 5

267. A 46-year-old woman with a 10-year history of diabetes mellitus presents to the emergency room with nausea, vomiting, and abdominal pain. Family members state that the patient has recently been taking over-the-counter medications for an upper respiratory tract infection. The blood pressure is 90/60 mmHg and the pulse is 120 beats per minute. The patient is lethargic but follows commands. Pupils are 3 mm bilaterally and reactive to light and accommodation. Abdominal examination reveals diffuse tenderness but no rebound tenderness. Neurologic examination reveals no focal deficits. Finger stick glucose is higher than 800 mg/dL, and arterial blood gas reveals a pH of 7.36. Which of the following is the most likely diagnosis?

a. Hyperosmolar state
b. Gestational diabetes
c. Barbiturate overdose
d. Impaired glucose tolerance
e. Diabetic ketoacidosis

268. A 52-year-old woman with a 20-year history of insulin-dependent diabetes mellitus presents complaining of a rash that has developed on her legs and ankles. Physical examination reveals several oval-shaped plaques with demarcated borders and a glistening yellow surface located on the anterior surface of the legs and dorsum of the ankles. Which of the following is the most likely diagnosis?

a. Peripheral neuropathy
b. Amyotrophy
c. Mononeuropathy
d. Acanthosis nigricans
e. Necrobiosis lipoidica diabeticorum

269. A 24-year-old man is referred to your practice for elevated cholesterol level. The patient has a father and two siblings with high cholesterol levels who are on medications. His 31-year-old brother recently had a myocardial infarction. On physical examination, the patient has bilateral arcus senilis. His extremities are remarkable for diffuse and nodular thickenings of the Achilles tendon. Which of the following is the most likely diagnosis?

a. Hypothyroidism
b. Nephrotic syndrome
c. Liver disease
d. Type 2A hyperlipoproteinemia
e. Type 3 dysbetalipoproteinemia

270. A 44-year-old woman with a 20-year history of poorly controlled diabetes mellitus presents with headache and unilateral proptosis. The patient is febrile and appears toxic. Her serum glucose level is 640 mg/dL. An urgent CT scan of the head reveals a retroorbital abscess and severe opacification of the frontal and ethmoid sinuses. Which of the following organisms is most likely responsible for this infection?

a. *Cryptococcus neoformans*
b. Mucormycosis
c. *Mycobacterium tuberculosis*
d. *Toxoplasma gondii*
e. *Listeria monocytogenes*
f. *Staphylococcus epidermis*

271. A 41-year-old woman presents with amenorrhea for nine months. She is found to have a prolactin-secreting pituitary adenoma. Laboratory data reveal a serum calcium level of 12.0 mg/dL and hypoglycemia (serum glucose of 49 mg/dL). Which of the following is the most likely diagnosis?

a. MEN 1 syndrome
b. MEN 2A syndrome
c. MEN 2B syndrome
d. Sipple's syndrome

272. A 42-year-old nursing student presents to the emergency room with confusion, diaphoresis, and dizziness. She is tremulous and tachycardic. Her serum glucose level is found to be 20 mg/dL, and she responds immediately to intravenous dextrose infusion. The patient states that she has been eating well. After the hypoglycemia is corrected, the physical examination is normal. Bloodwork reveals that insulin levels are high but C-peptide level is low. The rest of the laboratory data are normal. Which of the following is the most likely diagnosis?

a. Insulinoma
b. Surreptitious insulin injection
c. Hypopituitarism
d. Adrenal insufficiency
e. Glucagon deficiency

273. A 15-year-old girl has noticed that she has developed straight, barely pigmented hair along the medial border of her labia. Which of the following would best describe her Tanner stage of development?

a. Tanner 1
b. Tanner 2
c. Tanner 3
d. Tanner 4
e. Tanner 5

274. A 49-year-old man with a 25-year history of diabetes mellitus presents with a painful right foot. He denies a history of trauma. On physical examination, the patient has loss of pain and vibration in both feet. His Achilles deep tendon reflexes are absent bilaterally. Peripheral pulses are palpable, and there are no skin lesions. The right foot is erythematous with some edema. The patient's gait reveals a limp due to foot pain. Radiograph of the ankle reveals osteopenia and multiple fractures of the tarsal bones. Which of the following is the most likely diagnosis?

a. Somogyi effect
b. Dawn phenomenon
c. Whipple triad
d. Charcot joint
e. MODY
f. Charcot triad

275. A 60-year-old man is involved in a head-on motor vehicle accident and sustains significant head trauma. He is awake and oriented to person, place, and time but complains of dizziness. Physical examination reveals normal vital signs, no orthostasis, and no neurologic findings. Heart and lung exams are normal. Overnight in the surgical intensive care unit, the patient develops excessive thirst, polydypsia, and polyuria. He develops orthostatic changes on physical examination. His serum sodium rises to 160 meq/L (normal is ≤145 meq/L), and his serum glucose is normal. Which of the following is the most likely diagnosis?

a. Impaired glucose intolerance
b. Nephrogenic diabetes insipidus
c. Central diabetes insipidus
d. Syndrome of inappropriate antidiuretic hormone secretion (SIADH)
e. Iatrogenic saline infusion

DIRECTIONS: Each group of questions below consists of lettered options followed by a set of numbered items. For each numbered item, select the **one** lettered option with which it is **most** closely associated. Each lettered option may be used once, more than once, or not at all.

Questions 276–277

For each man with erectile dysfunction (ED), select the most likely mechanism causing the symptoms.

a. Neuropathic impotence
b. Vascular impotence
c. Psychogenic impotence
d. Endocrine impotence

276. A previously healthy 42-year-old man presents with impotence. He takes no medications and does not smoke, drink alcohol, or use illicit drugs. He attains nocturnal erections but is impotent with his sexual partner.

277. A 53-year-old diabetic man with a history of gastroparesis and peripheral neuropathy presents with erectile dysfunction. He drinks alcohol daily.

Endocrinology

Answers

248. The answer is b. (*Tierney, pp 1132–1133.*) **Cushing's syndrome** occurs secondary to corticosteroid use, nonpituitary neoplasms (i.e., small cell carcinoma of the lung), adrenal adenomas, adrenal carcinomas, and bilateral adrenal nodular hyperplasia. **Cushing's disease** is hypercortisolism due to adrenocorticotropic hormone (ACTH) hypersecretion by the pituitary gland, usually because of a small (<1 cm) benign pituitary microadenoma. Symptoms include central obesity, striae, hirsutism, easy bruisability, proximal myopathy, osteoporosis, amenorrhea, hypertension, glucose intolerance, and hypokalemia. Urinary cortisol is a good screening test for Cushing's syndrome. Alcoholic patients and depressed patients may have hypercortisolism (pseudo-Cushing state). **Polycystic ovary disease** (Stein-Leventhal syndrome) causes increased levels of testosterone, hirsutism, infertility, and menstrual irregularity.

249. The answer is a. (*Tierney, pp 1079–1080.*) **Acromegaly** (hypersecretion of growth hormone after closure of the epiphyses) is almost always caused by a pituitary adenoma (benign 99% of the time). Patients present with tall stature, large hands, large feet, prominent mandible, prognathism, coarse facial features, wide tooth spacing, deep voice, macroglossia, and carpal tunnel syndrome. Patients may have headache, visual field defects, hypertrophy of the laryngeal tissue causing obstructive sleep apnea, hypertension, cardiomegaly, multiple skin tags, premalignant colonic polyps, and diabetes mellitus. **Gigantism** occurs before the closure of the epiphyses. **Amyloidosis** is a group of disorders characterized by infiltration of various organs (kidney, heart, intestine, endocrine) by protein fibrils. Patients with amyloidosis may have macroglossia and carpal tunnel syndrome. Macroglossia is also seen in hypothyroidism. Coarse features may run in families (familial prognathism).

250. The answer is b. (*Goldman, pp 1396–1398.*) The patient who presents with redness and itchiness of the skin of the neck overlying the thyroid gland (**Marañón's sign**) most likely has Graves' disease. Serum T$_3$, T$_4$, free thyroxine, and thyroid resin uptake are all usually increased. A reliable sensitive TSH assay is the best test for thyrotoxicosis.

251. The answer is a. (*Tierney, pp 1102–1105.*) The patient most likely has **Graves' disease** (Basedow's disease), which is the most common cause of thyrotoxicosis or hyperthyroidism. Other signs of Graves' disease are heat intolerance, menstrual irregularity, weight loss, and pretibial myxedema. Patients present between the ages of 20 and 40, and women are affected more than men. The disorder is due to antibodies that bind to the TSH receptor, causing it to stimulate the thyroid gland to hyperfunction. **Plummer's disease** is an autonomous toxic adenomatous disease of the thyroid; patients do not present with ophthalmopathy or dermapathy. **Hashimoto's thyroiditis,** or **chronic lymphocytic thyroiditis,** is a common autoimmune disease (positive antimicrosomal antibodies and antithyroid peroxidase antibodies) that causes hypothyroidism. Patients present with a diffuse, firm, nontender goiter. Patients with Hashimoto's thyroiditis are susceptible to **postpartum thyroiditis.** **Struma ovarii** is thyroid tissue contained in a dermoid ovarian tumor. **Granulomatous,** or **subacute** (**de Quervain's**), **thyroiditis** is due to release of preformed thyroglobulin and follows a viral infection; the thyroid gland is painful and tender to palpation. The treatment for subacute thyroiditis is aspirin or nonsteroidal anti-inflammatory agents.

252. The answer is d. (*Tierney, pp 1098–1100.*) Symptoms of hypothyroidism include constipation, depression, edema, tongue thickening, cold intolerance, Queen Anne sign (missing lateral one-third of eyebrows), muscle cramps, weight gain, goiter, amenorrhea, galactorrhea, pleural effusion, pericardial effusion, cardiomegaly, bradycardia, hypothermia, hyponatremia, anemia, and hypertension. Patients are said to have **hung-up reflexes** (a prolonged relaxation phase). Amiodarone has high iodine content and causes hypothyroidism in 8% of patients. **Myxedema** is a rare complication of hypothyroidism; patients present with coma, severe hypotension, hypothermia, hypoventilation, and hypoxemia. **Cretinism** is congenital (infantile) hypothyroidism.

253. The answer is a. (*Seidel, p 311.*) A pituitary tumor may impinge on the optic chiasm. The temporal field fibers are damaged as they decussate at the optic chiasm, and the result is a **bitemporal hemianopsia.**

254. The answer is d. *(Seidel, p 1160.)* Tapping on cranial nerve VII as it exits the parotid gland will cause spasm or contraction of the facial muscles on the same side of the face that is being tapped in states of **hypocalcemia** (**tetany**). This is called **Chvostek's sign.** Clinical signs of hypocalcemia include paresthesias, neuromuscular irritability, a positive **Trousseau's phenomenon** (carpal spasm after application of a blood pressure cuff), and a prolonged QT interval on electrocardiogram. Hypocalcemia causes rickets in children and osteomalacia in adults. Parathyroidectomy can lead to hypocalcemia. The clinical presentation of hypercalcemia consists of **bones** (fractures, osteitis fibrosa), **stones** (renal calculi), **abdominal groans** (anorexia, constipation, vomiting, peptic ulcers, pancreatitis), and **psychic overtones** (anxiety, depression, and insomnia). Patients with **hypokalemia** present with muscle weakness, muscle cramps, and flaccid paralysis. **Hyperkalemia** may lead to areflexia, flaccid paralysis, and electrocardiographic abnormalities such as peaked T waves, prolongation of the PR interval, widening of the QRS complex, and ventricular tachycardia.

255. The answer is b. *(Seidel, p 273.)* A **thyroglossal ductal cyst** is a midline neck structure and is a remnant of the passage of the thyroid gland from the base of the tongue into the neck. A **carotid body tumor** arises from the carotid body at the bifurcation of the common carotid artery. A lipoma is a fatty tumor that can be found anywhere in the subcutaneous tissue. A **thyroid bruit,** usually seen with **Graves' disease** (hyperthyroidism), is turbulent blood flow heard with a stethoscope. A goiter is an enlarged thyroid gland. A **brachial cleft cyst** is a lateral neck structure, usually located near the upper third of the sternocleidomastoid muscle, and is a remnant of embryologic development. **Laryngoceles** are lateral neck swellings that increase in size with Valsalva maneuver.

256. The answer is c. *(Tierney, pp 1128–1131.)* Ninety percent of the adrenal gland must be destroyed for **Addison's disease** (hypoadrenalism) to develop; glucocorticoids, mineralocorticoids, and androgens are affected. Etiologies include tuberculosis, malignancy, sarcoidosis, trauma, histoplasmosis, hemochromatosis, amyloidosis, sepsis, cytomegalovirus infection, and medications (ketoconazole, rifampin, anticoagulants, and anticonvulsants). Patients without a clear etiology have idiopathic hypoadrenalism. Symptoms include weakness, hypotension, anorexia, weight loss, and hyperpigmentation of the skin. Patients may have hyponatremia, hyperkalemia, and eosinophilia. Adults with **craniopharyngioma** present with headache, visual problems, papilledema, personality changes, and hypopituitarism. **Sheehan's syndrome** is postpartum hemorrhage and necrosis of the pituitary gland. **Empty sella syndrome** occurs when cerebrospinal fluid (CSF) fills the sella space and flattens the pituitary gland, which continues to function normally. The disorder is seen in obese, hypertensive, multiparous women. Insulinoma causes hypoglycemia, which is often a feature of hypoadrenalism. **Schmidt's syndrome** is the combination of Hashimoto's thyroiditis with Addison's disease. **Pituitary apoplexy** occurs in less than 5% of patients with a pituitary macroadenoma (>1 cm); patients complain of headache, neck stiffness, fever, and visual disturbance and may present with acute adrenal insufficiency.

257. The answer is b. *(Tierney, pp 1120–1126.)* **Premature osteoporosis** is not caused by menopause-induced estrogen deficiency and may be secondary to medication use (diphenylhydantoin, corticosteroids, heparin), hyperthyroidism, anorexia nervosa, malabsorptive disease, hyperparathyroidism, multiple myeloma, immobilization, tobacco use, or alcoholism. Patients have a reduced bone mass with a normal mineral matrix. **Osteomalacia** is a disorder with reduced mineralization of the matrix; patients need to be evaluated for vitamin D deficiency. **Scleromalacia** is an inflammatory disorder often seen in patients with rheumatoid arthritis associated with chemosis and scleral-conjunctival inflammation. Patients with **Paget's disease** (increased bone turnover with the formation of disorganized bone) present with pain, enlarging skull bones (increasing hat size and hearing loss), skeletal deformities (bowing of the lower extremities), and increased warmth of the skin overlying the tibias.

258. The answer is c. *(Tierney, pp 850–852.)* **Hypercalcemia** is treated with intensive hydration using intravenous saline. **Bisphosphonates** (inhibitors of bone resorption) would be the initial pharmacotherapy for hypercalcemia. These agents take several days to work, however. Hydrochlorothiazide diuretics should be avoided in patients with hypercalcemia.

259. The answer is b. *(Tierney, pp 1134–1135.)* **Hirsutism** is growth of coarse, male-pattern hair in a woman. It is a sign of androgen excess, and patients must be evaluated for ovarian or adrenal tumors. The typical workup for hirsutism includes testosterone level, LH, follicle-stimulating hormone (FSH), 17-OH progesterone, and prolactin. The patient described most likely has **21-hydroxylase deficiency,** which is the most common form of **congenital adrenal hyperplasia.** The highly elevated 17-OH progesterone concentration (which will be even higher after stimulation with synthetic ACTH) supports the diagnosis. Cushing's syndrome seems unlikely in a patient without cushingoid features (central obesity). **Idiopathic hirsutism** applies to patients who have normal adrenal glands and ovaries. Seventy percent of patients with polycystic ovary disease (PCOD) present with hirsutism. They have elevated serum testosterone levels and elevated LH values. Patients with PCOD have slightly elevated levels of 17-OH progesterone after ACTH stimulation. Medications such as bodybuilding steroids, minoxidil, cyclosporine, oral contraceptives, and phenytoin can cause hirsutism.

260. The answer is d. (Tierney, p 1070.) **Gynecomastia** is seen in 50 to 60% of adolescent boys and usually occurs during Tanner stages 2 or 3. It is usually painful and may be unilateral or bilateral. It gradually appears and gradually disappears within one year of onset. Pubertal changes that occur during Tanner stages 2 and 3 include growth spurt, growth of testes and penis, spermarche, acne, axillary perspiration, and appearance of pubic hair. The boy in this case should be reassured and followed monthly. If the gynecomastia does not resolve, it will be necessary to rule out Klinefelter's syndrome, adrenal tumors, gonadal tumors, hyperthyroidism, hepatic disorders, and the use of drugs, especially marijuana and bodybuilding steroids.

261. The answer is c. (Tierney, pp 1081–1083.) Patients may use anabolic steroids to improve athletic performance. The risks associated with use of these agents include mood swings, aggressiveness, paranoid delusions, psychosis, gynecomastia, infertility, testicular atrophy, hepatic tumors, peliosis hepatis, hypertension, and decreased HDL cholesterol levels. Patients with **prolactinomas** (pituitary tumors) generally present with galactorrhea, reduced libido, erectile dysfunction, amenorrhea, infertility, and visual field defects. Chronic **cocaine** use may cause hyperprolactinemia. **Kallmann's syndrome** is characterized by cleft palate, impaired sense of smell, short fourth metacarpal bones, hypogonadism, and infertility.

262. The answer is c. (*Tierney, pp 1147–1148.*) **Pregnancy** (secondary amenorrhea) must always be considered in any patient who presents with amenorrhea. It is normal for prolactin levels to be elevated during pregnancy.

263. The answer is c. (*Tierney, pp 1138–1140.*) **Pheochromocytoma** is a life-threatening disease if left undiagnosed. Patients present with episodic symptoms of headache, sweating, and palpitations. Pheochromocytoma may be associated with von Recklinghausen's syndrome, neurofibromatosis, and von Hippel-Lindau disease. The diagnosis is made by 24-hour urine for catecholeamines and metanephrines. Ten percent of pheochromocytomas are bilateral, and 10% are extraadrenal. Increased levels of **5-HIAA** are associated with carcinoid syndrome (facial flushing and diarrhea) from a tumor usually located in the lung or ileum. Patients with **thyroid storm** present with nausea, diarrhea, jaundice, fever, dyspnea, shortness of breath, diaphoresis, delirium, and tachycardia. The combination of diabetes mellitus, hypertension, obesity, insulin resistance, and dyslipidemia (increased VLDL, increased triglyceride, and decreased HDL) is called **syndrome X** or **C**oronary artery disease, **H**ypertension, **A**therosclerosis, **O**besity, and **S**troke (**CHAOS**) or **metabolic syndrome.**

264. The answer is d. (*Tierney, pp 1088–1089.*) Simple goiter, if sufficiently large, may be accompanied by tracheal compression, esophageal compression, dysphagia, odynophagia, mediastinal obstruction, and superior vena cava syndrome. Retrosternal goiter may cause mediastinal obstruction and superior vena cava syndrome. **Pemberton's sign** is a reversible superior vena cava syndrome; when a patient elevates the arms above the head (obstructing the thoracic inlet and preventing venous return), facial plethora and dizziness occur.

265. The answer is e. (*Tierney, pp 850–851.*) **Primary hyperparathyroidism** is the most common cause of hypercalcemia in the outpatient setting. It is seen more frequently in women than in men and is usually due to one parathyroid adenoma (usually in the inferior lobe). Patients often have a history of hypophosphatemia, fatigue, hypertension, depression, peptic ulcer disease, pancreatitis, bone pain, hypercalciuria, and nephrolithiasis from calcium oxalate stones. The most common cause of hypercalcemia in hospitalized patients is malignancy (i.e., breast, lung, multiple myeloma, head and neck, and renal cell) due to the secretion of **parathyroid hormone (PTH)–related peptide (PTHrp)**. Patients with **familial hypocalciuric hypercalcemia (FHH)** have hypocalciuria, a positive family history, and no end organ damage. Other causes of hypercalcemia include sarcoidosis, mycobacteria, milk-alkali syndrome, and medications (i.e., thiazide diuretics). **Osteitis fibrosa cystica** (replacement by fibrous tissue) is the bone abnormality seen with hyperparathyroidism.

266. The answer is c. (*Seidel, pp 122–123.*) There are five Tanner stages:

Tanner 1 = young child penis, scrotum, and testes; no pubic hair
Tanner 2 = enlargement of scrotum and testes; penis the same; scrotal skin becomes more red, thinner, and wrinkled; some straight pubic hair at base of penis
Tanner 3 = enlargement of penis and testes; scrotum descends; dark, curly pubic hair
Tanner 4 = further penile enlargement; increased pigmentation of scrotum; sculpturing of the glans; adult pubic hair but not beyond inguinal fold
Tanner 5 = ample scrotum; penis reaches to bottom of scrotum; hair spreads to medial surface of thighs

267. The answer is a. (*Tierney, pp 1190–1195.*) **Hyperosmolar hyperglycemic nonketotic state (HHNKS)** is seen in patients with non-insulin-dependent diabetes mellitus (NIDDM) and is usually precipitated by an illness. The patient's residual insulin prevents lipolysis and ketogenesis. **Diabetic ketoacidosis (DKA)** is due to an absolute deficiency of insulin relative to the counterregulatory hormones. The result is gluconeogenesis, ketogenesis, lipolysis, and decreased glucose uptake, causing hyperglycemia and a metabolic acidosis. **Kussmaul respiration** is a respiration pattern of increased tidal volume seen in patients with metabolic acidosis (i.e., DKA). **Gestational diabetes** occurs in 3% of pregnancies; all women should be screened between the twenty-fourth and twenty-eighth weeks of pregnancy. Complications of undiagnosed gestational diabetes include macrosomia and neonatal hypoglycemia. **Impaired glucose tolerance** is defined as a two-hour plasma glucose of 140 to 200 mg/dL after a glucose load of 75 g in a patient whose fasting blood glucose is normal. Glucose intolerance is due to a combination of insulin resistance and impaired insulin secretion. Patients with barbiturate overdose generally present with hypoglycemia.

268. The answer is e. *(Tierney, p 1188.)* The patient most likely has a rash seen in diabetic patients called **necrobiosis lipoidica diabeticorum.** Acanthosis nigricans is a velvety, hyperpigmented, thickened skin lesion over the dorsum of the neck, axillae, and groin and often precedes the diagnosis of an endocrine (insulin-resistant) disorder. Patients with DM must be evaluated for both macrovascular and microvascular complications.

Macrovascular complications:

1. Coronary artery disease
2. Cerebral vascular disease
3. Peripheral vascular disease

Microvascular complications:

1. Retinopathy
2. Nephropathy
3. Neuropathy

Neuropathy in diabetic patients may be:

1. Autonomic: fixed tachycardia, inability of heart rate to increase when the patient stands, orthostatic hypotension, delayed gastric emptying, impotence, diarrhea, bladder dysfunction
2. Peripheral neuropathy: stocking-glove pattern, absent ankle jerk, Charcot joint
3. Mononeuropathy: involvement in distribution of one or several nerves
4. Amyotrophy: muscle atrophy and asymmetric motor neuropathy

269. The answer is d. *(Tierney, pp 1202–1204.)* The most common type of familial hyperlipoproteinemia is **type 2A** (elevated LDL). Heterozygous carriers present with a family history of coronary events and often have tendon xanthomas. Patients with **type 3** dysbetalipoproteinemia (normal LDL with elevated IDL and VLDL) often present with palmar xanthomas and tuberous xanthomas. Hypothyroidism, diabetes mellitus, nephrotic syndrome, and liver disease are secondary causes of hyperlipidemia. **Arcus senilis** before the age of 40 is consistent with hyperlipidemia. Physicians should be able to calculate different cholesterol levels (mg/dL) using the following simple formulas:

1. Total cholesterol = HDL + VLDL + LDL
2. VLDL = Triglycerides/5
3. LDL = Total cholesterol − HDL − (Triglycerides/5)

270. The answer is b. (*Tierney, p 1494.*) **Mucormycosis** is a rare fungal disease limited to persons with preexisting illness and may be seen in poorly controlled diabetic patients. Patients present with fever, nasal congestion, sinus pain, diplopia, and coma. Physical examination may reveal a necrotic nasal turbinate, reduced ocular motion, proptosis, and blindness. CT scan or MRI will reveal the extent of sinus involvement prior to surgery.

271. The answer is a. (*Tierney, pp 1154–1155.*) The patient most likely has multiple endocrine neoplasia or **MEN 1** (**Wermer's syndrome**), an autosomal dominant disorder consisting of tumors of the **P**ancreas, **P**ituitary, and **P**arathyroid gland (**PPP**). **MEN 2A** (**Sipple's syndrome**) consists of **P**heochromocytoma, hyper**P**arathyroidism, and medullary carcinoma of the **T**hyroid (**PPT**). Patients with **MEN 2B syndrome** present with **P**heochromocytoma, **N**euromas, and medullary carcinoma of the **T**hyroid (**PNT**).

272. The answer is b. (*Tierney, pp 1197–1201.*) The surreptitious injection of insulin is just as common as insulinoma. Patients have low C-peptide levels with high insulin levels. **Factitious disease** should be suspected when hypoglycemic symptoms appear in health professionals or in relatives of patients with diabetes mellitus. Patients with **insulinoma** have high levels of both C peptide and insulin. Finding high levels of circulating insulin antibodies may help to make the diagnosis of factitious hypoglycemia.

273. The answer is b. (*Seidel, p 124.*) There are five stages of **Tanner development:**

Tanner 1 = no growth of pubic hair
Tanner 2 = scarcely pigmented, straight pubic hair along medial border of labia
Tanner 3 = sparse, dark, curly pubic hair on labia
Tanner 4 = abundant coarse and curly pubic hair
Tanner 5 = lateral triangular spreading of adult hair to medial surfaces of thighs

274. The answer is d. *(Tierney, p 1186.)* Diabetics with peripheral neuropathy are susceptible to developing a **Charcot joint.** The insensitivity of the feet predisposes the patient to multiple silent fractures, causing a deformed joint. The **Somogyi effect** is nocturnal hypoglycemia, which stimulates a surge of counterregulatory hormones to produce a high fasting blood sugar in the morning. The **Dawn phenomenon** is morning hyperglycemia from reduced sensitivity to insulin in the morning hours evoked by spikes of growth hormone released during sleep. The **Whipple triad** is characteristic of hypoglycemia and consists of (1) hypoglycemic symptoms, (2) low fasting blood glucose, and (3) immediate recovery after administration of glucose. The Whipple triad is seen in any disorder that causes hypoglycemia (not only with insulinoma). **Mature-onset diabetes of the young (MODY)** is a rare autosomal dominant disorder characterized by impaired insulin secretion and the subsequent development of NIDDM in nonobese persons under the age of 25 years. The **Charcot triad** (fever, right upper quadrant pain, and jaundice) is seen in cholangitis.

275. The answer is c. *(Tierney, pp 1077–1078.)* The man had trauma to his posterior pituitary stalk from the car accident, resulting in **central diabetes insipidus (DI)** due to lack of vasopressin. The diagnosis may be made by raising the patient's serum osmolality through water restriction, then observing the urine osmolality response to injected vasopressin. **Nephrogenic DI** will not respond to the stimulation by vasopressin. Patients with the **syndrome of inappropriate antidiuretic hormone secretion (SIADH)** present with hyponatremia.

276–277. The answers are 276-c, 277-a. *(Tierney, pp 921–922.)* **Nocturnal penile tumescence** occurs during REM sleep, and if the man gives a history of rigid erections under any circumstances, the most likely etiology of his ED is psychological (i.e., depression, disinterest, anxiety). In patients with a history of neuropathy, further studies to evaluate impotence are not necessary. Patients with peripheral vascular disease should be evaluated with a **penile/brachial index.** An index of less than 0.06 suggests vascular impotence. Endocrine ED may be due to testicular failure (rare) or prolactinomas. Drugs that may cause impotence include antidepressants, anticholinergics, alcohol, methadone, heroin, tobacco, antihypertensives, and sedatives.

Hematology and Oncology

Questions

DIRECTIONS: Each item below contains a question followed by suggested responses. Select the **one best** response to each question.

278. A 55-year-old man presents with bone pain that is aggravated by movement or weight bearing. Physical examination is remarkable for pale conjunctivae. Laboratory results show a normocytic anemia and an increased serum globulin level. Peripheral blood smear is significant for rouleaux formation. Osteolytic bone lesions are seen on a radiograph of the pelvis. Bone scan is normal. Which of the following is the most likely diagnosis?

a. Multiple myeloma
b. Paget's disease
c. Metastatic bone disease
d. Monoclonal gammopathy of unknown significance (MGUS)
e. Waldenström's macroglobulinemia

279. A 56-year-old African American man presents with a 15-lb weight loss over the last six weeks. He states that food "gets stuck" in the middle of his chest. Initially, the patient had difficulty swallowing solids, but the symptoms have since progressed to the point where he has similar problems when swallowing liquids. He also complains of odynophagia. He denies hoarseness. He is a smoker and admits to heavily drinking alcohol. Physical examination reveals a left fixed supraclavicular node. Which of the following is the most likely diagnosis?

a. Achalasia
b. Squamous cell carcinoma of the esophagus
c. Adenocarcinoma of the esophagus
d. Esophageal stricture
e. Schatzki's ring

280. A 27-year-old man who is in excellent health presents for a routine physical examination. Family history reveals that the patient's mother died of colon cancer at the age of 40 years and a brother, who is 36 years old, was recently diagnosed with colon cancer. The patient also has two maternal aunts with ovarian cancer. Physical examination is normal, and fecal occult blood test (FOBT) is negative. Laboratory data are normal. Which of the following statements is true for this patient?

a.   He most likely has the *BRCA2* mutation
b.   He needs an annual colonoscopy beginning at age 36
c.   He should have a prophylactic colectomy
d.   If he develops colon cancer, it would most likely be in the proximal colon
e.   If he develops colon cancer, it would most likely be in the distal colon

281. A 61-year-old woman presents to the emergency room with dyspnea on exertion and facial swelling for nearly two weeks. She has smoked three packs of cigarettes per day for nearly 40 years but does not drink alcohol. Her blood pressure is 120/88 mmHg, pulse is 90 beats per minute, respirations are 16 breaths per minute, and she is afebrile. Heart and lung examinations are normal. She has dilated veins in the neck and upper chest area. Blood gases are normal. Which of the following is the most likely diagnosis?

a.   Tumor lysis syndrome
b.   Superior vena cava syndrome
c.   Cord compression
d.   Hypercalcemia
e.   Pericardial tamponade
f.   Pancoast's syndrome

282. A 19-year-old woman with a lifelong history of easy bruisability presents with menorrhagia. She also admits to occasional nosebleeds. She has no family history of bleeding disorders and takes no medications. Physical examination is normal. Laboratory investigation reveals a normal platelet count but a prolonged bleeding time. Which of the following is the most likely diagnosis?

a.   Hemophilia A
b.   Hemophilia B
c.   Type III von Willebrand's disease
d.   Type I von Willebrand's disease
e.   Christmas disease
f.   Bernard-Soulier syndrome

283. A 70-year-old woman was treated for infiltrating breast cancer with lumpectomy and radiotherapy. Her breast cancer did not involve any of her axillary nodes, and she had positive estrogen and progesterone receptors. She was started on tamoxifen to decrease the risk of recurrent disease. The patient now presents complaining of hot flashes. Eye examination reveals absence of the red light reflex bilaterally. The rest of the physical examination is normal. Which of the following is the most likely diagnosis?

a. Recurrence of breast cancer
b. Development of a new primary cancer
c. Menopause
d. Side effects of tamoxifen
e. Side effects of radiotherapy

284. A 43-year-old man presents with a two-month history of diarrhea and abdominal cramping. He has no nausea or vomiting. He denies melena and hematochezia. He has a 10-lb weight loss. Physical examination reveals edema of the head and neck. His face appears to be flushed. He has bilateral expiratory wheezes and a systolic murmur that increases with inspiration. Abdominal examination is normal. Rectal examination is FOBT negative. Which of the following is the most appropriate next step in diagnosis?

a. CT scan of the chest
b. Transthoracic echocardiogram
c. CT scan of the abdomen
d. 24-hour urine for 5-HIAA
e. Transesophageal echocardiogram

285. A 7-year-old boy with sickle cell disease presents with severe left upper quadrant pain that started suddenly two hours before he arrived at the emergency room. He has no previous history of pain in that area. Physical examination reveals a temperature of 37°C (98.6°F) and a normal blood pressure. Heart rate is 108 beats per minute. Heart and lung examinations are normal. There is fullness and tenderness in the left upper quadrant of the abdomen with palpation, but there is no audible rub. There is no hepatomegaly or rebound tenderness, and FOBT is negative. The rest of the physical examination is normal. Hemoglobin is 6.1 g/dL. Which of the following is the most likely diagnosis?

a. Vasoocclusive crisis
b. Splenic infarction
c. Splenic sequestration crisis
d. Left pleural effusion
e. Pulmonary infarction

286. A 37-year-old woman, G0P0, presents with an eczematous scaly eruption on her right nipple. She recently has taken up running and weight lifting and believes that the exercise has irritated her breast. Physical examination reveals a 1.5-cm erythematous and crusted lesion on her right nipple. The nipple is not inverted, and there are no masses or discharge. There are no axillary nodes, and the other breast is normal. Which of the following is the most appropriate next step in diagnosis?

a. Biopsy of the lesion
b. Mammogram
c. Topical steroid therapy
d. Topical antifungal therapy
e. Suggest the use of an athletic bra

287. A 42-year-old woman of Italian descent presents for a preemployment physical examination. She has no past medical problems and takes no medications. Her physical examination is normal except for pale conjunctivae. Fecal occult blood test (FOBT) is negative. Her complete blood count (CBC) is remarkable for a hemoglobin of 11.4 g/dL, a mean corpuscular volume (MCV) of 60 fL, and a reticulocyte count of 0.6%. Her white blood cell count and platelets are normal. Peripheral smear reveals microcytosis, hypochromia, acanthocytes (cells with irregularly spaced projections), and occasional target cells. Which of the following is the most likely diagnosis?

a. Iron-deficiency anemia
b. Sideroblastic anemia
c. Anemia of chronic disease
d. Thalassemia trait
e. Hemolytic anemia

288. A 23-year-old man with sickle cell disease presents with shortness of breath and pleuritic chest pain. His temperature is 38.5°C (101.3°F), and he is tachypneic and tachycardic. Heart examination is normal. Lung examination is notable for right basilar crackles. The patient's arterial saturation is 85%. He has a leukocytosis, and chest radiograph reveals an infiltrate. Which of the following is the most likely diagnosis?

a. Acute osteomyelitis
b. Acute chest syndrome
c. Myocardial infarction
d. Congestive heart failure
e. Parvovirus B19 infection

289. A 19-year-old woman in her second trimester of pregnancy presents with a deep venous thrombosis (DVT) of her left lower extremity. She has no previous history of DVT and has no family history of thromboembolism. Which of the following is the most likely reason for the patient developing a DVT?

a. Protein C deficiency
b. Protein S deficiency
c. Antithrombin III deficiency
d. Resistance to protein C
e. Hyperhomocysteinemia
f. Dysfibrinogenemia

290. A 31-year-old African American man presents to the emergency room and is diagnosed as having a community-acquired pneumonia. After two days of antibiotics, the patient becomes jaundiced. His hematocrit is 30% (decreased from 40% on admission), reticulocyte count is 6%, and indirect bilirubin value is 4.5 mg/dL (total bilirubin of 6.0 mg/dL). Peripheral blood smear demonstrates Heinz bodies. The patient recalls a similar problem when he was given antibiotics five years ago for an acute sinusitis. His three brothers have a similar reaction to antibiotics. Which of the following is the most likely diagnosis?

a. Sickle cell anemia
b. Sickle cell trait
c. Autoimmune hemolytic anemia
d. Glucose-6-phosphate dehydrogenase deficiency
e. Allergic reaction

291. A 32-year-old woman presents with the recent onset of petechiae of her lower extremities. She denies menorrhagia and gastrointestinal bleeding. She has no family history of a bleeding disorder and has been in excellent health her entire life. She takes no medications and does not drink alcohol. Physical examination is remarkable for petechiae of both legs. There is no hepatosplenomegaly. The rest of the physical examination is normal. Platelet count is 8000/μL. Hemoglobin and white blood cell count are normal. Peripheral smear reveals reduced platelets and an occasional megathrombocyte. Which of the following is the most likely diagnosis?

a. Thrombocytopenic thrombotic purpura (TTP)
b. Hemolytic-uremic syndrome (HUS)
c. Evans's syndrome
d. Disseminated intravascular coagulopathy (DIC)
e. Idiopathic thrombocytopenic purpura (ITP)
f. Henoch-Schönlein purpura (HSP)
g. "Cocktail thrombocytopenia"

292. A 52-year-old man presents with a painless neck mass. He states that after he drinks one to two glasses of wine, the neck mass becomes painful. He also complains of intermittent fever, night sweats, pruritus, and a 10-lb weight loss over the last month. Physical examination reveals a 3-cm mass in the left anterior cervical lymph node chain that is hard and tender to deep palpation. Several other cervical nodes and a left axillary node are palpable. The liver is enlarged, but there is no splenomegaly. Which of the following is the most likely diagnosis?

a. Non-Hodgkin's lymphoma
b. Hodgkin's lymphoma
c. Mononucleosis
d. Hairy cell leukemia
e. Sarcoidosis

293. A 62-year-old man presents for his annual health maintenance visit. The review of systems is positive for occasional fatigue and headache. The patient admits to generalized pruritus following a warm bath or shower. He has plethora and engorgement of the retinal veins. A spleen is palpated on abdominal examination. The patient's hematocrit is 63%, and he has a leukocytosis and thrombocytosis. Peripheral blood smear is normal. The patient does not smoke. Which of the following is the most likely diagnosis?

a. Spurious polycythemia
b. Essential thrombocytosis
c. Myelofibrosis
d. Polycythemia vera
e. Secondary polycythemia
f. Chronic myeloid leukemia
g. Erythropoietin-secreting renal tumor

294. A 42-year-old man develops fever and chills within a few hours after a blood transfusion. His temperature is 38.7°C (101.6°F), and his blood pressure is 120/80 mmHg. He is slightly tachycardic, but his respiratory rate is normal. His CBC is normal except for the anemia for which he was receiving the transfusion. Laboratory data including electrolytes, liver function tests, and urinalysis are normal. Which of the following is the most likely diagnosis?

a. Anaphylaxis to blood transfusion
b. Hemolytic reaction to blood transfusion
c. Febrile, nonhemolytic reaction to blood transfusion
d. Transfusion-associated circulatory overload
e. Urticarial reaction to blood transfusion

DIRECTIONS: Each group of questions below consists of lettered options followed by a set of numbered items. For each numbered item, select the **one** lettered option with which it is **most** closely associated. Each lettered option may be used once, more than once, or not at all.

Questions 295–299

For each patient with cancer, select the most likely risk factor for the malignancy.

a. *Helicobacter pylori* infection
b. Hepatitis C infection
c. Mutation to *BRCA1*
d. 9;22 translocation
e. Schistosomiasis
f. Vinyl chloride
g. Human papillomavirus
h. Tobacco use
i. Villous adenomatous polyp
j. Tubular adenomatous polyp
k. Radon gas
l. Epstein-Barr virus
m. Herpesvirus type 8 (HHV-8)
n. Human T cell lymphotrophic/leukemia virus type 1 (HTLV-1)

295. A previously healthy 49-year-old man presents with fever and night sweats. He has splenomegaly. His peripheral white blood cell count is 22,000/μL, and a peripheral smear shows immature leukocytes with an increase in the number of basophils. Leukocyte alkaline phosphatase score is low, and B$_{12}$ level is elevated.

296. A 29-year-old patient presents with squamous cell carcinoma of the anus. He is sexually promiscuous and is requesting an HIV test.

297. A 57-year-old patient presents with right upper quadrant abdominal pain. Serum α-fetoprotein level is higher than 1200 ng/mL. The patient does not drink alcohol and has no history of intravenous drug use or blood transfusions. A hepatic mass is present on CT scan of the abdomen.

298. A 62-year-old woman presents with jaundice, back pain, and weight loss. CT scan of the abdomen demonstrates a mass at the head of the pancreas.

299. A 44-year-old man presents with intermittent epigastric pain and is found to have a gastric lymphoma.

Questions 300–301

For each patient with a lung mass, select the most likely malignancy.
a. Adenocarcinoma of the lung
b. Hamartoma
c. Bronchial adenoma
d. Squamous cell carcinoma of the lung
e. Small cell carcinoma of the lung
f. Bronchioalveolar carcinoma of the lung
g. Mesothelioma

300. A 54-year-old woman presents with a lung mass. She has no history of tobacco use and has worked as a seamstress all her life. She has no family history of lung cancer.

301. A 39-year-old woman with a tobacco history has a centrally located lung mass and a serum sodium of 121 meq/L.

Questions 302–303

For each cell abnormality, select the most appropriate name of the abnormality.

a. Howell-Jolly bodies
b. Reed-Sternberg cells
c. Pelger-Hüet cells
d. Heinz bodies
e. Auer rods
f. Hypersegmented polymorphonuclear leukocytes
g. Schistocytes
h. Pappenheimer bodies
i. Döhle bodies
j. Toxic granulations

302. A 24-year-old man with a history of abdominal surgery following a motor vehicle accident presents with fever and bacteremia. Nuclear remnants are seen in circulating red blood cells.

303. A 7-year-old boy presents with epistaxis and gingival bleeding. He is pale and has petechiae over his lower extremities. Needle-like eosinophilic inclusions or precipitants from denaturing of oxidized hemoglobin are visible on bone marrow aspirate.

Questions 304–307

For each malignancy, select the most appropriate tumor marker.

a. CA-125
b. LDH
c. PSA
d. CEA
e. AFP
f. hCG
g. 5-HIAA
h. β_2-microglobulin

304. Hodgkin's disease

305. Multiple myeloma

306. Breast cancer

307. Carcinoid tumor

Questions 308–309

For each patient with a hematologic disorder, select the most appropriate diagnostic test.

a. Positive leukocyte alkaline phosphatase (LAP) test
b. Positive acid hemolysis (HAM) test
c. Positive osmotic fragility test

308. A patient has anemia and gallstones at the age of 20. The peripheral smear demonstrates spherocytosis.

309. A patient presents with hemolysis and recurrent venous thromboses. He has hemosiderinuria.

Hematology and Oncology

Answers

278. The answer is a. (*Tierney, pp 497–498.*) **Multiple myeloma** (**MM**) is a neoplasm characterized by proliferation of plasma cells ("fried-egg-appearing cells") seen typically in patients over the age of 50. The disorder may lead to bone pain, pathologic fracture, anemia, susceptibility to infections, renal failure, and hypercalcemia. The bone pain of MM worsens with movement (the pain of metastatic bone disease is typically worse at night). Patients have an increased serum globulin and a monoclonal IgA or IgG spike (M component) on electrophoresis. The monoclonal immunoglobulin causes rouleaux formation on blood smear. Urine examination reveals Bence-Jones proteinuria. Osteolytic lesions are seen in many bones on plain radiographic studies, but bone scan (technetium 99m) is normal (this would be positive in Paget's disease and in metastatic disease). **MGUS** is a monoclonal gammopathy that is more common than MM. However, these patients do not have anemia, renal failure, Bence-Jones proteinuria, lytic bone lesions, or hypercalcemia. Bone marrow aspirate is normal in MGUS. **Waldenström's macroglobulinemia** is a B cell malignancy (so is MM) with an IgM monoclonal protein and both lymphocytosis and plasmacytosis in the bone marrow. Patients present with bleeding, cytopenia, lymphadenopathy, and hyperviscosity crises.

279. The answer is b. (*Tierney, pp 559–562.*) Progressive (solids to liquids) difficulty swallowing or **dysphagia** accompanied by rapid weight loss and **odynophagia** (painful swallowing) often indicates esophageal carcinoma. Risk factors for **esophageal carcinoma** include tobacco and alcohol use, chronic gastric reflux causing a Barrett's esophagus, achalasia, and lye ingestion. Tumor involvement of the recurrent laryngeal nerve would cause hoarseness. The fixed supraclavicular node (**Virchow's node**) is consistent with the diagnosis. Adenocarcinoma is more common in white patients (commonly arising in the distal third of the esophogus due to Barrett's metaplasia), while squamous cell carcinoma is more common in black patients (also has a high incidence in China and southeast Asia). Patients with **Schatzki's ring** (lower esophageal web) have intermittent dysphagia to solids, and patients with strictures typically present with complaints of heartburn. **Achalasia** is a neuromuscular disorder of esophageal relaxation; patients often present with respiratory symptoms from aspiration. Esophagram in achalasia reveals a dilated esophagus with a beaklike tapering distal to the esophageal contraction.

280. The answer is d. *(Tierney, pp 617–618.)* The pedigree of the patient (multiple primary cancers) is most consistent with **hereditary nonpolyposis colon cancer (HNPCC).** The median age for adenocarcinoma of the colon is 50 years, and the most common site is the proximal colon. Inheritance is autosomal dominant, and members of the family should undergo biennial colonoscopy starting at age 25. Prophylactic colectomy is recommended for patients with familial adenomatous polyposis, an autosomal dominant disorder characterized by small polyps that develop during the second decade of life and undergo malignant transformation before the age of 40. Breast cancer is not associated with HNPCC (the genetic defect is in DNA mismatch repair genes).

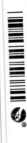

281. The answer is b. *(Tierney, pp 457–458.)* There are several life-threatening complications in cancer patients. **Superior vena cava (SVC) obstruction** is due to lung cancer in 85% of cases. Tumors that may cause SVC syndrome include small cell carcinoma of the lung, squamous cell carcinoma of the lung, lymphoma, thymoma, and germ cell tumor. Tissue diagnosis is preferable prior to starting any treatment. Some malignancies are so responsive to chemotherapy that **tumor lysis syndrome** occurs, resulting in hyperkalemia, hyperphosphatemia, hypocalcemia, hyperuricemia, and renal failure hours after receiving treatment (these tumors require allopurinol prophylaxis prior to chemotherapy to prevent hyperuricemia). Patients with **cord compression** may present with back pain, gait difficulty, weakness, sensory deficits, and incontinence. Patients with **hypercalcemia from malignancy-paraneoplastic syndrome** may present with lethargy, weakness, constipation, vomiting, and coma. Cancer patients may develop **cardiac tamponade** from pericardial metastasis; physical examination might demonstrate findings such as hypotension, jugular venous distention, distant heart sounds, and pulsus paradoxus. **Pancoast's syndrome** (superior sulcus tumor) is a complication of lung cancer when it extends into the apex. Patients have compression of the C8, T1, and T2 nerves and often complain of arm and shoulder pain.

282. The answer is d. *(Tierney, pp 505–506.)* **von Willebrand's disease** (**vWD**) is the most common inherited bleeding disorder (autosomal dominant). It is due to an abnormality in the quantity or quality of von Willebrand factor. The most common type is type I (80% of cases), caused by a quantitative decrease in vWF. Type IIA and IIB vWD are qualitative disorders; type III vWD is a rare autosomal recessive disorder in which vWF is nearly absent. Most bleeding from vWD is mucosal (epistaxis, gingival bleeding, menorrhagia) or gastrointestinal, and bleeding is exacerbated by aspirin use. Hemarthroses do not occur in vWD. The treatment for vWD types I and IIA is **desmopressin,** which stimulates the release of vWF from endothelial cells. Spontaneous hemarthroses are characteristic of **hemophilia A or factor VIII deficiency** (classic hemophilia); the diagnosis is made by finding a decreased level of factor VIII:C. Specific assays can distinguish between factor VIII and factor IX hemophilia (**hemophilia B or Christmas disease**). Hemophilia has an X-linked pattern of inheritance, and the symptoms and prognosis are similar for hemophilia A and B. **Bernard-Soulier syndrome** is a rare platelet disorder in which platelets cannot adhere to the endothelium because they lack receptors for vWF. Patients present with severe bleeding, especially postoperatively. Platelets appear abnormally large on peripheral smear. Measurements of vWF in Bernard-Soulier syndrome are normal.

283. The answer is d. *(Tierney, p 1619.)* **Tamoxifen** is one of the most commonly prescribed antineoplastic agents. It is considered to be an estrogen receptor blocker, but it has both estrogen receptor agonist and antagonist properties. The most common side effect is hot flashes, but patients may also develop deep venous thrombosis, pulmonary embolus, and cataracts. Tamoxifen is associated with an increased risk of endometrial carcinoma. Side effects of **radiotherapy** include short-term reactions (fatigue, skin reaction, nausea, vomiting, diarrhea, dysphagia, mucositis, and xerostomia) and long-term complications (pericarditis, pneumonitis, hepatitis, sterilization, and nephropathy).

284. The answer is d. *(Tierney, pp 592–593.)* **Carcinoid syndrome** is usually associated with primary carcinoid tumors of the lung or stomach and carcinoid tumors of the small bowel metastatic to the liver. Patients with **carcinoid tumor** often present with the carcinoid syndrome (cutaneous flushing, diarrhea, wheezing, telangiectasias, and paroxysmal hypotension) due to the production of **serotonin.** Patients often have cardiac lesions, such as tricuspid insufficiency and pulmonic stenosis. The best next step in this patient would be a 24-hour urine collection for 5-hydroxyindoleacetic acid (**5-HIAA**), a breakdown product of serotonin.

285. The answer is c. *(Tierney, pp 474–475.)* Patients with hemoglobin SC disease and children with sickle cell disease are at risk for **splenic sequestration** crisis when blood is trapped in the spleen (leading to further splenic enlargement and anemia). Splenic infarction is not associated with anemia or sudden splenomegaly; patients often have a **left upper quadrant rub** on physical examination. Episodes of **vasoocclusive crisis** (pain crises) are not associated with increased hemolysis, anemia, or splenomegaly.

286. The answer is a. *(Tierney, p 692.)* The basic lesion of **Paget's carcinoma** (<1% of all breast cancers) is an infiltrative ductal carcinoma, usually well differentiated, or a ductal carcinoma in situ (DCIS). A tumor mass may not be palpable, and there are few gross nipple changes. The diagnosis is established by biopsy of the erosion. The **risk factors for breast cancer** include age (80% of cases occur after age 50), family history of breast cancer, previous breast biopsy for benign disease, genetic mutations (*BRCA1* and *BRCA2*), increased breast tissue density on mammogram, early menarche (<12 years old), nulliparity, late menopause (>50 years old), and late age at birth of first child (>30 years old). Breast cancer should always be the primary consideration in any woman who presents with a breast lesion; delay in biopsy diagnosis by empirically treating with topical antibacterial, antifungal, and anti-inflammatory medications may delay cancer treatment.

287. The answer is d. *(Tierney, pp 462–468.)* The differential diagnosis for **microcytic hypochromic anemia** is **TICS** (**T**halassemia, **I**ron deficiency, **C**hronic disease, and **S**ideroblastic). This patient of Mediterranean descent most likely has thalassemia trait. **Thalassemia** generally produces a greater degree of microcytosis for any given level of anemia than does iron deficiency. **Target cells** are seen in this disorder, but these are also seen in lead poisoning, liver disease, hyposplenism, and hemoglobin C disease. The most common cause of a microcytic anemia is **iron deficiency,** but this is unlikely in this asymptomatic patient with a negative FOBT. The MCV in anemia of chronic disease is usually normal or slightly reduced, and patients typically have a history of chronic infection or inflammation, cancer, or liver disease. Alcoholics, patients taking antituberculosis medication or chloramphenicol, or those with lead poisoning may develop **sideroblastic anemia** (a failure to incorporate heme into protoporphyrin). Bone marrow staining will demonstrate iron deposits (**ringed sideroblasts**) encircling the nucleus in siderocytes. Coarse **basophilic stippling** of the red blood cells on peripheral smear would be characteristic of **lead poisoning.**

288. The answer is b. (*Goldman, pp 1034–1035.*) This patient with sickle cell disease most likely has **acute chest syndrome,** which is characterized by fever, dyspnea, leukocytosis, pulmonary infiltrate, and hypoxemia. The usual causes of acute chest syndrome are vasoocclusion, infection, and pulmonary fat embolus from infarcted marrow. Acute chest syndrome affects 30% of patients with sickle cell disease and is responsible for significant mortality. **Parvovirus B19** causes **aplastic anemia** in patients with sickle cell disease.

289. The answer is d. (*Goldman, p 1083.*) The most common reason for **DVT** in pregnancy is the **factor V Leiden mutation or activated protein C (APC) resistance.** The defect is a mutation in activated factor V, not in protein C, and is found in 8% of the general population (**exclusively in white populations**). Forty percent of all patients presenting with DVT have the mutation. All of the primary hypercoagulable states in the question may cause DVT, especially during pregnancy (due to the elevation in estrogen), but these are less common than APC resistance.

290. The answer is d. (*Tierney, p 474.*) The clinical picture strongly suggests **glucose-6-phosphate dehydrogenase (G6PD) deficiency,** in which red blood cells are unable to deal with oxidative stresses. Acute hemolysis occurs when affected patients are exposed to an infection or an **oxidizing drug** (dapsone, primaquine, sulfonamides, nitrofurantoin, quinine). The hemolytic episodes are **self-limited,** even if the offending agent is still present, because older red cells with low enzyme activity are removed and replaced by younger red cells with adequate levels of G6PD. Cells that survive a hemolytic episode have adequate amounts of G6PD, so testing is not useful during the acute illness. G6PD deficiency has an X-linked pattern of inheritance. G6PD deficiency is often called favism in the Mediterranean, as hemolysis can occur after patients eat fava beans.

291. The answer is e. *(Tierney, pp 500–504.)* **Idiopathic thrombocytopenic purpura (ITP)** is an autoimmune disorder in which an IgG autoantibody binds to platelets. Destruction of the platelets takes place in the spleen, where macrophages bind to the antibody-coated platelets. Fifty percent of patients with ITP have no associated disease, but HIV infection, SLE, or a lymphoproliferative disorder should be considered. ITP is a disease of persons between the ages of 20 and 50 years and occurs in women more than in men. There is no splenomegaly in ITP. The diagnosis is one of exclusion, but often megathrombocytes are seen on peripheral smear. **Evans's syndrome** is ITP with coexistent autoimmune hemolytic anemia. **DIC** is a systemic coagulation disorder that can be accompanied by thrombocytopenia. It may be secondary to transfusion, infection, malignancy, trauma, or obstetric complications. TTP is unlikely since the patient does not have the pentad of symptoms seen in 40% of patients (**FAT R.N.** = **F**ever, **A**utoimmune hemolytic anemia, **T**hrombocytopenia, **R**enal disease, **N**eurologic disease). **HUS** presents with three of the five symptoms seen in TTP (**RAT** = **R**enal disease, **A**utoimmune hemolytic anemia, and **T**hrombocytopenia). Fever and neurologic disease are lacking. **Henoch-Schönlein purpura** occurs in children; patients present with **AGAR** = **A**bdominal pain, **G**lomerulonephritis, **A**rthralgia, and a **R**ash that is purpuric. In the past, **quinine** (found in the **tonic water** used to make gin and tonics 20 years ago) was an agent that could induce thrombocytopenia ("**cocktail thrombocytopenia**"). Quinine is still found in some over-the-counter medicines for nocturnal leg cramps.

292. The answer is b. *(Tierney, pp 493–496.)* Patients with **Hodgkin's lymphoma** often present with painless regional lymphadenopathy and the constitutional symptoms of fever, drenching night sweats, and weight loss. Occasionally, patients may present with pruritus or pain in an involved lymph node after ingestion of alcohol. There is a bimodal age distribution with one peak in the twenties and a second peak at over age 50. The diagnosis of Hodgkin's disease is made by lymph node biopsy with the finding of **Reed-Sternberg cells** ("**owl eyes**"). Patients with **non-Hodgkin's lymphoma** (a group of cancers variable in presentation and course) often present with disseminated disease such as systemic adenopathy. Patients with **hairy cell leukemia** present with pancytopenia, massive splenomegaly, and hairy cells on peripheral blood smear.

293. The answer is d. (*Tierney, pp 482–489.*) The patient most likely has **polycythemia vera.** This is an acquired myeloproliferative disorder characterized by a primary erythrocytosis, but there is overproduction of all three cell lines. Hematocrits are more than 54% in males and less than 51% in females. Patients present with symptoms related to an increase in blood volume and viscosity. Pruritus after a warm bath or shower is due to **histamine release by basophils.** Splenomegaly exists in virtually every patient with polycythemia vera. The treatment of choice for polycythemia vera is phlebotomy. **Spurious polycythemia, or Gaisböck's syndrome,** is due to a contracted plasma volume (diuretic use); **secondary polycythemia** may be due to smoking, high altitudes, cardiac or pulmonary disease, or erythropoietin-secreting cysts or tumors. Patients with **chronic myelogenous leukemia** (**CML**) typically have a leukocytosis and the **Philadelphia chromosome.** Patients with **essential thrombocythemia** have platelet counts of more than 2 million/μL. Patients with **myelofibrosis** have splenomegaly, dry bone marrow taps, and peripheral blood smears showing abnormal and bizarre morphologies and immature forms.

294. The answer is c. (*Tierney, pp 514–515.*) The most common reaction to blood transfusion is the **febrile, nonhemolytic reaction.** Patients develop fever and chills several hours after receiving the transfusion because of recipient antibodies to donor leukocyte antigens. **Hemolytic reactions** (fever, chills, hemoglobinuria, back pain, flank pain, dyspnea, anxiety, renal failure, DIC, multiorgan failure, and death) are due to erythrocyte (ABO) incompatibility. Other transfusion reactions, such as urticaria (recipient antibodies to protein), anaphylaxis (anti-IgA in the recipient), and circulatory overload (pulmonary congestion), are unlikely in this patient.

295–299. The answers are 295-d, 296-g, 297-b, 298-h, 299-a. (*Tierney, pp 1589–1594.*) Most patients with CML have the **Philadelphia chromosome t(9;22)** and the **bcr/abl fusion protein.** **Mucosa-associated lymphoid tissue** (**MALT**) **tumor** has been shown to be secondary to

H. pylori. Squamous cell carcinomas of the anus, penis, and cervix have been linked to **human papillomavirus** (**HPV**). Hepatitis B and C and hemochromatosis are the major risk factors for **hepatocellular carcinoma.** Other risk factors include aflatoxin (peanuts) exposure and being from the Far East or Africa (high-incidence areas). Cigarette smoking is the most consistently observed risk factor for pancreatic cancer. **Schistosomiasis** is associated with squamous cell carcinoma of the bladder. Patients with the **BRCA1 gene on chromosome 17** present with breast cancer at a young age with a family history of breast or ovarian cancer. **Vinyl chloride** exposure is a risk factor for hemangiosarcoma of the liver. Patients with colonic polyps are at risk for developing colon cancer. **Villous adenomas** are more likely to be malignant, but tubular adenomas are four times more common. **Radon gas** is associated with lung cancer. **Epstein-Barr virus** is associated with Burkitt's lymphoma and nasopharyngeal cancer; patients often present with an enlarging neck mass. **HHV-8** is associated with Kaposi's sarcoma, and **HTLV-1** is associated with adult T-cell leukemia.

300–301. The answers are 300-a, 301-e. *(Tierney, pp 262–264.)* **Adenocarcinoma of the lung** (increasing in incidence in women) often occurs in the absence of a smoking history (although the role of second-hand smoke is still unknown). Adenocarcinoma is the most common lung cancer (usually found in the **periphery**). **Small cell carcinoma of the lung** (20% of all new cases of lung cancer) is usually found **centrally** and is associated with a history of tobacco use and the production of ectopic hormones, such as antidiuretic hormone (ADH), parathyroid hormone (PTH), and adrenocorticotropic hormone (ACTH). **Squamous cell carcinoma** (another **central** lesion) is associated with PTH production. Patients with **bronchioalveolar carcinoma** (a variant of adenocarcinoma) may present with an infiltrate on chest radiograph. **Hamartomas** and **bronchial adenomas** are benign lung tumors. Hamartomas are located **peripherally;** bronchial adenomas are located **centrally.** **Mesothelioma** is associated with asbestos exposure but not tobacco use.

302–303. The answers are 302-a, 303-d. *(Tierney, pp 476, 488, 490.)* **Howell-Jolly bodies** are found in asplenic or hyposplenic patients; **Heinz bodies** are the precipitants of denatured oxidized hemoglobin in G6PD deficiency. The **Reed-Sternberg cell** is the diagnostic tumor cell of Hodgkin's disease. The **Pelger-Hüet anomaly** is a benign inherited trait resulting in neutrophils with bilobed nuclei. **Hypersegmented polymorphonuclear cells** are seen in B_{12} or folic acid deficiency. Prominent cytoplasmic granules called **toxic granulations** and **Döhle bodies** representing fragments of ribosome-rich endoplasmic reticulum are seen in immature neutrophils in bacterial infections. **Auer rods** are eosinophilic inclusions seen in acute myelogenous leukemia (AML); **schistocytes** (as well as helmet cells, burr cells, triangular cells, and spherocytes) are seen in microangiopathic hemolytic anemia. **Pappenheimer cells** are often seen in thalassemia.

304–307. The answers are 304-b, 305-h, 306-d, 307-g. *(Tierney, pp 1635–1636.)* Tumor markers should not be used to diagnose cancer, but may be helpful in following patients for whom a diagnosis has already been made. **Carcinoembryonic antigen (CEA)** is associated with colon and breast cancer. **CA-125** is associated with ovarian cancer. **Lactate dehydrogenase (LDH)** is an important prognostic factor for Hodgkin's disease; β_2**-microglobulin** is the most important prognostic factor for multiple myeloma. **LDH, α-fetoprotein (AFP)**, and **human chorionic gonadotropin (hCG)** are associated with testicular cancer, and **5-HIAA** is associated with carcinoid syndrome (facial flushing and diarrhea from a tumor usually located in the lung or ileum). **AFP** is also associated with hepatocellular carcinoma. **Prostate-specific antigen (PSA)** is associated with prostate cancer. The most commonly used marker for pancreatic cancer is **CA 19-9.**

308–309. The answers are 308-c, 309-b. *(Tierney, pp 472–473.)* The **osmotic fragility test** is used to identify patients with red blood cell membrane defects (hereditary spherocytosis). The **acid hemolysis test** and the **sugar water test** are screening tests for **paroxysmal nocturnal hemoglobinuria (PNH)**. **Leukocyte alkaline phosphatase** is elevated in polycythemia vera, Hodgkin's lymphoma, hairy cell leukemia, aplastic anemia, myelofibrosis, and leukemoid reactions, but is decreased in CML.

Rheumatology

Questions

DIRECTIONS: Each item below contains a question followed by suggested responses. Select the **one best** response to each question.

310. A 60-year-old, mildly obese woman presents complaining of bilateral medial right knee pain that occurs with prolonged standing. The pain does not occur with sitting or climbing stairs but seems to be worse with other activity and at the end of the day. The patient denies morning stiffness. Examination of the knees reveals no deformity, but there are small effusions. Some mild pain and crepitus are produced with palpation of the medial aspect of the knees. Which of the following is the most likely diagnosis?

a. Rheumatoid arthritis
b. Gouty arthritis
c. Chondromalacia patellae
d. Osteoarthritis
e. Psoriatic arthritis

311. A 41-year-old woman with a three-year history of systemic lupus erythematosus (SLE) presents with right-sided hemiparesis. CT of the head reveals ischemia of the left parietotemporal area. The patient has a systolic murmur that radiates to the axilla. Which of the following is the most likely diagnosis?

a. Acute myocarditis causing cardiac failure
b. Stroke due to carotid artery disease
c. Polyarteritis nodosa
d. Atypical verrucous endocarditis
e. Bacterial endocarditis
f. Cranial neuropathy

312. A 17-month-old boy has a history of multiple fractures due to "brittle bones." The child is short in stature and has a deformed skull. Physical examination is normal except for the finding of blue scleras. Which of the following is the most likely diagnosis?

a. Osteoporosis
b. Achondroplasia
c. Osteomalacia
d. Osteitis deformans
e. Osteogenesis imperfecta

313. A 34-year-old woman has a 15-year history of Crohn's disease. She presents to your office with the acute onset of right ankle and left knee pain. She recalls a worsening of her gastrointestinal symptoms a few days before the joint symptoms developed. Radiographs of the knee and ankle demonstrate soft tissue swelling and small effusions but no bone destruction. Which of the following statements is true?

a. The patient is not HLA-B27 positive
b. The patient is experiencing the most common extraintestinal manifestation of inflammatory bowel disease
c. Controlling the intestinal symptoms will eliminate the knee and ankle arthritis
d. The patient will go on to develop bone erosion and destruction of the knee and ankle
e. The patient requires high-dose nonsteroidal anti-inflammatory drugs (NSAIDs)

314. A 24-year-old man with a two-year history of ankylosing spondylitis presents for his regularly scheduled appointment. An electrocardiogram reveals first-degree heart block. Which of the following heart sounds is most likely to be audible in this patient?

a. Systolic murmur that radiates to the carotid artery
b. Holosystolic murmur that radiates to the axilla
c. Diastolic rumbling murmur
d. Midsystolic click with systolic murmur
e. Pericardial friction rub
f. Diastolic murmur with an opening snap

315. A 25-year-old man presents with morning back pain and stiffness and tenderness over the sacroiliac joints. The patient denies any previous history of eye or genitourinary problems. On physical examination, there is diminished chest expansion with breathing. Which of the following is the most likely diagnosis?

a. Rheumatoid arthritis
b. Ankylosing spondylitis
c. Sjögren's syndrome
d. Systemic lupus erythematosus
e. Reiter's syndrome

316. A 28-year-old woman presents with her third episode of left lower extremity deep venous thrombosis. She has a history of two second-trimester miscarriages in the past. Laboratory data reveal an elevated activated partial thromboplastin time (PTT) that is not corrected by dilution with normal plasma and an abnormal dilute Russell's viper venom. Which of the following is the most likely diagnosis?

a. Libman-Sacks disease
b. Livedo reticularis
c. Antiphospholipid syndrome
d. Takayasu's arteritis
e. Sjögren's syndrome

317. A 61-year-old woman with a 10-year history of rheumatoid arthritis presents with painful swelling at the back of the knee that is visible on physical examination only when the knee is extended. Which of the following is the most likely diagnosis?

a. Anserine bursitis
b. Baker's cyst
c. Deep venous thrombosis
d. Prepatellar bursitis
e. Infrapatellar bursitis

318. A 28-year-old law student complains of blanching and cyanosis of her fingertips in cold weather and in times of emotional stress. She complains that her fingers become numb and painful during these episodes. She has a six-month history of dysphagia and arthralgias. She does not smoke or take any medications. On physical examination, the skin of her hands appears to be taut and atrophic, with a flexion deformity from the tight skin (sclerodactyly). Which of the following is the most likely diagnosis?

a. Rheumatoid arthritis
b. Progressive systemic sclerosis
c. Dermatomyositis
d. Ulcerative colitis
e. Sarcoidosis

319. A 9-year-old girl with no past medical history presents with the acute onset of fever, arthralgias, abdominal pain, hematochezia, and hematuria. Physical examination reveals purpura on the patient's lower extremities bilaterally. Which of the following is the most likely diagnosis?

a. Cryoglobulinemia
b. Kawasaki's disease
c. Wegener's granulomatosis
d. Goodpasture's disease
e. Henoch-Schönlein purpura

320. A 49-year-old man presents with painful, recurring episodes of swelling in his left great toe. He takes 25 mg of hydrochlorothiazide daily for blood pressure control but otherwise is in good health. On physical examination, the patient is afebrile, but his great toe is warm, swollen, erythematous, and exquisitely tender to palpation. He has several subcutaneous nodules in his pinna. Which of the following is the most likely diagnosis?

a. Calcium pyrophosphate dihydrate deposition disease
b. Calcium oxalate deposition disease
c. Monosodium urate deposition disease
d. Calcium phosphate deposition disease
e. Osteoarthritis of the great toe

321. A 41-year-old music teacher presents with a 10-month history of prolonged morning stiffness accompanied by swelling of her wrists and the proximal interphalangeal joints of both hands. Now she feels that her knees are also swollen and painful. Physical examination reveals synovial tenderness and swelling of her knees, wrists, and proximal interphalangeal joints. She has subcutaneous nodules in the extensor area of her right forearm. The right knee has a positive bulge sign consistent with an effusion. Which of the following is the most likely diagnosis?

a. Osteoarthritis
b. Rheumatoid arthritis
c. Septic arthritis
d. Chondrocalcinosis
e. Scleroderma

322. A 43-year-old man presents with fever and arthritis. During the past two months he has been treated four times for a maxillary sinus infection. He also complains of the recent onset of hematuria. Which of the following is the most likely diagnosis?

a. Churg-Strauss syndrome
b. Wegener's granulomatosis
c. Lofgren's syndrome
d. Sjögren's syndrome
e. Sarcoidosis

323. A 31-year-old man presents with fever and arthralgias for one day. He complains of diffuse abdominal pain and inability to move his left foot due to weakness. He also states he has had hematuria for several hours. On physical examination, the patient has a temperature of 38.4°C (101.2°F). He has diffuse abdominal tenderness on palpation but has no rebound tenderness. Testicular exam reveals marked tenderness of the testes but no urethral discharge. Neurologic examination reveals a left footdrop. Which of the following is the most likely diagnosis?

a. Polyarteritis nodosa
b. Behçet's syndrome
c. Whipple's disease
d. Osteonecrosis

324. A 46-year-old woman with SLE presents with episodic swelling of her ears and nose. On physical examination, her nose is swollen and tender to palpation. Her ears are not acutely inflamed but are atrophic and deformed. This patient is at increased risk for which of the following conditions?

a. Bacteremia
b. Embolus
c. Asphyxiation
d. Myocarditis
e. Blindness

325. A 44-year-old woman presents with diffuse myalgias and excessive fatigue. She has morning stiffness and pain of all her joints, especially her wrists, elbows, shoulders, hips, knees, and neck. She does not sleep well at night. Her symptoms have been progressing for over four years. On physical examination, the patient has 13 tender points at the elbows, knees, shoulders, and hips. Which of the following is the most likely diagnosis?

a. Polymyalgia rheumatica
b. Fibromyalgia syndrome
c. Rheumatoid arthritis
d. Scleroderma
e. Polymyositis

DIRECTIONS: Each group of questions below consists of lettered options followed by a set of numbered items. For each numbered item, select the **one** lettered option with which it is **most** closely associated. Each lettered option may be used once, more than once, or not at all.

Questions 326–327

For each patient with joint pain, select the most likely diagnosis.

a. Behçet's syndrome
b. Drug-induced lupus
c. Systemic lupus erythematosus
d. Thromboangiitis obliterans

326. A 69-year-old man taking hydralazine for hypertension presents with joint pain and chest pain. On cardiac examination, the patient has a pericardial rub.

327. A 17-year-old woman complains of intermittent ankle pain and swelling, photosensitivity, and oral ulcers. On physical examination, joints are normal but a pericardial rub is audible.

Questions 328–330

For each patient with rheumatologic complaints, select the most likely diagnosis.

a. Dermatomyositis
b. Polymyositis
c. Polymyalgia rheumatica
d. Felty's syndrome
e. Scleroderma

328. A 75-year-old woman presents with malaise and myalgias for the last several months. She is chronically tired and has one hour of morning stiffness in the cervical, shoulder, and hip areas. She often has a low-grade temperature and has lost approximately 8 lb during this period. Neurologic exam reveals normal sensation, strength, and reflexes.

329. A 53-year-old woman presents with a two-month history of difficulty climbing stairs and arising from the seated position. On physical examination, she has a purplish discoloration of the skin over the forehead, eyelids, and cheeks. She has tenderness on palpation of the quadriceps muscles.

330. A patient with a 15-year history of rheumatoid arthritis develops splenomegaly and neutropenia.

Rheumatology

Answers

310. The answer is d. (*Tierney, pp 781–783.*) **Osteoarthritis** most often affects the weight-bearing joints and is associated with obesity or other forms of mechanical stress. It has no systemic manifestations. It is more common in women, and onset is usually after the age of 50. Pain often occurs on exertion and is relieved with rest, after which the joint may become stiff. Distal interphalangeal joints may be involved, with the production of **Heberden nodes. Bouchard nodes** are often found at the proximal interphalangeal joint. Crepitus (the sensation of bone rubbing against bone) is often felt on examination of the involved joint. **Rheumatoid arthritis** is a systemic disease of women under the age of 40. Joint involvement is usually symmetric, involving the proximal interphalangeal and metacarpophalangeal joints. Ninety-five percent of **gouty arthritis** occurs in men and often involves the great toe. *Chondromalacia patellae,* or **chondromalacia,** means softening of the cartilage. Patients present with anterior knee pain and tenderness over the undersurface of the patella. Pain is worse when sitting for long periods of time or when climbing stairs. **Psoriatic arthritis** is an asymmetric oligoarthritis that involves the knees, ankles, shoulders, or digits of the hands and feet and occurs in 50% of patients with psoriasis.

311. The answer is d. (*Tierney, pp 807–809.*) **Libman-Sacks endocarditis** may occur on any valve (not just the tricuspid valve, as previously thought) but rarely causes any valvular insufficiency. It is a nonbacterial atypical verrucous endocarditis probably associated with the antiphospholipid antibody syndrome. It is a source of cerebral emboli.

312. The answer is e. (*Tierney, pp 1123–1126.*) **Osteogenesis imperfecta** is inherited as an autosomal dominant trait and is characterized by brittle bones that often lead to multiple fractures. Other characteristics include blue scleras, short stature, deformed skull, hearing loss, and dental abnormalities. **Osteomalacia** (rickets in children) is a disorder of defective mineralization of the organic matrix of the skeleton. It is due to inadequate intake or metabolism of vitamin D. Patients are susceptible to fractures, weakness, disturbances in growth, and skeletal deformities, but the disorder does not affect the eyes. **Paget's disease** of the bone, or osteitis deformans, is due to excessive resorption of bone by osteoclasts; patients present after the age of 40 with swelling or deformity of a long bone or enlargement of the skull. **Achondroplasia** results from a decrease in the proliferation of cartilage in the growth plate and causes dwarfism.

313. The answer is c. *(Tierney, pp 824–827.)* **HLA-B27** diseases are easy to remember with the mnemonic **PAIR** (**P**soriasis, **A**nkylosing spondylitis, **I**nflammatory bowel disease, and **R**eiter's syndrome). These are called the **seronegative spondylarthropathies.** Reiter's syndrome preceded by a bacterial infection (*Yersinia, Salmonella,* or gonococcus) has a high association with a positive HLA-B27. Ankylosing spondylitis has a 90% association with HLA-B27; overall, Reiter's syndrome and inflammatory bowel disease (IBD) have an 80% HLA-B27 association. Patients with IBD (Crohn's disease and ulcerative colitis) may develop a nonerosive oligoarthritis of the large peripheral joints that is usually eliminated after controlling the gastrointestinal symptoms. Arthritis is the second most common extraintestinal manifestation in patients with IBD (anemia is the most common extraintestinal manifestation). Patients with IBD must use NSAIDs with caution.

314. The answer is c. *(Tierney, p 825.)* Aortitis in ankylosing spondylitis may cause **aortic insufficiency.** The AI manifests itself early in the course of the spinal disease and may lead to congestive heart failure.

315. The answer is b. *(Tierney, pp 824–825.)* **Ankylosing spondylitis** (**Marie-Strümpell arthritis**) is a chronic and progressive inflammatory disease that most commonly affects the spinal, sacroiliac, and hip joints. All patients have symptomatic sacroiliitis. Other symptoms may include uveitis and aortitis. Men in the third decade of life are most frequently affected, and there is a strong association with **HLA-B27** (90%) in white patients. Patients with advanced disease present with a bent-over posture. A positive **Schober test** indicates diminished anterior flexion of the lumbar spine. Involvement of the costovertebral joints limits chest expansion, and eye involvement may cause an iritis. Patients with Reiter's syndrome may present with a history of conjunctivitis, urethritis, arthritis, and enthesopathy (Achilles tendinitis).

316. The answer is c. (*Tierney, p 514.*) The patient most likely has **antiphospholipid syndrome.** Patients with this antibody are at risk for venous and arterial thrombotic events, probably due to antibody reactivity with platelets or endothelial cell phospholipids. Patients often have a history of miscarriages, leg ulcers, Raynaud's phenomenon, and livedo reticularis. Laboratory data often reveal a positive lupus anticoagulant, thrombocytopenia, a prolonged partial thromboplastin time (PTT; not corrected by adding normal plasma; a clotting factor deficiency would correct with normal plasma), elevated titers of anticardiolipin antibodies, and an abnormal dilute **Russell's viper venom. Takayasu's arteritis** (pulseless disease) is a granulomatous arteritis that affects women more than men. Patients are usually in their fourth decade of life. The disease typically affects the aorta and its major branches, including the arteries that supply the upper extremities. Patients have absent pulses in the upper arm and complain of arm claudication. **Livedo reticularis** is characterized by reddish or bluish mottling of the extremities and is usually idiopathic and requires no treatment. Livedo reticularis may be secondary to atheroembolism-induced emboli following an intraarterial procedure. **Libman-Sacks disease** is endocarditis in patients with SLE and may be associated with antiphospholipid antibodies.

317. The answer is b. (*Tierney, pp 453–454.*) A **Baker's cyst** occurs in the midline of the popliteal fossa and is often a complication of rheumatoid arthritis. The cyst represents a diverticulum of the synovial sac that protrudes through the joint capsule of the knee. The knee is composed of **12** different bursae. **Anserine bursitis** occurs with inflammation of the bursa on the medial side of the proximal tibia. There is localized tenderness and swelling over the knee. Prepatellar bursitis is called **housemaid's knee** (i.e., associated with scrubbing floors) and is characterized by inflammation of the bursa anterior to the patella. Usually, the history supports the diagnosis. Inflammation of the infrapatellar bursa is called **clergyman's** or **carpet-layer's knee.** Deep venous thrombosis (DVT) is due to partial or complete occlusion of a vein by a thrombus and may be characterized by a painful, swollen calf or thigh. Occasionally there is a positive **Homan's sign** (pain with dorsiflexion of the foot), but often a DVT is asymptomatic.

318. The answer is b. (*Tierney, pp 811–812.*) The patient presents with symptoms suggestive of **scleroderma** or **progressive systemic sclerosis** (**PSS**). This disease, when diffuse, involves the skin, joints, lungs, heart, and gastrointestinal system. **Limited systemic sclerosis** (**LSSc**) was formerly known as the **CREST** syndrome (**C**alcinosis cutis, **R**aynaud's phenomenon, **E**sophageal dysfunction, **S**clerodactyly, and **T**elangiectasia). **Raynaud's phenomenon** may be associated with tobacco use, medication use (β-adrenergic blockers), or diseases such as SLE, rheumatoid arthritis, carpal tunnel syndrome, or thromboangiitis obliterans. **Dermatomyositis** is a systemic disease characterized by a violaceous rash of the eyelids and periorbital areas (**heliotrope**) and flat, violaceous papules over the knuckles (**Gottron's sign**). The rash seen in ulcerative colitis is **pyoderma gangrenosum**. These painful ulcers are large and irregular and drain a purulent, hemorrhagic exudate. **Sarcoidosis** is a systemic disease with skin manifestations, bilateral hilar adenopathy, and pulmonary disease. Patients with sarcoidosis may present with **erythema nodosum,** which typically takes the form of multiple firm, red, painful plaques that are bilateral and most frequently distributed on the legs. Musculoskeletal findings in sarcoidosis include arthritis and tenosynovitis.

319. The answer is e. (*Tierney, p 823.*) The multisystem disease described in this patient is most likely **Henoch-Schönlein purpura** (**HSP**), which is a small-vessel vasculitis that affects mostly children. The purpura and all of the symptoms described are a result of the vasculitis. Histopathology of the vasculitic lesions reveals the deposition of IgA in the walls of the small vessels (postcapillary venules). The mnemonic for HSP is **AGAR** (**A**bdominal pain, **G**lomerulonephritis, **A**rthralgia, and **R**ash). The prognosis for HSP is excellent. **Kawasaki's disease** (**KD**), or mucocutaneous lymph node syndrome, is uncommon in children over the age of 8 years and is characterized by fever, a desquamating, edematous, blotchy-appearing, mucocutaneous erythema, cervical lymphadenitis, and aneurysms of the coronary arteries. It is idiopathic. **Wegener's disease** and **Goodpasture's syndrome** usually have pulmonary involvement. **Cryoglobulinemia** does cause palpable purpura, abdominal pain, and glomerulonephritis, but it does not cause any gastrointestinal bleeding. Cryoglobulinemia is associated with hepatitis B or C virus.

320. The answer is c. (*Tierney, pp 784–788.*) Tophaceous **gout** is characterized by the finding in synovial fluid of monosodium urate crystals that are needle-shaped and strongly negative birefringent (bright yellow when parallel to the axis). Gouty attacks may be precipitated by trauma, medications that inhibit tubular secretion of uric acid (aspirin, hydrochlorothiazide), surgery, stress, alcohol, or a high-protein diet. The patient may have an accumulation of tophi in and around the joints and earlobe. Radiographs may show "**rat bite**" erosions. **Pseudogout** is due to calcium pyrophosphate dihydrate (CPPD) deposition disease; the crystals here are rhomboid-shaped and weakly positive birefringent (blue when parallel to the axis). Calcium oxalate deposition disease is usually seen in patients with end-stage renal disease; calcium phosphate deposition disease causes **calcific tendinitis** or **Milwaukee shoulder.**

321. The answer is b. *(Tierney, pp 828–830.)* A **septic joint** will usually produce systemic symptoms such as fever. **Osteoarthritis** produces a short period of morning stiffness and often affects the distal interphalangeal joints. **Chondrocalcinosis** is a radiologic finding (destructive arthropathy) associated with pseudogout or CPPD crystals. The patient most likely has **rheumatoid arthritis,** since she meets four of the seven criteria as classified by the American College of Rheumatology:

1. Symmetric polyarthritis for over three months
2. Morning stiffness lasting more than one hour
3. Rheumatoid nodules
4. Arthritis of more than three joint areas
5. Involvement of the joints of the hands and wrists; patients may have **swan-neck deformity** (hyperextension of the proximal interphalangeal joints with compensatory flexion of the distal joint), **boutonnière deformity** (extension of the distal interphalangeal joint), or **ulnar deviation** of the digits
6. A positive rheumatoid factor (RF)
7. Erosions or decalcification on radiographs

322. The answer is b. *(Tierney, pp 820–821.)* **Wegener's granulomatosis** involves the upper airways (nasopharynx and sinuses) and the lungs, kidneys, and joints. The diagnosis is made by the clinical picture, a positive antineutrophil cytoplasmic antibody with a cytoplasmic staining pattern (C-ANCA), and biopsy showing necrotizing granulomas. The disease causes a systemic necrotizing arteritis and is fatal without treatment. The typical history for **Churg-Strauss syndrome** (allergic angiitis and granulomatosis) is asthma followed by systemic vasculitis with eosinophilia (mnemonic is **RAVE: R**hinitis, **A**sthma, **V**asculitis, and **E**osinophilia). **Lofgren's syndrome** is a benign form of sarcoidosis that causes bilateral hilar adenopathy, periarthritis of the ankles, and erythema nodosum of the anterior tibial regions of the lower extremities. **Sjögren's syndrome** is a slowly progressive autoimmune disease that primarily affects middle-aged women; it affects the lacrimal and salivary glands, resulting in xerostomia and dry eyes. It may occur alone (primary) or in association with other autoimmune diseases such as rheumatoid arthritis or SLE.

323. The answer is a. *(Tierney, pp 817–818.)* The most probable diagnosis is **polyarteritis nodosa (PAN)**, a life-threatening vasculitis of the medium-sized vessel that causes visceral ischemia, especially in the gastrointestinal tract. Other systems, such as the genitourinary system (kidney and testes) and neurologic system (**mononeuritis multiplex manifesting itself as wristdrop or footdrop**), may also be involved. **Hepatitis B** has been shown to be present in 50% of patients with PAN. Whipple's disease causes a synovitis of the hands, feet, and knees. Often, the patient exhibits fever, lymphadenopathy, and signs of malabsorption, such as diarrhea. **Whipple's disease** is caused by the infectious agent *Tropheryma whippelii.* Osteonecrosis is usually found in patients with sickle cell disease.

324. The answer is c. *(Tierney, p 823.)* The patient has **relapsing polychondritis,** which is associated with SLE, rheumatoid arthritis, cancer (especially multiple myeloma), and Hashimoto's thyroiditis. Skin biopsy reveals inflammation and chondrolysis. Noncartilaginous manifestations include fever, uveitis, deafness, aortic insufficiency, and glomerulonephritis. Patients present with destructive lesions of the cartilaginous structures (nose, ears, and trachea). Patients may require immediate tracheostomy if they present with tracheal swelling.

325. The answer is b. *(Tierney, pp 794–795.)* The history and physical examination revealing tender points make **fibromyalgia** syndrome the most likely diagnosis. This is a disorder predominantly of females; patients complain of insomnia, easy fatigability, and widespread musculoskeletal pain and stiffness. There are up to **18** symmetrical bilateral tender points occurring in the same locations on all patients. Laboratory data are normal in primary fibromyalgia syndrome.

326–327. The answers are 326-b, 327-c. *(Tierney, p 808.)* The 69-year-old man has **drug-induced lupus.** Drugs that may cause lupus are Dilantin, procainamide, quinidine, hydralazine, and isoniazid. Patients are usually older, and renal involvement is rare. The 17-year-old woman has 4 of the 11 criteria (see below) for systemic lupus erythematosus. **Behçet's syndrome** is a multisystem disorder that involves the eye and causes painful oral and genital ulcerations. The nondeforming arthritis of Behçet's syndrome affects the knees and ankles. **Thromboangiitis obliterans,** or **Buerger's disease,** is an inflammatory peripheral vascular disease of the upper and lower extremities that usually affects men under the age of 40 who smoke. Patients may complain of extremity claudication or Raynaud's phenomenon. The treatment of Buerger's disease is to quit smoking cigarettes.

The American College of Rheumatology criteria for SLE (need 4 of the 11: **BRAIN SOAP M.D.**) are the following:

1. **B**lood or hematologic (hemolytic anemia, thrombocytopenia, or lymphopenia)
2. **R**enal (proteinuria or casts)
3. **A**NA (antinuclear antibody)
4. **I**mmunologic (+VDRL or anti-dsDNA Ab or anti-Sm Ab or LE prep)
5. **N**eurologic (seizures or psychosis)
6. **S**erositis (pericarditis, pleuritis)
7. **O**ral ulcers
8. **A**rthritis that is nonerosive and involves more than two joints
9. **P**hotosensitivity
10. **M**alar rash
11. **D**iscoid rash

328–330. The answers are 328-c, 329-a, 330-d. *(Tierney, pp 818–819.)* **Polymyalgia rheumatica** affects older patients. They present with weight loss, profound fatigue, and pain and stiffness of the neck, shoulders, thighs, and hips. Physical examination is typically normal. **Temporal arteritis** may be seen in patients with polymyalgia rheumatica and must always be ruled out. **Dermatomyositis** is an autoimmune disease that causes proximal muscle weakness that involves the skin; polymyositis spares the skin. Patients with rheumatoid arthritis who develop splenomegaly and neutropenia are said to have **Felty's syndrome.**

Musculoskeletal System

Questions

DIRECTIONS: Each item below contains a question followed by suggested responses. Select the **one best** response to each question.

331. A 52-year-old nurse has a history of low back pain for two months. She states that the pain started after she lifted a heavy patient at work. It is a nagging pain that worsens with bed rest. She has tried nonsteroidal anti-inflammatory agents (NSAIDs) without any relief and has continued to work. She has a past medical history significant for breast cancer eight years ago and, except for a recent 10-lb weight loss, has been well since her lumpectomy. Her neurologic exam and straight-leg raising test are normal. The rest of her physical examination is unremarkable. Which of the following is the most likely diagnosis?

a. Lumbosacral strain
b. Metastatic breast cancer
c. Disk herniation of L5–S1
d. Spondylolysis
e. Spondylolisthesis

332. A 33-year-old graduate student complains of low back pain after carrying heavy suitcases on a recent vacation in Europe. Because of his pain, he went to a neurologist in London who recommended bed rest and NSAIDs. After 10 days, the back pain resolved, but the patient comes to see you because of new weakness of his right anterior tibialis. The rest of the physical examination is normal. Which of the following is the most likely diagnosis?

a. Nerve root impingement
b. Tibial stress fracture
c. Anterior compartment syndrome
d. Gastrocnemius muscle tear
e. Popliteal cyst

333. A 45-year-old swimmer presents with a sore right shoulder for nearly two months. He was taking NSAIDs throughout this period with minimal relief. Over the last several days, he has developed pain with elevation of his arm above the horizontal and has some loss of passive motion in external rotation and with abduction. The pain is relieved after you inject 2 mL of lidocaine into the subacromial space. Which of the following is the most likely diagnosis?

a. Fracture of the surgical neck of the humerus
b. Bicipital tendinitis due to snapping
c. Cervical radiculopathy due to a herniated disk
d. Calcific tendinitis
e. Frozen shoulder due to a rotator cuff injury

334. A 7-year-old boy presents with a one-year history of pain of the left anterior thigh. He has no history of trauma. On physical examination, he has limited hip motion, especially with abduction and internal rotation. A slight limp is noticeable with ambulation. Pain is brought on by activity and improves with rest. Which of the following is the most likely diagnosis?

a. Legg-Calvé-Perthes disease
b. Osgood-Schlatter disease
c. Muscular dystrophy
d. Rickets
e. Juvenile rheumatoid arthritis

335. A 20-year-old college student develops left shoulder pain after jumping into a lake from a swinging rope. She presents holding her arm beside her body (adducted) and avoiding any shoulder movement. On examination, the rounded contour of the shoulder is lost and the head of the humerus is felt under the coracoid process. Which of the following is the most likely diagnosis?

a. Inferior glenohumeral dislocation
b. Rupture of the long head of the biceps
c. Posterior glenohumeral dislocation
d. Anterior glenohumeral dislocation

336. A 47-year-old man fell on his outstretched right hand while roller-blading. Several days later, he develops right wrist pain that is constant and progressive. Pain is in the area of the anatomical snuffbox and is worse with wrist flexion, extension, and ulnar deviation. The anatomical snuffbox is tender to palpation but there is no swelling. Finkelstein test is negative. Which of the following is the most likely diagnosis?

a. Cervical radiculopathy
b. Scaphoid fracture
c. Compartment syndrome
d. de Quervain's disease
e. Boxer's fracture

337. A 31-year-old man develops left ankle pain after stepping off a curb. He treated the injury with ice overnight, but the next day he cannot walk due to the pain. On examination of the ankle, you notice that it is swollen and ecchymotic. The anterior and lateral aspects of the ankle are tender to palpation. Inversion of the ankle is painful. Which of the following is the most likely diagnosis?

a. Ankle sprain
b. Rupture of the Achilles tendon
c. Metatarsal stress fracture
d. Plantar fasciitis
e. Tarsal tunnel syndrome

338. An 81-year-old woman has recurrent back pain in her lumbar area. The pain radiates to her buttocks but is worse on the right side than the left. Both sitting and walking aggravate the pain. She denies bladder dysfunction. On physical examination, the patient has diminished sensation and decreased reflexes of the right lower limb. Straight-leg raising and cross-leg raising tests are positive for reproduction of right lower limb symptoms. The patient has no spinal deformities. Which of the following is the most likely diagnosis?

a. Sciatica
b. Osteomyelitis
c. Cauda equina syndrome
d. Kyphosis
e. Epidural abscess

339. A 12-year-old boy is brought to your office two days after a fracture of the humerus in its distal third. The patient complains that he is unable to extend the wrist. Which of the following structures was most likely damaged?

a. Median nerve
b. Ulnar nerve
c. Radial nerve
d. Axillary nerve
e. Artery supplying the brachial plexus

340. A 60-year-old man was involved in a motor vehicle accident and suffered multiple long bone fractures and a severe injury to the pelvis. Two days following admission to the hospital, he develops fever, tachypnea, and tachycardia. The rest of his physical examination reveals chest, neck, and conjunctival petechiae. Respiratory exam reveals scattered crackles bilaterally but no wheezes. Pulse oximetry reveals a hemoglobin saturation of 80% on room air. Which of the following is the most likely diagnosis?

a. Pneumothorax
b. Pneumonia
c. Exacerbation of chronic obstructive pulmonary disease (COPD)
d. Anemia from traumatic blood loss
e. Fat embolism syndrome

341. An 18-year-old gymnast heard a popping sound in her left knee while practicing for the Olympic Games. Her knee immediately became swollen and painful. On physical examination, it is obvious that the left knee has an effusion. The anterior drawer test and Lachman test are positive. McMurray test is negative. Which of the following is the most likely diagnosis?

a. Anterior cruciate ligament tear
b. Posterior cruciate ligament tear
c. Torn medial meniscus
d. Torn lateral meniscus

342. A 20-year-old man presents with complaints of pain in the left hip and left proximal femur. The pain has been present for approximately three weeks and is increasing in severity. It is worse at night and is relieved by aspirin. There is no history of trauma or previous hip or leg problems. Which of the following is the most likely diagnosis?

a. Osteosarcoma
b. Paget's disease
c. Osteoid osteoma
d. Chondrosarcoma
e. Muscle strain

343. A 17-year-old football player with his foot planted is tackled from the side, causing a forced valgus bending of the knee. On physical examination, there is tenderness over the medial femoral condyle. McMurray test is negative for any palpable clicks. Which of the following is the most likely diagnosis?

a. Tear of the lateral meniscus
b. Rupture of the lateral collateral ligament
c. Rupture of the medial collateral ligament
d. Dislocation of the patella
e. Subluxation of the patella

344. A 30-year-old woman with a history of diabetes mellitus presents with a three-week history of hand numbness that often awakens her from sleep. The symptoms resolve after she shakes her hands for a few minutes. On physical examination, there is no sensory or motor deficit of her hands but there is a positive Tinel's sign. Which of the following is the most likely diagnosis?

a. Thoracic outlet syndrome
b. Carpal tunnel syndrome
c. Dupuytren's contracture
d. Mallet finger
e. Ganglion
f. Trigger finger

345. A 41-year-old construction worker complains of the sudden onset of severe back pain after lifting some heavy equipment. He describes the pain as being in his right lower back and radiating down the posterior aspect of his right buttock to the knee area. He has no bladder or bowel dysfunction. The pain has improved with bed rest. On physical examination, the patient has tenderness in his lumbar area with palpation. The straight-leg maneuver with the right leg increases the back pain at 80°. The straight-leg maneuver with the left leg also causes thigh pain. Sensation, strength, and reflexes are normal. Which of the following is the most likely diagnosis?

a. Nerve root compression
b. Paravertebral abscess
c. Lumbosacral strain
d. Osteoporosis compression fracture
e. Paget's disease

346. A 73-year-old man presents complaining of right lateral hip pain that worsens when he lies on his right side or when he is standing. He has no other complaints. Physical examination is normal. He has a negative Faber test. Which of the following is the most likely diagnosis?

a. Ischial bursitis
b. Osteoarthritis of the hip
c. Avascular necrosis of the hip
d. Trochanteric bursitis
e. Fracture of the proximal femur

347. A 2-year-old child cannot raise his arm completely on the right side and has torticollis. He has no other congenital abnormalities. Which of the following is the most likely diagnosis?

a. Slipped capital femoral epiphysis
b. Juvenile rheumatoid arthritis
c. Sprengel's deformity
d. Arnold-Chiari malformation
e. Cerebral palsy

348. A 67-year-old musician presents with a long history of low back pain. Pain is worsened with prolonged standing and with exercise. For the last several months, the patient has noticed that the back pain comes on with walking less than one block and radiates to the buttocks. The pain is relieved by sitting for several minutes. On physical examination, there are no neurologic deficits and bilateral straight-leg raising maneuvers are normal. Peripheral pulses are strong and bilaterally equal. Which of the following is the most likely diagnosis?

a. Lumbar spinal stenosis
b. Peripheral vascular disease
c. Lumbosacral sprain
d. Disk herniation
e. Diffuse idiopathic skeletal hyperostosis

349. A 42-year-old man presents with a crush injury to his left lower extremity. He complains of severe leg pain that seems out of proportion to his injury. He also complains of paresthesias of the injured extremity. Leg examination is significant for pallor and coldness. The dorsalis pedis and posterior tibialis pulses are not palpable. Which of the following is the most likely diagnosis?

a. Arterial insufficiency
b. Pelvic fracture
c. Aortic insufficiency
d. Aortic dissection
e. Compartment syndrome

350. A 20-year-old woman presents complaining of proximal forearm pain exacerbated by extension of the wrist against resistance with the elbow extended. She denies trauma but is an avid racquetball player. Which of the following is the most likely diagnosis?

a. Lateral epicondylar tendinitis
b. Medial epicondylar tendinitis
c. Olecranon bursitis
d. Biceps tendinitis
e. Long thoracic nerve early paralysis

351. A 41-year-old man was recently in a motor vehicle accident (MVA) in which he was the driver. He states that he was wearing his seat belt at the time of the accident. A day after the accident, he developed neck pain that has now continued for 10 days. He notices crunching on extension and lateral bending of the neck. Physical examination reveals no neurologic deficits. His neck has no areas of tenderness and there are no areas of spasm. He has normal lateral bend, extension, and flexion of the neck. Which of the following is the most likely diagnosis?

a. Ankylosing spondylitis
b. Osteoarthritis
c. Reiter's syndrome
d. Whiplash
e. Wry neck

DIRECTIONS: Each group of questions below consists of lettered options followed by a set of numbered items. For each numbered item, select the **one** lettered option with which it is **most** closely associated. Each lettered option may be used once, more than once, or not at all.

Questions 352–354

For each patient with a foot problem, select the most likely diagnosis.

a. Hammertoe
b. March fracture
c. Genu valgum
d. Genu varum
e. Bunion
f. Genu recurvatum
g. Gout
h. Genu impressum
i. Pes planus
j. Morton's neuroma

352. A patient with hallux valgus develops lateral displacement of the extensor and flexor hallucis longus tendons.

353. A long-distance runner develops foot pain with exercise.

354. A patient develops painful swelling of the first metatarsophalangeal joint.

Questions 355–356

For each patient with a joint complaint, select the most likely diagnosis.

a. Reflex sympathetic dystrophy
b. Ankylosing spondylitis
c. Reiter's syndrome
d. Hypertrophic osteoarthropathy
e. Charcot joint

355. A 67-year-old man with lung cancer presents with metacarpopha-langeal joint pain. On physical examination, there is pain on moving his fingers and a spongy sensation when palpating the proximal aspects of the fingernails.

356. An 18-year-old man presents with a history of low back pain that awakens him from sleep. He also complains of morning stiffness and decreased mobility. The pain does not improve with activity. Schober test is positive.

Questions 357–358

For each patient described, select the most likely root that is affected.

a. S1 nerve root
b. L5 nerve root
c. L4 nerve root
d. L2 nerve root

357. A 37-year-old man presents complaining of difficulty walking. On physical examination, he is unable to walk on his heels.

358. A 71-year-old woman has difficulty squatting or rising out of a chair.

Questions 359–360

For each description of a maneuver, sign, or test, choose the most appropriate name of the maneuver, sign, or test.

a. Ballottement procedure
b. Bulge sign
c. Apley test

359. The patient lies prone with knee flexed to 90°, and the leg is externally and internally rotated.

360. With the knee extended, the medial aspect of the knee is milked upward two to three times and the lateral side of the patella is tapped.

Musculoskeletal System

Answers

331. The answer is b. *(Tierney, pp 791–794.)* **Lower back pain** is a very common complaint. The differential diagnosis includes soft tissue problems (muscles and ligaments), disk problems (prolapse), facet problems (degenerative joint disease), spinal canal disease (spinal stenosis), and vertebral body diseases (osteoporosis causing a compression fracture, infection, metastatic disease, spondylolisthesis). Patients with **disk herniation** at L5–S1 may present with S1 nerve root compression (the herniated disk affects the nerve root below the lesion). The patient is unable to stand on his or her toes and has an absent Achilles reflex (S1). The **straight-leg raising test** is positive. **Spondylolysis** is a defect of a lumbar vertebra (lack of ossification of the articular processes) and rarely causes symptoms. **Spondylolisthesis** occurs when the vertebra slips forward from its position and is generally a consequence of spondylolysis or degenerative joint disease (DJD) without spondylolysis. It, too, is usually asymptomatic. A back strain is an injury to a ligament or muscle; it may mimic disk disease, but the neurologic exam and straight-leg raising test generally remain normal. Although radiologic studies are needed in this patient to make a definitive diagnosis, the leading diagnosis with her history of breast cancer and weight loss is metastatic disease to the lumbosacral area. Pain made worse by lying down or at night may be a sign of malignancy or infection.

332. The answer is a. *(Goldman, p 2235.)* **Lumbar disk herniation** may occur rapidly after lifting heavy objects awkwardly or with poor technique but usually resolves with a short period of rest ("unloading the spine") and NSAIDs. Surgery is rarely needed. If a patient develops significant neurologic deficit after the initial pain has resolved, the diagnosis is most likely nerve impingement due to a herniation of the disk. **Tibial stress fractures (shin splints)** may occur due to weight-bearing exercises or training errors. These injuries cause anterior tibial pain after exercise, but not weakness. **Anterior compartment syndrome** occurring after weight-bearing exercise may cause a neuropraxia of the peroneal nerve, leading to footdrop. A **gastrocnemius muscle tear** usually occurs suddenly after rapid dorsiflexion of the ankle and causes severe midcalf pain. In a few days, the calf characteristically develops a bluish discoloration. A popliteal cyst (**Baker's cyst**) causes calf pain, swelling, and knee effusion. It is often a complication of rheumatoid arthritis and represents a diverticulum of the synovial sac that protrudes through the posterior joint capsule of the knee.

333. The answer is e. *(Tierney, p 797.)* **Passive range of motion (ROM) tests** are performed by the examiner, while **active ROM tests** are performed by the patient. Passive ROM tests need not be done if active ROM tests are performed adequately. The loss of passive range of motion indicates a stiffening shoulder (**frozen shoulder or adhesive capsulitis**). The most likely etiology in this patient would be impingement of the rotator cuff, causing inflammation, degeneration, and possibly a tear. The rotator cuff, which is formed by the **SITS** tendons of the **S**upraspinatus, **I**nfraspinatus, **T**eres minor, and **S**ubscapularis muscles, stabilizes the glenohumeral joint and prevents upward movement of the head of the humerus. Injuries may occur from overhead activities including freestyle and butterfly-style swimming. The **drop arm sign** may be positive in rotator cuff tear (abduct the arm to 180° and ask the patient to bring it down slowly; at 90° the arm will drop quickly due to weakness). An injection of lidocaine often relieves the inflammation in the subacromial space in patients with rotator cuff tendinitis and alleviates the symptoms. Fracture of the surgical head of the humerus is usually seen in the elderly after a fall. Swelling and ecchymosis are visible. **Cervical radiculopathy** typically results in decreased sensation, strength, and reflexes all matching one root level of the upper extremity. **Bicipital tendinitis** may be seen with overuse and trauma, but pain is typically felt over the anterior aspect of the shoulder, and palpation of the biceps tendon in the bicipital groove elicits tenderness. Pain produced on supination of the forearm against resistance (**Yergason's sign**) confirms bicipital tendinitis. Lidocaine injection into the synovial sheath of the long head of the biceps relieves pain. **Calcific tendinitis** is due to calcium deposits in the subacromial region and is especially common in the supraspinatus tendon near its insertion.

334. The answer is a. *(Seidel, p 762.)* **Legg-Calvé-Perthes disease** (osteochondrosis) is an uncommon disorder that affects boys more than girls between the ages of 2 and 12. The hallmark is avascular necrosis of the capital femoral epiphysis, which has the potential to regenerate new bone. Consequently, children with Legg-Calvé-Perthes disease are of short stature and present with a painless limp. **Osgood-Schlatter disease** occurs in adolescence and is usually self-limiting. It is due to patellar tendon stress, which causes pain in the region of the tibial tuberosity, especially when the patient extends the knee against resistance. **Rickets** is attributed to vitamin D deficiency and is manifested by bowing of the long bones, enlargement of the epiphyses of the long bones, delayed closure of the fontanels, and enlargement of the costochondral junctions of the ribs (rachitic rosary). **Juvenile rheumatoid arthritis** is an inflammatory disorder that begins in childhood and may produce extraarticular symptoms, including iridocyclitis, fever, rash, anemia, and pericarditis. Muscular dystrophy is characterized by progressive weakness and muscle atrophy.

335. The answer is d. *(Seidel, p 720.)* **Glenohumeral dislocations** may be anterior, posterior, or inferior, depending on the position of the head of the humerus in relation to the glenoid. The most common dislocation is anterior (>90%) and is due to forceful abduction, external rotation, or extension. There is typically flattening of the deltoid and loss of the greater tuberosity, causing a **squared-off appearance** of the shoulder. The patient is usually in severe pain and holds the arm in slight abduction and external rotation. Posterior dislocations are typically seen following a seizure. Possible complications of shoulder dislocation include damage to the axillary artery, axillary nerve (deltoid paralysis), and brachial plexus. First-time dislocation requires orthopedic management (surgery or therapeutic exercise), since 80% of patients will have a recurrence. Rupture of the long head of the biceps causes a bulge in the lower half of the arm and pain on elbow flexion.

336. The answer is b. *(Seidel, p 733.)* **Scaphoid fractures** occur as a result of a fall on an outstretched hand. These fractures heal poorly due to a poor blood supply in this area. Radiographs done early may be negative, but later radiographs may show evidence of healing (callus fracture). Cervical (C6–C8) radiculopathy causes pain, numbness, and tingling from the neck to the hand. **de Quervain's disease,** or tenosynovitis of the tendon sheath of the extensor pollicis brevis and abductor pollicis longus, causes swelling and tenderness of the anatomic snuffbox. This disorder is usually found in middle-aged women who perform repetitive activity. The **Finkelstein test** is positive (patient makes a fist around his or her own thumb; pain is produced with adduction toward the ulnar side) in de Quervain's disease. **Compartment syndrome** is a surgical emergency and is due to a tight cast or swelling, causing compression of the blood vessels and nerves in the forearm. A **boxer's fracture** causes flattening or loss of the fifth knuckle prominence due to displacement of the metacarpal toward the palm. It is usually the result of striking an object with a clenched fist.

337. The answer is a. *(Tierney, pp 799–800.)* Ligament injuries of the ankle are common and may occur in sports requiring jumping and running. These injuries occur when the foot twists as it lands on the ground and can even be a consequence of walking on uneven ground. The **medial ligament** is typically injured with eversion and the **lateral ligament** (the ligament most commonly affected by injuries) with inversion. The lateral ligament is composed of three parts: the anterior talofibular ligament, the calcaneofibular ligament, and the posterior talofibular ligament. The injured ligament is tender to palpation, ecchymotic, and swollen. Metatarsal stress fractures (**march fractures**) occur after long periods of running or walking; pain is typically in the middle of the forefoot. **Rupture of the Achilles tendon** may occur with running and jumping. It causes a palpable defect, swelling, and tenderness over the tendon. The **Thompson test** is positive (patient lies with knee flexed to 90° and the examiner squeezes the calf muscle; if the Achilles tendon is ruptured, the foot will not move, but if the tendon is intact, the foot will plantarflex). **Plantar fasciitis** causes pain over the medial aspect of the plantar fascia. It usually starts slowly and is of long duration. The **windlass test** is positive (pain increases with ankle and great toe dorsiflexion). **Tarsal tunnel syndrome** occurs with entrapment of the posterior tibial nerve. The patient complains of burning and numbness that extends from the sole of the foot and toes to the medial malleolus.

338. The answer is a. *(Seidel, p 736.)* The sciatic nerve is located between the ischial tuberosity and the greater trochanter; tenderness over the nerve indicates irritation of the nerve roots forming the nerve. The most common cause of **sciatica** is a herniated disk, usually occurring at the L4–L5 or L5–S1 levels. The **straight-leg raising test** is usually positive in sciatic nerve irritation (pain is produced with elevation of less than 70° and worsened with dorsiflexion of foot or **Lasègue's sign**). A pulling or tight sensation in the hamstring is not a positive straight-leg raising test. The **cross-leg raising test** (elevation of unaffected leg causes pain in affected leg) may also be positive. Osteomyelitis and epidural abscesses are usually accompanied by systemic symptoms (i.e., fever) and are found in patients who are immunocompromised. The typical presentation for **cauda equina syndrome** is progressive weakness and numbness of the lower extremities bilaterally with urinary retention. There is perineal and perianal sensory loss (**saddle anesthesia**) and a lax anal sphincter. The cauda equina syndrome is a true surgical emergency. Kyphosis (hunchback) is a smooth and rounded backward convexity of the thoracic region.

339. The answer is c. *(Tierney, p 997.)* The radial nerve lies next to the shaft of the humerus in the spiral groove. It may be injured as a result of humeral fractures, especially those involving the distal third of the humerus. The radial nerve (C6–C8) supplies the extensor muscles of the wrist; damage to it results in **wristdrop,** a condition in which the patient is unable to extend the wrist. **Clawhand** is due to paralyzed interosseous and lumbrical muscles from an ulnar nerve (C8–T1) injury. The median nerve (C6–T1) supplies most of the flexors in the forearm (motor branches) and supplies sensory branches to the radial part of the hand; an injury will cause thenar atrophy.

340. The answer is e. *(Goldman, p 567.)* The signs and symptoms of **fat embolism** syndrome are those of adult respiratory distress syndrome (ARDS) in association with musculoskeletal trauma. It usually occurs two to four days after the injury. The dominant feature is respiratory failure. Petechiae are found in 50 to 60% of patients, generally on the anterior chest and neck, axillae, and conjunctiva. Although fractures of the pelvis may cause life-threatening blood loss and subsequent hypovolemic shock, the patient will probably have other symptoms, such as oliguria, hypotension, pale conjunctiva, clouded sensorium, and cool extremities.

341. The answer is a. *(Seidel, pp 737–738.)* The anterior and posterior cruciate ligaments are intraarticular ligaments and contribute to the stability of the knee. The most likely diagnosis in this gymnast is tear of the **anterior cruciate ligament** (**ACL**). Both the **Lachman test** (the patient is placed in the supine position with the knee flexed at 15° while the examiner stabilizes the distal thigh with one hand and grasps the patient's leg distal to the tibiofemoral joint with the other hand; the test is positive if the examiner is able to move the tibia anteriorly) and the **anterior drawer**

test (the foot is immobilized while the hip and knee are flexed, then the tibia is moved anterior relative to the femur; a positive test occurs with forward displacement of the tibia of more than 0.5 cm) are positive in this kind of injury. The Lachman test is more sensitive than the drawer test. Aspirated joint fluid is usually bloody in ACL injuries. An MRI is helpful in diagnosing this injury. A **posterior cruciate ligament** (**PCL**) tear would have a positive **posterior drawer test** whereby posterior displacement of the tibia is elicited on physical examination. A **torn medial meniscus** often causes the patient to complain of knee catching, locking, and clicking. The **McMurray test** (with the patient supine, flex the knee and hold the foot in one hand; rotate the leg and slowly extend the knee while palpating the posteromedial margins of the joint for a palpable click as the femur passes over the torn meniscus) is positive for a torn medial meniscus. A **torn lateral meniscus** is tested by palpating the posterolateral margin of the knee joint with the leg in full internal rotation as the knee is extended. Medial meniscus tears are more common than lateral meniscus tears and are usually due to twisting injuries. Unlike the immediate swelling seen with tears of vascular structures such as the ACL, the relatively avascular meniscus (cartilage) causes more gradual swelling.

342. The answer is c. (*Tierney, p 834.*) A history of pain that increases in severity, worsens at night, and is relieved by aspirin suggests the diagnosis of **osteoid osteoma**. This benign tumor is more common in males than females, and patients present between 20 and 30 years of age. The proximal femur is the most common site for this tumor. Other benign tumors of bone include giant cell tumor (osteoclastoma), osteochondroma, chondroblastoma, and osteoblastoma. The most common malignant tumors of bone include osteosarcoma (45%), chondrosarcoma (25%), Ewing's sarcoma (15%), and malignant fibrous histiocytoma. Osteosarcomas commonly involve the distal femur. Chondrosarcomas are seen in older patients (40 to 50 years old). Osteosarcomas may be seen later in life as a complication of Paget's disease.

343. The answer is c. (*Seidel, pp 737–738.*) The lateral and medial collateral ligaments are on either side of the knee. Forced valgus bending of the knee may rupture the **medial collateral ligament** (**MCL**), also called the tibial collateral ligament. This is the most frequently injured ligament of the knee. Patients present with pain over the medial aspect of the knee.

Injuries to the MCL may in turn tear the medial meniscus, since the MCL is attached to the medial meniscus. Patients with medial meniscal tears may complain of locking of the knee in flexion with activity while walking. Injuries of the lateral (fibular) collateral ligament cause tenderness over the lateral knee with palpation, but these injuries are not common. Dislocation or subluxation of the patella is due to a great force. Locking is common, and the patella is usually displaced laterally. Subluxation reduces by itself, while dislocation requires reduction.

344. The answer is b. *(Seidel, p 735.)* **Carpal tunnel syndrome (CTS)** is the most likely diagnosis. It is due to median nerve compression by the transverse carpal ligament. Risk factors for this disorder include diabetes mellitus, pregnancy, hypothyroidism, rheumatoid arthritis, repetitive activity, and acromegaly. **Tinel's sign** (paresthesias or pain reproduced with percussion of the volar surface of the wrist) and **Phalen's sign** (symptoms are reproduced by holding the wrist in passive flexion for one minute) may be positive. Patients may complain of pain in the forearm, the thenar eminence, and the first three digits. **Thoracic outlet syndrome** usually causes medial arm pain and paresthesia when using the arms. The presence of a cervical rib is a risk factor for this disorder. **Dupuytren's contracture** is a fibrotic process of the palmar fascia that causes fixed flexion of the ring finger. **Mallet finger** is a flexion deformity of the distal interphalangeal joint and is generally the result of traumatic rupture of the extensor tendon of the distal phalanx. A **ganglion** is a painless, firm cystic mass arising from any joint or tendon sheath. A **trigger finger** may be seen in patients with rheumatoid arthritis. It occurs when an enlarged flexor tendon sheath passes through the pulleys of the digits, causing locking or catching.

345. The answer is c. *(Tierney, pp 793–795.)* Since the patient has no neurologic compromise, the most likely diagnosis is **back strain.** Strain is common in people in their 40s. It is exacerbated by activity and improves with rest. A **straight-leg maneuver** is positive for nerve root compression from disk herniation when pain is produced at less than 70° of elevation. **Crossover pain** (straight-leg maneuver of nonpainful leg worsens pain of involved leg) is also a strong indicator of nerve root compression, but only if pain is produced below the knee. **Paravertebral abscess** usually presents with fever and tenderness with percussion of the affected back area. Risk factors for **osteoporosis** include female gender, menopause, lack of activity, slim body habitus, older age, inadequate calcium intake, medications such as corticosteroids, and racial-ethnic background (Asian and northern European descent). **Paget's disease** (osteitis deformans) is a slowly progressing disease of bone that may be asymptomatic or may cause bone pain, deformities (such as a large skull or leg bowing), hearing loss, and fractures. It begins in middle-aged men and is thought to be due to an inborn error of metabolism causing the formation of poorly organized bone.

346. The answer is d. *(Goldman, p 1643.)* **Trochanteric bursitis** is a common cause of hip pain in the elderly but may be seen in bicyclists and runners. Pain is exacerbated by standing and by external rotation. Lying on the affected side compresses the inflamed bursa. **Ischial bursitis (weaver's bottom,** so named because weavers had to sit for long periods of time, which led to ischial bursitis) causes pain in the buttock made worse with sitting and with hip flexion. Today, it is usually a problem for workers who operate heavy equipment on rough roads. **Avascular necrosis (AVN)** of the hip may be due to trauma or to medications such as corticosteroids. Patients are usually between the ages of 30 and 60 years and often complain of groin pain made worse with weight bearing. Fracture of the proximal femur usually follows trauma. On inspection, the affected lower extremity lies in external rotation and is shorter than the normal side. Hip osteoarthritis presents with groin pain exacerbated by the **FABER maneuver** (also called the **Patrick test**), which is a mnemonic for **F**lexion, **AB**duction, and **E**xternal **R**otation.

347. The answer is c. *(Seidel, p 762.)* A child with **Sprengel's deformity** cannot raise one arm completely due to a small and elevated scapula. **Torticollis** (wry neck due to shortening of the sternocleidomastoid muscle) often accompanies the deformity. Adolescents with **slipped capital femoral epiphysis (SCFE)** are often obese African American males who present with thigh or knee pain. SCFE is a disorder of unknown etiology that causes posterior and medial displacement of the femoral head. Children with **juvenile rheumatoid arthritis (JRA)** present with fever, salmon-colored rash, arthritis, hepatosplenomegaly, nodules, pericarditis, and iridocyclitis (may lead to blindness). There is no diagnostic test for JRA, but the disease resolves by puberty in the majority of children. **Arnold-Chiari malformation** is an abnormality of neural tube closure.

Cerebral palsy (**CP**) is a nonprogressive disorder resulting from a perinatal insult; it causes either a spastic paresis of the limbs or extrapyramidal symptoms (chorea, athetosis, ataxia). Patients with CP often have an associated seizure disorder, mental retardation, and speech or sensory deficits.

348. The answer is a. *(Tierney, p 794.)* The patient is describing **pseudoclaudication,** which is characteristic of lumbar spinal stenosis. This arises from compression of the exiting nerve roots by a disk, osteophyte, or narrow canal. The leg pain is most pronounced when walking downhill or descending stairs and takes several minutes of sitting or flexing forward before resolution. Often, patients who continue to walk with pain will stoop over to relieve the symptoms (**stoop sign**). **Claudication** is seen in peripheral vascular disease, but the pain that occurs with walking resolves immediately upon stopping or standing without sitting. Peripheral pulses may be compromised. **Diffuse idiopathic skeletal hyperostosis** (**DISH**) causes calcification of the longitudinal ligaments of the spine and is usually found in patients with diabetes mellitus.

349. The answer is e. *(Tierney, p 444.)* The patient most likely has **compartment syndrome** from elevated pressure in a confined space compromising nerve, soft tissue, and muscle perfusion. Etiologies include burn injuries, crush injuries, and fractures. Compartment syndrome is often referred to as the disorder of **Six P's** (**P**ain, **P**allor, **P**aralysis, **P**aresthesias, **P**oikilothermia, and **P**ulselessness). Immediate fasciotomy and restoration of tissue perfusion is the treatment for compartment syndrome.

350. The answer is a. *(Tierney, p 798.)* **Tennis elbow,** or **lateral epicondylar tendinitis,** is most commonly characterized by tenderness of the common extensor muscles at their origin (the lateral epicondyle of the humerus). Passive flexion of the fingers and wrist and having the patient extend the wrist against resistance causes pain. **Golfer's elbow,** or **medial epicondylar tendinitis,** is a similar disorder of the common flexor muscle group at its origin, the medial epicondyle of the humerus. **Olecranon bursitis** is an inflammation of the bursa over the olecranon process caused by acute or chronic trauma (**student's elbow**) or secondary to gout, rheumatoid arthritis, or infection. Clinically, there is swelling or pain on palpation of the posterior elbow. Paralysis of the serratus anterior muscle (innervated by the long thoracic nerve) causes the scapula to protrude posteriorly from the posterior thoracic wall when the patient is asked to push against a wall (**winged scapula**).

351. The answer is d. *(Tierney, p 789.)* The most likely diagnosis in this patient is **whiplash**, or cervical musculoligamental sprain or strain. Whiplash-associated disorders begin after a symptom-free period following a hyperextension or hyperflexion injury, usually in an MVA. It is vital to perform a complete neurologic examination to exclude other causes of neck pain. **Ankylosing spondylitis** is a chronic and progressive inflammatory disease that most commonly affects spinal, sacroiliac, and hip joints. Osteoarthritis most often affects the weight-bearing joints. **Reiter's syndrome** usually causes an arthritis of the hips, and there is often a history of urethritis, conjunctivitis, and foot involvement.

352–354. The answers are 352-e, 353-b, 354-g. *(Seidel, p 732.)* Improper footwear results in lateral deviations of the great toe, extensor, and flexor hallucis longus tendons (**bunion formation**). **Hammertoe** often affects the second toe. The metatarsophalangeal joint is dorsiflexed, and the proximal interphalangeal joint displays plantar flexion. A stress fracture of a metatarsal is called a **march fracture. Stress fractures** result in bone resorption followed by insufficient remodeling due to continued activity. Stress fractures occur in the tibia as well as the metatarsal; examination typically reveals point tenderness and swelling. In **genu varum (bowleg)**, the lateral femoral condyles are widely separated when the feet are placed together in the extended position. In **genu recurvatum,** the knee hyperextends, and in **genu impressum,** there is flattening and bending of the knee to one side with displacement of the patella. **Pes planus** is a flattened longitudinal arch of the foot, often called flat foot. **Morton's neuroma** causes pain in the forefoot that radiates to one or two toes with tenderness between the two metatarsals. The pain may be further aggravated by squeezing the metatarsals together. Painful swelling and erythema of the first metatarsophalangeal joint is the typical presentation of **gout.**

355–356. The answers are 355-d, 356-b. *(Goldman, pp 219, 835.)* **Hypertrophic osteoarthropathy** is nail clubbing accompanied by a symmetrical polyarthritis involving the large joints and occasionally the metacarpophalangeal joints. Hypertrophic osteoarthropathy may be seen secondary to malignancy, endocarditis, vasculitis, and other pulmonary and cardiac diseases. **Ankylosing spondylitis (AS)** is a chronic and progressive inflammatory disease, seen mostly in men in their thirties, that most commonly affects the spinal, sacroiliac, and hip joints. It may go undiagnosed for many years, and bilateral hip pain due to sacroiliac involvement may be clinically undetectable. It is strongly associated with HLA-B27. Examination of the spine usually reveals limitation in movement; patients in advanced stages may have a characteristic bent-over posture. Patients with AS may present with an acute nongranulomatous uveitis and limited chest expansion due to involvement of the costovertebral joints. The **Schober test** is positive in AS (with the patient erect, marks are made 5 cm below and 10 cm above the lumbosacral junction between the posterior superior iliac spines; the patient bends, marks are measured, and if the distance between the two marks increases by less than 4 cm there is spinal immobility). The pathogenesis of **reflex sympathetic dystrophy** is unknown. The presentation may be seen after peripheral limb injury; early symptoms include pain in the limb and edema. This disorder may lead to contractures. **Charcot joint** is a complication of peripheral neuropathy seen in diabetic patients. Repetitive minor trauma to the foot causes deformities, which may lead to skin breakdown, erythema, edema, and callus formation.

357–358. The answers are 357-b, 358-c. *(Seidel, p 755.)* Ninety percent of radiculopathies involve the L5 or S1 nerve roots.

L5 motor: assessed by asking the patient to walk on the heels
L5 sensory: medial forefoot and lateral aspect of the leg
S1 motor: assessed by asking the patient to walk on the toes
S1 sensory: lateral foot
S1 reflex: Achilles reflex
L4 motor: assessed by asking the patient to squat and rise (knee flexion and extension)
L4 sensory: medial aspect of the leg
L4 reflex: patella
L2 motor: assessed by hip adduction

359–360. The answers are 359-c, 360-b. *(Seidel, pp 737–739.)* The **Apley test** is used to detect a torn meniscus. A positive test occurs when there is pain, clicking, or locking of the knee with rotation. Both the **ballottement test** and the **bulge sign** (sometimes called the **balloon sign**) detect a knee effusion. The ballottement procedure is performed with the knee extended. Downward pressure is applied on the suprapatellar pouch, and the patella is pushed backward against the femur. Pressure on the patella is then released, and the patella floats out (fluid wave) with an effusion. A positive bulge test occurs when a bulge of fluid returns to the medial aspect of the knee with lateral tapping.

Neurology

Questions

DIRECTIONS: Each item below contains a question followed by suggested responses. Select the **one best** response to each question.

361. A 31-year-old man complains of daily throbbing headaches for the last two weeks. He has approximately eight episodes per day, each lasting 20 minutes. The headaches are localized to the left periorbital area and are accompanied by tearing of the left eye, left ptosis, rhinorrhea, and left facial redness. The patient remembers having a similar problem two years ago that lasted for three weeks. He did not seek medical help at that time. The patient thinks that the headaches are often precipitated by drinking a glass of wine. Which of the following is the most likely diagnosis?

a. Migraine headache
b. Cluster headache
c. Tension headache
d. Trigeminal neuralgia
e. Sinusitis

362. A 22-year-old woman presents with the chief complaint of diplopia for several weeks. She admits to occasional vertigo and ataxia. Six months ago, she had urinary incontinence for one month. Examination of the eyes reveals nystagmus, and funduscopic exam reveals swelling of the optic nerve (papillitis). The patient has increased muscle tone of the lower extremities and is hyperreflexic. She has bilateral extensor plantar reflexes and loss of position sense. Which of the following is the most likely diagnosis?

a. Multiple sclerosis (MS)
b. Friedreich's ataxia
c. Acute transverse myelitis
d. Brown-Séquard syndrome
e. Syringomyelia

363. A 49-year-old woman is brought to the emergency room after suddenly losing consciousness. Her husband states that the patient was in good health until two hours ago, when she suddenly complained of a severe headache. After one episode of vomiting, the patient lost consciousness. The husband states that there were no seizure-like movements and no incontinence. The patient did not take any medications, smoke, drink, or use illicit drugs. On physical examination, the patient has a regular heart rate of 100 beats per minute, respiratory rate of 16 breaths per minute, and blood pressure of 120/80 mmHg, and is afebrile. Heart and lung examinations are normal. On neurologic exam, the patient responds only to painful stimuli and her deep tendon reflexes are bilaterally equal. She has bilateral flexor plantar responses. She has neck stiffness and attempts to resist forward flexion. Which of the following is the most likely diagnosis?

a. Carotid artery thrombosis
b. Embolic infarction of the brain
c. Frontal lobe hemorrhage
d. Subarachnoid hemorrhage
e. Complicated migraine

364. A 39-year-old man presents with progressive weakness of his arms and legs. He noticed difficulty in performing tasks such as buttoning his shirt several months ago, and his symptoms have continued to worsen. On physical examination, cranial nerve and sensory findings are normal. Severe atrophy and fasciculations are seen in the legs, arms, and tongue. The patient has a spastic muscle tone, hyperactive reflexes, and bilateral extensor plantar reflexes. Which of the following is the most likely diagnosis?

a. Werdnig-Hoffmann disease
b. Multiple sclerosis
c. Pott's disease
d. Amyotrophic lateral sclerosis
e. Todd's paralysis
f. Poliomyelitis
g. Guillain-Barré syndrome

365. When testing a patient's extraocular muscle movements, you detect that the right eye cannot adduct past the midline. However, when you move a fingertip toward the patient's nose, convergence does occur. Additionally, the patient has nystagmus. Which of the following is the most likely diagnosis?

a. Paralysis of cranial nerve VI
b. Paralysis of cranial nerve III
c. Internuclear ophthalmoplegia
d. Retrobulbar optic neuritis
e. Paralysis of cranial nerve II

366. A 30-year-old obese woman presents with a two-month history of a nonthrobbing headache that is constant and dull in nature. The headache is worsened with bending over or sneezing and on awakening in the morning. The patient also complains of blurred vision and occasional diplopia. Funduscopic examination reveals blurring of the optic discs bilaterally and no other neurologic deficit. Which of the following is the most likely diagnosis?

a. Infratentorial brain tumor
b. Pseudotumor cerebri
c. Supratentorial brain tumor
d. Pituitary adenoma
e. Metastatic brain tumor

367. A 44-year-old man presents with facial asymmetry. On physical examination, touching the cornea of either eye with a cotton swab results in blinking of only the left eye. The patient states that he feels the cotton swab touch in both eyes. Which of the following is the most likely diagnosis?

a. Left trigeminal palsy
b. Right trigeminal palsy
c. Right facial nerve palsy
d. Left facial nerve palsy
e. Left oculomotor nerve palsy

368. A 52-year-old pedestrian is brought to the emergency room after being struck by a speeding automobile. He is intubated and stabilized by paramedics. On physical examination, the oculocephalic maneuver reveals the eyes to move when the head is moved rapidly from side to side but disconjugately. Which of the following is the most likely cause of these findings?

a. The brainstem is intact
b. The brainstem is partially intact
c. The brainstem is not intact
d. The patient has locked-in syndrome
e. The patient is in a vegetative state

369. A 51-year-old alcoholic presents to the emergency room with horizontal nystagmus, ataxic gait, and confusion. Which of the following is the most likely diagnosis?

a. Wernicke's syndrome
b. Niacin deficiency
c. Korsakoff's syndrome
d. Klüver-Bucy syndrome
e. Delirium tremens

370. An 18-year-old presents with bilateral leg weakness that has progressed over the last several days. He noticed some numbness and tingling of the toes and feet that has now progressed to his thigh and pelvic areas. He has no bladder or bowel incontinence. He denies use of tobacco, alcohol, or drugs and takes no medications. Past medical history is unremarkable except for an upper respiratory tract infection two weeks ago. On physical examination, the vital signs are normal. Neurologic examination reveals an inability to move the muscles of facial expression on the left side of the face. There is bilateral symmetric weakness and deficit to pinprick and vibration of the lower extremities. Deep tendon reflexes are absent in the lower extremities (0). Which of the following is the most likely diagnosis?

a. Myasthenia gravis
b. Multiple sclerosis
c. Poliomyelitis
d. Charcot-Marie-Tooth disease
e. Guillain-Barré syndrome

371. A 76-year-old woman has deviation of her tongue to the left after a recent stroke. Which of the following is the most likely cause for these findings?

a. Right hypoglossal nerve paralysis
b. Left hypoglossal nerve paralysis
c. Left vagus nerve paralysis
d. Right glossopharyngeal nerve paralysis
e. Left glossopharyngeal nerve paralysis
f. Right vagus nerve paralysis

372. A 37-year-old woman who works as a computer data analyst presents with intermittent numbness and tingling of her right thumb, middle finger, and index finger. The sensation awakens her from sleep and is worse when she is knitting or driving. She denies back, neck, arm, or shoulder pain. There is no history of trauma. On physical examination, there is atrophy and weakness of the muscles of abduction of the right thumb. Flexion of the wrist or percussion of the wrist intensifies the tingling sensation. Which of the following is the most likely diagnosis?

a. Wristdrop
b. Ulnar neuropathy
c. Erb-Duchenne palsy
d. Klumpke-Déjérine palsy
e. Carpal tunnel syndrome
f. Cervical radiculopathy

373. A 46-year-old woman has a one-month history of headache. She has no past medical history of headache and no family history of headache. She does not use illicit drugs, drink alcohol, or smoke cigarettes. Physical examination reveals alexia, agraphia, acalculia, right-left confusion, and finger agnosia. An MRI of the brain with gadolinium is most likely to show which of the following?

a. Frontal lobe lesion
b. Parietal lobe lesion
c. Temporal lobe lesion
d. Occipital lobe lesion
e. Cerebellar lesion

374. A 66-year-old man has the chief complaint of pain and numbness over the lateral aspect of the right thigh. He has no back pain or difficulty ambulating. The symptoms are relieved by sitting. Physical examination is normal except for impaired cutaneous sensation over the affected lateral aspect of the right thigh. There is a negative straight-leg raise maneuver; motor strength and deep tendon reflexes are normal. Romberg test is negative. Which of the following is the most likely diagnosis?

a. Peroneal nerve palsy
b. Meralgia paresthetica
c. Vitamin B_{12} deficiency
d. Sciatic nerve palsy
e. Femoral neuropathy

375. A 14-year-old boy presents with a history of intermittent facial grimacing, twitching, and eye blinking since childhood. The movements are repetitive and often move from one part of the face to another. On physical examination, cranial nerve, sensory, and cerebellar examinations are normal. Motor examination reveals frequent and quick repetitive eye blinking, nasal twitching, and facial grimacing accompanied by an occasional snort or grunt. Which of the following is the most likely diagnosis?

a. Tardive dyskinesia
b. Gilles de la Tourette's syndrome
c. Asterixis
d. Sydenham's chorea
e. Huntington's chorea
f. Wilson's disease

376. A 26-year-old woman presents with the chief complaint of weakness that worsens throughout the day. She especially notices weakness and feeling tired when chewing food. The patient states that she feels strong on arising in the morning but the weakness develops over the course of the day. She also complains of her eyelids drooping and occasional diplopia. Neurologic examination reveals ptosis after one minute of sustained upward gaze. Which of the following is the most likely diagnosis?

a. Lambert-Eaton syndrome
b. Botulism
c. Myasthenia gravis
d. Multiple sclerosis
e. Friedreich's ataxia

377. Examination of a patient's visual fields reveals complete blindness in the left eye. Ophthalmoscopic examination is normal. Which of the following lesions is most likely causing this abnormality?

a. A lesion between the optic chiasm and the lateral geniculate body
b. A lesion between the retina and the optic chiasm
c. A lesion between the lateral geniculate body and the visual cortex
d. A lesion at the medial longitudinal fasciculus
e. A lesion of one occipital lobe
f. Bilateral lesions of the occipital lobes

378. A 32-year-old previously healthy man is brought to the emergency room after having a seizure. He has no family history of seizure and denies alcohol use, illicit drug use, and trauma. A family member states that recently the patient has been complaining of a headache and has been acting bizarre, which is a change in his personality. Physical examination reveals a temperature of 38.3°C (100.9°F). Blood pressure and heart rate are normal. During examination, the patient has a partial complex seizure. CT scan of the head reveals hemorrhagic necrosis of the temporal lobes. Which of the following is the most likely diagnosis?

a. Lyme disease
b. Cysticercosis
c. Progressive multifocal leukoencephalopathy
d. Herpes encephalitis
e. Rabies
f. Waterhouse-Friderichsen syndrome

DIRECTIONS: Each group of questions below consists of lettered options followed by a set of numbered items. For each numbered item, select the **one** lettered option with which it is **most** closely associated. Each lettered option may be used once, more than once, or not at all.

Questions 379–382

For each patient with neurologic deficit, select the most likely diagnosis.

a. Basilar artery stroke
b. Middle cerebral stroke
c. Anterior cerebral stroke
d. Transient ischemic attack
e. Posterior cerebral stroke
f. Persistent vegetative state
g. Wallenberg's syndrome
h. Lacunar infarct

379. A 52-year-old man presents with locked-in syndrome. On neurologic examination, the patient is quadriplegic with sensory loss and cranial nerve involvement. He is able to respond to questions using his eyes.

380. A 71-year-old woman presents with aphasia and severe right-sided hemiparesis greater in the arm than the leg. Her eyes deviate to the left.

381. A 67-year-old man presents with an episode of right face, arm, and leg weakness that resolved on arrival at the emergency room.

382. A 31-year-old woman is resuscitated after a motor vehicle accident but does not respond to painful stimuli. She occasionally yawns, coughs, and has spontaneous eye opening and movement. She maintains a sleep-wake cycle.

Questions 383–386

For each patient with neurologic deficit, select the most likely diagnosis.

a. Upper motor neuron disease
b. Lower motor neuron disease
c. Myelopathy
d. Radiculopathy
e. Broca's aphasia
f. Wernicke's aphasia

383. A 61-year-old man presents with flaccid paralysis, atrophy, fasciculations, and hyporeflexia.

384. A 48-year-old man presents with spastic paralysis, hyperreflexia, and an extensor plantar reflex.

385. A 41-year-old man presents with spastic legs, bilateral extensor plantar reflexes, hyperreflexia, and loss of sensation (position sense and vibration) of the lower extremities.

386. A 70-year-old woman presents with poorly articulated phrases but understands commands.

Questions 387–388

For each patient with headache, select the most likely kind of headache.
a. Complicated migraine
b. Basilar artery migraine
c. Classic migraine
d. Common migraine
e. Sinus headache
f. Temporal arteritis

387. A 24-year-old woman has a two-year history of recurrent right-sided headaches that are throbbing in nature and are preceded by 30 minutes of scintillating scotomas and fortifications.

388. A 23-year-old woman complains of periodic, throbbing, right-sided headaches accompanied by nausea and vomiting. On physical examination during the time of headache, the patient demonstrates a right oculomotor nerve palsy. MRI is normal.

Questions 389–392

For each patient with a gait disturbance, select the most likely kind of gait disturbance.

a. Ataxic gait
b. Parkinsonian gait
c. Spastic hemiplegic gait
d. Steppage gait
e. Scissor gait

389. A 60-year-old man ambulates with his upper torso stooped forward. His feet shuffle and he has lost his arm swing.

390. A 55-year-old woman walks by lifting one foot farther off the ground than the other.

391. A 62-year-old man walks with his feet widely spaced; steps occur with each foot lifted abruptly and too high and brought down in a stamping manner.

392. A 49-year-old woman walks by moving her right leg forward by abduction and circumduction.

Neurology

Answers

361. The answer is b. *(Tierney, pp 944–948.)* **Cluster headaches** are often referred to as "**suicide headaches**" because of the severity of the symptoms. These recurring headaches are accompanied by facial flushing, nasal stuffiness, tearing, and a partial Horner's syndrome (there is no anhidrosis). They are more common in men (the usual age range is 20 to 50) than women and are exacerbated by alcohol use. First-line treatment is often high-flow **oxygen**. **Migraine headaches** do not have this timing or duration. **Tension headaches** are bilateral, nonthrobbing, and symmetric. They are usually located in the frontal or occipital areas of the skull and are thought to be related to muscle contraction. They are often described as being viselike. The **headache of sinusitis** is not abrupt in onset or cessation, and patients often have tenderness with percussion of the sinuses. **Trigeminal neuralgia** (**tic douloureux**) is a paroxysmal severe facial pain over the distribution of the trigeminal nerve. Women are affected more than men, and patients are usually over the age of 40. The pain of trigeminal neuralgia can be triggered by simply touching the skin near the nostril.

362. The answer is a. *(Tierney, pp 983–984.)* The patient most likely has **multiple sclerosis,** a demyelinating disease characterized by visual impairment, an afferent pupillary defect (**Marcus Gunn pupil**), diplopia, nystagmus, limb weakness, spasticity, hyperreflexia, extensor plantar reflexes, vertigo, ataxia, dysarthria, scanning speech, emotional lability, and bladder dysfunction. Patients with optic neuritis are at risk for developing blindness. **Friedreich's ataxia** is an autosomal recessive disease in which young patients present with pes cavus foot deformity, spasticity, areflexia, ataxia, and cardiomyopathy. Patients with **acute transverse myelitis** initially present with back pain followed by weakness and loss of sensation below the level of the pain. Often, there may be bladder and bowel incontinence. Transverse myelitis may be seen after vaccination or infections. **Brown-Séquard syndrome** (**cord hemisection**) is characterized by contralateral loss of pain and temperature and ipsilateral spasticity, weakness, hyperreflexia, extensor plantar reflex, and loss of proprioception (vibration and position sense). Patients with **syringomyelia** have bilateral paralysis, muscle atrophy, and fasciculations, along with pain and temperature sensory loss in a shawl-like or capelike distribution.

363. The answer is d. (*Tierney, pp 960–967.*) There are three types of stroke: subarachnoid hemorrhage, cerebral infarction, and intracerebral hemorrhage. This patient presented after complaining of a severe headache. She has neck stiffness and no focal deficit on neurologic exam. The loss of consciousness requires bihemispheral dysfunction, and this along with the abrupt history is most consistent with a **subarachnoid hemorrhage (SAH)**. Common causes of SAH include ruptured aneurysm (i.e., berry) and arteriovenous malformation (AVM). **Intracerebral hemorrhage (ICH)** rarely produces coma (must be significantly large to do so), and patients do not complain of headache (does not involve the meninges). Patients with ICH have focal deficits that appear abruptly and slowly progress over hours. An **embolic stroke** can involve any cerebral artery but must be bilateral to cause loss of consciousness. Patients often have a history of atrial fibrillation or cardiac problems.

364. The answer is d. (*Tierney, pp 991–992.*) **Amyotrophic lateral sclerosis (ALS)** is a degenerative disease that is the result of lower (anterior horn cells) and upper (corticospinal tracts) motor neuron loss. Patients present with asymmetric muscle weakness, atrophy, fasciculations, spasticity, hyperactive reflexes, and extensor plantar reflexes. Patients may complain of dysphagia and difficulty holding the head up. **Pott's disease** is tuberculosis of the thoracic vertebral bodies. **Todd's paralysis** is a transient paralysis following a seizure. **Werdnig-Hoffmann disease** is floppy baby disease; infants present with fasciculations. **Poliomyelitis** is a lower motor neuron disease.

365. The answer is c. (*Goldman, pp 2425–2426.*) **Internuclear ophthalmoplegia (INO)** is caused by a lesion in the medial longitudinal fasciculus (MLF) and may be due to glioma in children, multiple sclerosis in young adults, or vascular infarction in the geriatric age group. INO commonly causes paresis of adduction of the ipsilateral eye (patients cannot look medially), horizontal nystagmus in the contralateral abducting eye, and vertical nystagmus with upward gaze, but convergence is intact.

366. The answer is b. (*Tierney, p 975.*) Patients with **pseudotumor cerebri** (idiopathic intracranial hypertension) present with headache and papilledema. They are often obese women in their childbearing years. Other possible causes include hypervitaminosis A and the use of oral contraceptives or antibiotics (tetracycline). Lumbar puncture will reveal an elevated opening pressure. Treatment includes weight reduction and repeated lumbar punctures to reduce intracranial pressure. A complication of pseudotumor cerebri is blindness; patients with visual changes may require emergency optic nerve sheath decompression. **Pituitary adenomas** are benign tumors that may cause a bitemporal hemianopsia and endocrine disturbances, such as hyperprolactinemia (galactorrhea), acromegaly or gigantism, and Cushing's disease. A ruptured berry aneurysm causes a subarachnoid hemorrhage (SAH). Patients present with the acute onset of severe headache, photophobia, and neck stiffness. **Adults** commonly have supratentorial primary brain tumors (**astrocytoma including glioblastoma multiforme is the most common**), while **children** have infratentorial primary brain tumors (**medulloblastoma is the most common**). Overall, metastatic brain tumors are more common than primary brain tumors. The most common metastatic brain tumors come from the **L**ung, **B**reast, **S**kin, **K**idney, or **G**I tract (**mnemonic: Lots of Bad Stuff Kills Glia**). The headache of tumor is often continuous; exacerbated by coughing, sneezing, movement, or the Valsalva maneuver; and worse in the morning.

367. The answer is c. *(Seidel, p 785.)* The **corneal reflex** is normal when touching the cornea (trigeminal nerve provides sensation) causes bilateral eye closure (facial nerve provides motor). This reflex will not occur on the side of a facial nerve paralysis.

368. The answer is c. *(Goldman, p 2274.)* The test for the **oculocephalic,** or **doll's eyes, reflex** is performed by rapidly rotating the head from side to side. If the brainstem is intact in a comatose patient, the eyes will move conjugately in the direction opposite to the head rotation. If the brainstem is not intact, the eyes will move disconjugately or not at all. The **oculovestibular,** or **caloric, reflex** is performed by introducing ice water into the external auditory canal. The comatose patient with an intact brainstem will respond with deviation of the eyes to the side of the irrigation. If the brainstem is not intact, the reflex will be absent or the eyes will move disconjugately.

369. The answer is a. *(Tierney, p 986.)* The triad of nystagmus and paralysis of eye muscles, ataxia, and confusion is associated with **Wernicke's syn-**

drome. **Korsakoff's syndrome** consists of confabulation, confusion, and recent memory loss. These disorders are often found in thiamine (B_1)–deficient malnourished alcoholics and are secondary to lesions in the mammillary bodies. **Niacin deficiency** (pellagra or vitamin B_3 deficiency) causes the **triad of D's** (**D**ementia, **D**ermatitis, and **D**iarrhea). **Klüver-Bucy syndrome** is due to lesions in the amygdala; patients present with hypersexuality, compulsive attention to detail, docile behavior, and an inability to recognize objects visually (agnosia). **Delirium tremens** is seen 48 to 96 hours following abstinence from alcohol; patients present with insomnia, confusion, tremors, delusions, visual hallucinations, and hyperactivity of the autonomic nervous system (i.e., sweating, tachycardia, fever, and dilated pupils).

370. The answer is e. (*Tierney, pp 993–996.*) **Acute inflammatory polyneuropathy,** or **Guillain-Barré syndrome,** is a progressive, symmetrical, autoimmune demyelinating disorder that affects distal areas first (legs) and marches proximally to involve the arms, trunk, and intercostal, neck, and cranial muscles. Patients often have an antecedent viral infection (respiratory or gastrointestinal) or a history of a recent immunization. Patients are areflexic and have sensory and motor deficits with cranial nerve involvement. **Poliomyelitis** is a viral meningoencephalitis that destroys the anterior horn cells and causes an asymmetric flaccid weakness with fasciculations and hyporeflexia (lower motor neuron). **Charcot-Marie-Tooth disease** (**CMT**) is an inherited, slowly progressive peripheral sensorimotor neuropathy causing distal muscle atrophy ("**inverted champagne bottle legs**" or "**stork legs**") and sensory loss. Patients with CMT typically have pes cavus or hammertoe foot deformities. Deep tendon reflex (DTR) response is graded on a scale from 0 to 4+:

0 = no response
1+ = sluggish or diminished response
2+ = active or expected response
3+ = more brisk than expected and slightly hyperactive response
4+ = intermittent or transient clonus; hyperactive and brisk response

371. The answer is b. (*Seidel, pp 787–788.*) The **tongue** will deviate to the left with a left hypoglossal nerve palsy. The nerve is purely motor.

372. The answer is e. (*Tierney, pp 795–796.*) The patient most likely has **carpal tunnel syndrome** (**CTS**), which is compression of the median nerve by the transverse volar ligament of the wrist. Patients complain of pain and paresthesias of the hand and weakness and atrophy of the thenar muscles. **Tinel's sign** (tapping the median nerve at the wrist) and **Phalen's sign** (forced wrist flexion) intensify the symptoms. Risk factors for CTS include pregnancy, diabetes mellitus, hypothyroidism, rheumatoid arthritis, amyloid infiltration as seen in patients with multiple myeloma, acromegaly, and repetitive trauma. **Ulnar nerve paralysis** causes a **claw-hand** deformity. **Radial nerve palsy** causes **wristdrop**. **Erb-Duchenne palsy** (C5–C6) causes weakness of the shoulder and elbow and results in the **waiter's tip position** (arm dangles at the side with palm in a backward position with fingers flexed). **Klumpke-Déjérine palsy** (C8–T1) is a triad of clawhand deformity, absent triceps reflex, and Horner's syndrome. Patients with **cervical radiculopathy** (C6 or C7 root) complain of neck pain that radiates to the arm (radicular pain), dermatomal sensory loss, and decreased reflexes.

373. The answer is b. (*Tierney, pp 969–971.*) MRI will most likely reveal a lesion of the parietal lobe. Parietal lobe lesions may produce contralateral hyperpathia and pain (**thalamic syndrome**) and **Gerstmann syndrome** (alexia, agraphia, acalculia, right-left confusion, and finger agnosia). **Occipital lobe** lesions produce partial field defects. **Temporal lobe** lesions produce seizures, lip smacking, olfactory or gustatory hallucinations, and behavioral changes. **Frontal lobe** lesions lead to intellectual decline and personality changes. The most common adult primary tumors are gliomas.

374. The answer is b. (*Tierney, p 998.*) The patient describes symptoms due to compression of the lateral femoral cutaneous nerve arising from the L2 and L3 roots (**meralgia paresthetica**). Entrapment of the nerve at any point from hyperextension of the hip may cause symptoms. Symptoms are usually mild, but patients may require hydrocortisone injections medial to the iliac spine. Patients with **femoral neuropathy** present with weakness and wasting of the quadriceps muscle, sensory impairment, and an absent patellar reflex. The **Romberg test** is performed by having the patient stand with feet together, head erect, and eyes open. The patient is examined for steadiness and then asked to close his or her eyes. A positive test occurs when the patient displays increased unsteadiness with the eyes closed but not with the eyes open. A positive Romberg test may be seen in diseases that affect the dorsal columns, such as tabes dorsalis and vitamin B_{12} deficiency.

375. The answer is b. (*Tierney, pp 980–983.*) **Tourette's syndrome** is a disorder of repetitive progressive multiple tics involving the face, head, and shoulders and is often accompanied by vocal tics (i.e., grunts, snorts, involuntary swearing, or coprolalia). **Huntington's disease** is an autosomal dominant disorder characterized by abrupt, involuntary, nonrepetitive, jerky movements (chorea) and dementia. Patients with **tardive dyskinesia** have developed purposeless movements, such as mouth smacking and tongue protrusion, after use of a dopamine-blocking neuroleptic drug. **Asterixis** is seen in patients with hepatic encephalopathy (liver flap) or renal failure and is characterized by frequent inability to sustain wrist extension (bye-bye gesture). **Wilson's disease** (hepatolenticular degeneration) is an autosomal recessive disorder of copper metabolism characterized by choreoathetosis, ataxia, cirrhosis, and corneal deposits called **Kayser-Fleischer rings.** A low serum ceruloplasmin or a high urinary copper level is found in Wilson's disease. **Sydenham's chorea** is seen in rheumatic fever.

376. The answer is c. (*Tierney, pp 1002–1004.*) **Myasthenia gravis** is fatigable weakness that primarily affects the respiratory, bulbar, and ocular muscles. The etiology of the disorder is autoimmune, causing destruction of the acetylcholine receptors in the affected muscles. Thymic abnormalities often accompany the disorder, and the tensilon test (injection of edrophonium, which is an acetylcholinesterase inhibitor) often results in improvement of symptoms. **Lambert-Eaton myasthenic syndrome** (**LEMS**) is a progressive generalized weakness that improves with exercise and is associated with small cell carcinoma of the lung. Ocular and bulbar muscles are spared, but patients often have autonomic dysfunction. **Botulism** causes rapid progressive paralysis of the bulbar (nonreactive dilated pupils) and extraocular muscles and eventually causes skeletal and respiratory muscle weakness. The disorder is caused by ingestion of the exotoxin produced by *Clostridium botulinum,* which blocks acetylcholine release from nerve terminals. Recently, patients receiving unregulated botox injections for wrinkles have developed botulism. **Aminoglycosides** should be avoided in patients with neuromuscular disturbances, since they prevent the release of acetylcholine from nerve endings.

377. The answer is b. (*Seidel, p 311.*) When defects are detected in only one eye, the lesion must be anterior to the optic chiasm. Lesions at the optic chiasm produce a bitemporal hemianopsia because this is where the nasal retinal fibers decussate. The **medial longitudinal fasciculus (MLF)** is involved with extraocular muscle contraction; a lesion to the MLF bilaterally will not allow either eye to look medially. Lesions between the geniculate body and the visual cortex produce a contralateral upper homonymous quadrantanopsia. A lesion in the visual cortex (occipital lobe) produces similar defects in each eye. Bilateral lesions of the occipital lobes result in complete loss of vision, but pupillary reflexes (fibers end in the midbrain) and extraocular muscle movements remain intact.

378. The answer is d. *(Tierney, p 1306.)* Patients with **herpes simplex encephalitis** present with a subacute course consisting of personality changes, fever, headaches, and seizures. Temporal lobes are primarily affected, and the disease is fatal without treatment. **Progressive multifocal leukoencephalopathy (PML)** is a human papovavirus (JC virus) seen in patients with AIDS. Patients present with dementia, visual field defects, weakness, and spasticity. **Rabies** causes personality changes, headache, dysphagia to even water (hydrophobia), and pharyngeal muscle spasm that makes patients appear to be frothing at the mouth. **Lyme disease** can produce an encephalitis or demyelination that mimics multiple sclerosis, but infection follows a tick bite. **Waterhouse-Friderichsen syndrome** is hemorrhagic infarction of the adrenal glands due to fulminant menigococcemia. **Cysticercosis** is characterized by multiple brain cysts produced by the larval form of the pork tapeworm (*Taenia solium*). Patients coming from endemic areas will present with seizures or other new neurologic deficit.

379–382. The answers are 379-a, 380-b, 381-d, 382-f. *(Tierney, pp 961–963.)* **Basilar artery stroke** causes quadriplegia, sensory loss, and cranial nerve involvement; patients may present with coma or locked-in syndrome. **Wallenberg's syndrome,** or lateral medullary syndrome, causes an ipsilateral weakness of the palate and vocal cords, ipsilateral ataxia, ipsilateral Horner's syndrome, and ipsilateral loss of facial pain and temperature but contralateral loss of body pain and temperature sensation. There is no limb weakness in Wallenberg's syndrome. **Anterior cerebral stroke** causes unilateral leg weakness and sensory loss. **Posterior cerebral artery stroke** causes an occipital stroke and a homonymous hemianopsia. **Middle cerebral artery stroke** causes hemiplegia or hemiparesis greater in the arm than the leg, aphasia, unilateral sensory loss, and eyes that deviate to the side of the hemispheric lesion. Patients with **lacunar infarcts** may present with different syndromes, such as dysarthria and mild hemiparesis (**clumsy-hand dysarthria**). Lacunar infarcts represent small artery occlusions; hypertension and diabetes are risk factors for these infarcts. Patients in a **vegetative state** from diffuse cortical damage have spontaneous eye opening and movement without evidence of awareness.

383–386. The answers are 383-b, 384-a, 385-c, 386-e. (*Seidel, p 798.*) Upper motor neuron (UMN) disease (above the level of the corticospinal synapses in the gray matter) is characterized by spastic paralysis, hyperreflexia, and a positive Babinski reflex (**everything is up in UMN disease**). Lower motor neuron (LMN) disease (below the level of synapse) is characterized by flaccid paralysis, significant atrophy, fasciculations, hyporeflexia, and a flexor (normal) Babinski reflex (**everything is down in LMN disease**). A **radiculopathy** occurs with root compression from a protruded disk that causes sensory loss, weakness, and hyporeflexia in the distribution of the nerve root. **Myelopathy** causes severe sensory loss of posterior column sensation (position sense and vibration), spasticity, hyperreflexia, and positive Babinski reflexes. **Broca's aphasia** (left inferior frontal gyrus) is a nonfluent expressive aphasia (**Broca's should remind you of broken speech**); **Wernicke's aphasia** (left posterior-superior temporal gyri) is a receptive aphasia because patients lack auditory comprehension (**Wernicke's should remind you of wordy speech that makes no sense**).

387–388. The answers are 387-c, 388-a. (*Tierney, pp 945–948.*) **Classic migraine** is a unilateral headache that is pulsatile and throbbing in nature and is preceded by a prodromal aura consisting of scotomas (black spots), scintillations (light flashes), or hemianopsia. **Common migraines** lack a prodromal aura. **Complicated migraines** may be preceded by aura and are headaches accompanied by sensory or motor deficits or muscle palsies. The patient described is having a specific kind of complicated migraine called an **ophthalmoplegic migraine**. A mnemonic for migraine is **POUND** (**P**ulsatile, lasts **O**ne day, **U**nilateral, **N**ausea, and interferes with **D**aily activities). **Basilar artery migraine** is a variant of classic migraine in which the aura consists of drop attacks, confusion, blindness, and vertigo (all signs of basilar artery ischemia). Patients with **temporal arteritis** are older (>50 years old) and have headaches along with jaw claudication and tenderness over the temporal artery.

389–392. The answers are 389-b, 390-d, 391-a, 392-c. *(Seidel, pp 791–792.)* **Ataxic gait** is often characterized by clumsiness; when steps are taken, the advancing foot is lifted high. The foot is then brought down in a slapping or stamping manner. **Spastic hemiplegic gait** is the result of spasticity of the involved limb. The limb is moved forward by abduction and circumduction. **Parkinsonian gait** is noted for the forward stoop of the head and shoulders, with arms slightly abducted and forearms partially flexed; there is decreased arm swing as the feet shuffle. **Steppage gait** occurs with footdrop (paralysis of the peroneal nerve); the affected foot is raised higher than normal to prevent dragging of the toe. Bilateral footdrop results in a gait resembling that of a **high-stepping horse.** Spastic diplegia gait, or **scissor gait,** occurs with extrapyramidal disorders. The patient uses short steps and drags the foot; the legs are extended and stiff and cross on each other.

Miscellaneous Topics

Geriatrics

Questions

DIRECTIONS: Each item below contains a question followed by suggested responses. Select the **one best** response to each question.

393. A daughter brings her 81-year-old mother to your office and states that over the last six months her mother has become forgetful. The mother has difficulty remembering recent events and often forgets to pay her bills. The patient has been in good health all her life and takes no medications. Vital signs and physical examination are normal. Which of the following is the best first step in diagnosing this patient?

a. Imaging study of the brain
b. Mini–mental status examination (MMSE)
c. Thyroid function tests
d. Lumbar puncture
e. Vitamin levels

394. A 77-year-old nursing home patient is brought to the emergency room because of low-grade fever. She has no vomiting or diarrhea. She has no cough or foul-smelling urine. Her chest radiograph and urinalysis are normal. A 2.5-cm stage 3 pressure ulcer is visible over her sacrum. Antibiotics are started, and the patient is transferred back to the nursing home. Which of the following is the most effective method to prevent further skin lesions?

a. Wet to dry dressings
b. Dry to wet dressings
c. Frequent turning
d. Whirlpool therapy
e. Surgical debridement

395. A 76-year-old woman is admitted to the hospital for a urinary tract infection. The patient takes no medications and does not drink alcohol. During the evening hours the patient suddenly becomes anxious, restless, and combative. The nurses report that the woman is diaphoretic, with a heart rate of 120 beats per minute. They think the patient is hallucinating and has waxing and waning levels of consciousness. Which of the following is the most likely diagnosis?

a. Dementia
b. Delirium
c. Mania
d. Schizophrenia
e. Depression

396. A 74-year-old man presents with no visual symptoms. On funduscopic examination, the cup/disc ratio is greater than 0.5 in the left eye but normal in the right eye. Flame hemorrhages are visible at the disc edge. Which of the following is the most likely diagnosis?

a. Macular degeneration
b. Glaucoma
c. Cataracts
d. Pterygium
e. Chemosis

397. A 74-year-old woman presents complaining of a severe right-sided headache for one day. She states that the vision in her right eye has diminished, and she complains of claudication of her jaw when she is chewing food. On physical examination, her right temple is tender to palpation. Which of the following is the most likely diagnosis?

a. Acute frontal sinusitis
b. Giant cell arteritis
c. Migraine headache
d. Cluster headache
e. Trigeminal neuralgia

398. A 66-year-old woman presents with several weeks of unsteady gait, forgetfulness, and urinary incontinence. She denies headache or any recent trauma. Her past medical history is significant only for meningitis as a child. On physical examination, her blood pressure is 130/85 mmHg and her heart rate is 82 beats per minute. Her neurologic examination is normal except for a stiff, "magnetic" gait. The patient scores a 22 on the MMSE. After a lumbar puncture, the gait disturbance improves. Which of the following is the most likely diagnosis?

a. Multi-infarct dementia
b. Pick's disease
c. Alzheimer's disease
d. Normal pressure hydrocephalus
e. Pseudodementia
f. Binswanger's disease
g. Creutzfeldt-Jakob disease

399. An 81-year-old woman comes to your office for an overdue checkup. She last saw a doctor three years ago. She has no complaints other than some forgetfulness that she feels is normal aging. Physical examination reveals mild hypertension, which you plan to control with diet and exercise. MMSE score is 25. Thyroid function tests are normal. Which of the following is the most appropriate next step?

a. A determination of cerebral atrophy by CT scan of the head
b. A determination of arrhythmias by Holter monitor
c. A determination of hearing loss by referral to an audiologist
d. A determination of who will help the patient in case of emergency
e. A determination of alcohol use by the CAGE questionnaire

400. A 76-year-old woman presents with the sudden onset of severe left-sided chest pain that radiates in a bandlike fashion to her left side and back. Heart and lung examinations are normal. The patient complains of excruciating pain when the area is lightly touched with a cotton swab. No rash is visible. Electrocardiogram is normal. Which of the following is the most likely diagnosis?

a. Myocardial infarction
b. Gastroesophageal reflux disease
c. Costochondritis
d. Dissecting aortic aneurysm
e. Herpes zoster

401. A 71-year-old woman presents with the chief complaint of distorted central vision. Funduscopic examination reveals the presence of subretinal neovascularization, and there are depigmented areas in the macula. Distinct yellow-white lesions are seen in the posterior pole surrounding the macula. The patient reports wavy lines during Amsler grid testing. Which of the following is the most likely diagnosis?

a. Cataract formation
b. Macular degeneration
c. Open-angle glaucoma
d. Angle-closure glaucoma
e. Narrow-angle glaucoma

402. A 62-year-old man presents with a two-year history of tremors of the right hand that disappear with voluntary movement. He has no past medical history and takes no medications. Review of systems is positive for anhidrosis and a five-year history of impotence. On physical examination, the patient is alert and oriented. He has a resting tremor of his hands that has a pill-rolling quality. His face is expressionless (masklike), and his movements are slow. He has difficulty getting out of a chair and is unable to complete the get-up-and-go test in under 15 seconds. There is a decrease in tone and strength of the extremities. Deep tendon reflexes are diminished. The Babinski reflex is normal (flexor). Which of the following is the most likely diagnosis?

a. Benign essential tremor
b. Parkinson's disease
c. Shy-Drager syndrome
d. Creutzfeldt-Jakob disease
e. Cerebellar tremor
f. Progressive supranuclear palsy

403. A 67-year-old woman presents with back pain for several months. She denies recent trauma. She has no weight loss or loss of appetite. She has no fever, chills, or night sweats. Physical examination reveals a dowager hump and mild kyphotic bowing of the spine. Serum calcium, phosphorus, alkaline phosphatase, and parathyroid hormone levels are normal. Which of the following is the most appropriate next step in diagnosis?

a. Lumbar spine radiographs
b. MRI of the spine
c. CT densitometry of the lumbar spine
d. Dual-energy x-ray absorptiometry
e. Bone scan

404. A 74-year-old woman presents with paresthesias of the feet and an unsteady gait for several months. Other than a previous history of anemia, the patient has no past medical history. She takes no medications and does not smoke cigarettes or drink alcohol. On physical examination, the patient is alert and oriented but cannot recall three objects after five minutes. Her gait is unsteady and broad-based, and she has increased muscle tone in the lower extremities. Muscle strength is normal, but the patient has diminished sensation to vibration from the midcalf areas to the feet. Patellar and ankle reflexes are absent bilaterally. The patient has bilateral extensor Babinski reflexes and a positive Romberg test. Laboratory data reveal a macrocytic anemia. Which of the following is the most likely diagnosis?

a. Vitamin B_{12} deficiency
b. Tabes dorsalis
c. Lead poisoning
d. Vitamin B_6 deficiency
e. Vitamin E deficiency

405. A 68-year-old asymptomatic man is found on routine testing to have a peripheral white blood count of 79,000/μL with 20% neutrophils, 75% lymphocytes, and 5% monocytes. His hemoglobin is 14.2 g/dL and his platelet count is 210,000/μL. Peripheral smear reveals well-differentiated lymphocytes and the presence of smudge cells. Physical examination reveals no lymphadenopathy and no hepatosplenomegaly. Which of the following statements is most likely to be true regarding disease in this patient?

a. His disease is a clonal proliferation of B cells
b. His disease is a clonal proliferation of T cells
c. He is likely to have hypogammaglobulinemia
d. He is not expected to survive more than five years
e. His disease will most likely transform into an acute leukemia

406. A 79-year-old man presents with the chief complaint of insomnia. He states that he wakes up frequently at night and feels tired most of the day. He has no difficulty falling asleep and is not an early riser. He denies headache and has no symptoms of depression. He does not smoke or drink alcohol. He denies stress and avoids caffeine. Which of the following is the most likely cause of these findings?

a. Depression
b. Narcolepsy
c. Sleep apnea
d. Normal aging
e. Kleine-Levin syndrome
f. Nocturnal myoclonus

407. A 67-year-old man, with a past medical history significant only for moderate bilateral hearing loss, presents with the chief complaint of leg pain. He states that he has started to limp. On physical examination, the patient has bowing of the lower extremities, and the right lower extremity is longer than the left lower extremity. Both legs are warm to the touch anteriorly. The rest of the physical examination is normal. Laboratory data reveal an isolated elevated serum alkaline phosphatase level. Which of the following is the most likely diagnosis in this patient?

a. Cerebral vascular accident
b. Paget's disease
c. Parkinson's disease
d. Metastatic bone disease
e. Vitamin D deficiency

408. A 74-year-old woman presents with an inability to walk after a fall in her home. On physical examination, the left lower extremity is shorter than the right lower extremity. The injured extremity is in abduction and is slightly externally rotated. Which of the following is the most likely diagnosis?

a. Tibial fracture
b. Fibular fracture
c. Bursitis of the hip
d. Fracture of the femoral neck
e. Quadriceps muscle rupture

409. A 76-year-old man, who has been healthy all of his life, presents to the emergency room after a syncopal episode. He was strolling through the supermarket when he suddenly lost consciousness. He denies chest pain, dizziness, or palpitations. He has no previous history of syncope and takes no medications. He was not incontinent of bladder or bowel and had no tonic-clonic movements. When he awoke in the ambulance, he was oriented and asymptomatic. Vital signs and physical examination are normal. The patient has no orthostatic changes. The electrocardiogram is normal. Which of the following is the most likely diagnosis?

a. Vasovagal syncope
b. Hyperventilation syncope
c. Cardiac syncope
d. Cerebral transient ischemia attack
e. Carotid sinus syncope
f. Subclavian steal syndrome
g. Seizure disorder

410. A 73-year-old woman is undergoing rehabilitation after a recent hip fracture. She is on calcium and vitamin D replacement therapy. She has lost 10 lb since the hip fracture and fatigues easily. She has periods of wakefulness while sleeping and occasional bladder incontinence. Physical examination indicates that she has poor personal hygiene and mild peripheral edema. The family is concerned that the patient will fall again once she returns to her home. Which of the following is the most likely cause of her frequent falling?

a. History of weight loss
b. Poor personal hygiene
c. Urinary incontinence
d. Peripheral edema
e. Poor sleep pattern
f. Low energy level

411. An 80-year-old woman presents to the emergency room with cough, pleuritic chest pain, and shortness of breath. Her cough is productive of purulent sputum. The patient had been ill for one week with what her private physician had diagnosed as influenza, but for the last two days she has been afebrile and asymptomatic and thought the flu was over. The patient is febrile, tachycardic, and tachypneic. Lung auscultation reveals increased fremitus, egophony, dullness, and crackles at the right base. Chest radiograph reveals a right lower lobe area of consolidation. Which of the following is the most likely diagnosis?

a. Bacterial pneumonia
b. Pulmonary embolus
c. Lung abscess
d. Bronchiectasis
e. Asthma

412. A 72-year-old man was recently admitted to a nursing home after having had a stroke. For the last two weeks, the patient has exhibited a depressed mood. He eats very little and has no interest in the social activities of the nursing home. He sleeps most of the day and refuses to get out of bed. He lacks energy and seems uninterested in participating in daily rehabilitation. Most of the time, he states that he wishes to be left alone. When he speaks, he remarks how little he has accomplished in his life. Which of the following is the most likely diagnosis?

a. Schizrenia
b. Depression
c. Dementia
d. Delirium
e. Parkinson's disease

413. An 87-year-old man has been living alone. He has no chore worker or caregiver. His neighbor is concerned because the patient is often disheveled and forgetful. He has been late paying his rent and appears to have difficulty ambulating. Which of the following is the most likely intervention for this patient?

a. Assisted living situation
b. Nursing home placement
c. Arrange for a chore worker
d. Arrange for a day program
e. Arrange for a boarding home situation

DIRECTIONS: Each group of questions below consists of lettered options followed by a set of numbered items. For each numbered item, select the **one** lettered option with which it is **most** closely associated. Each lettered option may be used once, more than once, or not at all.

Questions 414–416

For each patient with incontinence, select the most likely explanation for the symptoms.

a. Urge incontinence
b. Stress incontinence
c. Overflow incontinence
d. Functional incontinence

414. A 71-year-old woman with a history of stroke is incontinent of large amounts of urine. She is ambulatory with a walker and takes no medications. The incontinence is not associated with activity. Her postvoid residual urine volume is 75 mL.

415. A 74-year-old man with benign prostrate hyperplasia (BPH) presents with urgency (strong desire to void) immediately followed by incontinence. He is active and takes no medications. His postvoid residual urine volume is 65 mL.

416. A 66-year-old man with a 15-year history of diabetes mellitus presents with dribbling of his urine. He has a sensation of fullness in his abdomen and inadequate emptying. Palpation of the abdomen reveals a smooth, round, tense mass. Prostate exam reveals an enlarged (50 g) symmetric gland. There are no nodules palpated. The patient's postvoid residual urine volume is 800 mL.

Geriatrics

Answers

393. The answer is b. (*Tierney, pp 1008–1009.*) The best first test to evaluate changes in mental status in elderly patients is the **Folstein mini-mental status examination** (**MMSE**). A score of 23 or less out of a possible 30 is consistent with dementia. The differential diagnosis for dementia includes Alzheimer's disease (the most common etiology), but other causes must be considered, such as multi-infarct dementia (stepwise decline), normal pressure hydrocephalus (NPH), hypothyroidism, vitamin B_{12} deficiency, folic acid deficiency, depression (pseudodementia), neurosyphilis, HIV, and subdural hematoma.

394. The answer is c. (*Seidel, p 198.*) **Pressure ulcers** can be prevented by frequent turning. The grading system for pressure ulcers is as follows:

Stage 1 = skin is red but not broken
Stage 2 = damage through the epidermis and dermis
Stage 3 = damage through to the subcutaneous tissue
Stage 4 = muscle and possible bone involvement

395. The answer is b. (*Goldman, pp 1060–1063.*) **Delirium** is a transient global disorder characterized by waxing and waning levels of consciousness, hallucinations, anxiety, restlessness, combative behavior, paranoia, short attention span, autonomic disturbances (tachycardia and diaphoresis), and decreased short-term memory. Patients often worsen in the evening hours (**sundowning**). Risk factors for delirium include **H**ypoxemia, **I**nfection, **D**rugs, and **E**lectrolyte abnormalities (**HIDE**); the mainstay of treatment is to treat the underlying cause.

396. The answer is b. (*Tierney, pp 157–163.*) **Glaucoma** may occur without visual symptoms, and patients at risk for the disease should be screened carefully. Patients at risk include the elderly, African Americans, those with a family history of glaucoma, and those with a history of hypertension, diabetes mellitus, or myopia. Signs of glaucoma include asymmetry of the cup/disc ratios (even if normal), **cup/disc ratio greater than**

0.5, and flame hemorrhages at the edge of the disc. The disc of glaucoma is pale, not hyperemic. **Macular degeneration,** etiology unknown, is the leading cause of blindness in older persons. Patients complain of a progressive loss of central vision, and funduscopic exam reveals small, yellow-white **drusen deposits** around the macula and posterior pole of the eye. **Cataracts** are opacities of the lens; patients often complain of glare and the inability to see well in reduced light (contrast sensitivity). Eye examination reveals a reduced red reflex. A **pterygium** is an abnormal triangular fold of membrane extending from the conjunctiva to the cornea that occurs because of irritation secondary to sand, dust, or ultraviolet light. **Chemosis** is conjunctival edema.

397. The answer is b. *(Tierney, pp 818–819.)* **Giant cell arteritis,** or **temporal arteritis,** usually appears after the age of 55 and is more common in women than in men. Patients typically present with severe headache, malaise, fever, and tenderness over the involved temporal artery. Patients may have ocular symptoms due to ischemic optic neuropathy (blindness is an irreversible complication) and complain of jaw pain when chewing (jaw claudication). **Polymyalgia rheumatica** (limb girdle stiffness and pain, weight loss, malaise) may be seen in up to 30% of patients with temporal arteritis. Patients suspected of having temporal arteritis require immediate corticosteroids; diagnosis is confirmed by temporal artery biopsy. **Trigeminal neuralgia** (tic douloureux) causes severe unilateral facial pain but is not associated with vision changes or claudication. **Cluster headaches** occur mostly in men and are characterized by periorbital or temporal pain lasting up to two hours and accompanied by lacrimation and ptosis. Patients complain of several attacks a day for several weeks, followed by a period of remission.

398. The answer is d. *(Tierney, p 989.)* The patient has **normal pressure hydrocephalus (NPH),** which is characterized by a triad of dementia, incontinence, and ataxia in a patient with a past history of meningitis or subarachnoid hemorrhage. CT scan will show large ventricles. In **Alzheimer's disease** (dementia of the senile type), patients have motor signs and incontinence, but usually late in the disease. **MMSE** score is typically 20 or less out of a possible score of 30. Patients with **pseudodementia** or depression have vegetative signs, such as sleep disturbances and lack of energy. **Multi-infarct dementia** (vascular dementia) causes a stair-step progression of symptoms; patients often have a history of hypertension, cardiac emboli, or atherosclerosis. **Binswanger's disease** is a specific kind of vascular dementia associated with demyelination of the cerebral white matter. Patients with **Pick's disease** have dementia with alterations in emotion and personality. **Creutzfeldt-Jakob disease** (spongiform encephalopathy) is due to a transmissible prion and is related to **mad cow disease.** It is a rare disorder characterized by dementia, ataxia, myoclonus, and death within 6 to 12 months of onset.

399. The answer is d. *(Tierney, pp 49–51.)* Physicians must determine the degree of functional incapacity of the elderly patient based on both medical and psychosocial evaluations. Determining the **activities of daily living (ADLs),** the **instrumental activities of daily living (IADLs),** and the socioeconomic circumstances and social support system (who will help the patient in case of illness or in an emergency) are integral in the functional assessment of an elderly patient. The **ADLs** are **D**ressing, **E**ating, **A**mbulating, **T**oileting, and **H**ygiene **(DEATH).** The **IADLs** are **S**hopping, **H**ousekeeping, **A**ccounting, **F**ood preparation, and **T**ransportation **(SHAFT).**

400. The answer is e. *(Tierney, pp 107–108.)* **Herpes zoster** is due to reactivation of latent varicella virus; patients typically present with a history of pain, tingling, or itching of the affected area, followed by an eruption of vesicles overlying an erythematous base. Although the disease can disseminate and produce diffuse eruptions, it typically presents with involvement of a single dermatome. The disease is not limited to adults or immunocompromised patients and may be seen in children.

401. The answer is b. *(Tierney, pp 157–162.)* Macular changes include the formation of **drusen,** subretinal neovascularization, and degenerative changes (depigmentation and atrophy) of the retinal epithelium. Drusen are hyaline nodules or colloid bodies deposited in Bruch's membrane. **Amsler grid testing** is a method of evaluating the function of the entire macula. The patient looks at a square grid pattern; if he or she sees irregularities in the grid in the form of wavy or fuzzy lines, this indicates macular involvement. **Open-angle glaucoma** is an insidious form of glaucoma in which the chamber angle remains open. **Acute angle-closure glau-**

coma (also called **narrow-angle glaucoma**) is an ocular emergency in which the trabeculum suddenly becomes completely occluded by iris tissue. Patients complain of severe eye pain, nausea, and the presence of halos or rainbows around light. The pupil may be fixed and dilated secondary to the abrupt rise in intraocular pressure.

402. The answer is c. *(Tierney, p 977.)* **Shy-Drager syndrome** (also called multiple system atrophy, or MSA) is parkinsonism associated with autonomic dysfunction; patients may present with anhidrosis, disturbance of sphincter control, impotence, and orthostatic hypotension. Patients typically have signs of LMN involvement (everything is down or low, meaning flaccid paralysis, diminished reflexes, and flexor Babinski reflex). **Parkinson's disease** (**PD**) is a triad of resting asymmetric tremor, rigidity (cogwheel in nature), and bradykinesia. Patients have difficulty getting out of a chair, and gait, which is slow at first, becomes faster (festination) with ambulation. The **get-up-and-go test** (patient gets out of a chair, walks 10 ft, turns around, and returns to chair in under 15 seconds) is a good test for assessing gait and will be abnormal in patients with parkinsonism. PD is an idiopathic progressive disease in which there is **Lewy body inclusion** and degeneration of neurons in the substantia nigra. **Benign essential tremor** is also called senile tremor or familial tremor (autosomal dominant) and is reduced by alcohol use. **Cerebellar tremor** occurs with intention and is absent at rest. Patients usually have other signs of cerebellar disease, such as ataxia. **Progressive supranuclear palsy** is a disorder of bradykinesia and rigidity with dementia and loss of voluntary control of eye movements. **Creutzfeldt-Jakob disease** is accompanied by parkinsonian features, but patients typically have dementia and myoclonic jerky movements.

403. The answer is d. *(Tierney, pp 1120–1123.)* Risk factors for **osteoporosis** include white, Asian–Pacific Islander, and Native American race; Northwestern European descent; blonde or red hair; freckles; thin body frame; nulliparity; early menopause; family history of osteoporosis; postmenopause; constant dieting; calcium intake less than 500 mg/day; scoliosis; rheumatoid arthritis; poor teeth; previous fractures; cigarette smoking; heavy alcohol use; medications (heparin, steroids, thyroxine); and metabolic disorders (diabetes, hyperthyroidism, hypercortisolism). **CT densitometry** of vertebrae is highly accurate and reproducible. **Dual-energy x-ray**

absorptiometry (**DEXA**) can determine the density of any bone and is accurate without significant radiation. It is a good screening test and allows assessment of response to therapy.

404. The answer is a. (*Tierney, pp 468–470.*) The patient most likely has vitamin B_{12} deficiency due to **pernicious anemia** (lack of intrinsic factor). Patients show loss of posterior column sensation (vibration and position sense), positive Romberg test, mild spasticity, and bilateral extensor plantar reflexes (upper motor neuron). Patients may also present with mild dementia or psychiatric symptoms. The polyneuropathy associated with B_6 (**pyridoxine**) **deficiency** is associated with isoniazid use. **Lead poisoning** causes a motor neuropathy (i.e., wristdrop, footdrop) and requires chronic exposure to lead as an adult. **Tabes dorsalis** due to tertiary syphilis causes progressive sensory loss, ataxia, and a positive Romberg test, but patients complain of severe lancinating leg pain. Patients are not spastic and do not have a positive Babinski sign. **Vitamin E deficiency** is seen in liver disease, cystic fibrosis, and other malabsorption syndromes; patients present with ataxia and peripheral neuropathy.

405. The answer is a. (*Tierney, pp 492–493.*) The peripheral blood results are highly suggestive of **chronic lymphocytic leukemia** (**CLL**), which is primarily a clonal proliferation of B cells. Often, smudge cells are seen in the peripheral blood smear. The life expectancy of this patient (stage 0 since he has no lymphadenopathy, hepatosplenomegaly, anemia, or thrombocytopenia) is greater than 10 years. **Hypogammaglobulinemia** with subsequent infections from encapsulated organisms is a late manifestation of CLL. Patients with CLL almost never undergo transformation into acute lymphoblastic leukemia.

406. The answer is d. (*Tierney, pp 1048–1050.*) Elderly patients may suffer from age-related sleep problems such as a decrease in delta (deep) sleep and periods of wakefulness at night. Early bedtimes and daytime naps play a role in complaints of insomnia in the elderly. **Kleine-Levin syndrome** occurs in young men and is characterized by hypersomnic attacks that may last for up to two days, accompanied by hypersexuality and confusion on awakening. **Age-related physiologic changes** include increase in body fat, decrease in total body water, decrease in thyroxine clearance and production, decrease in gastric acidity, decrease in colonic motility, and decrease in lean body mass. The process of aging produces important physiologic changes in the central nervous system, which cause age-related symptoms. The elderly may experience the following changes:

Cognitive: forgetfulness, declining processing speed, decreased verbal
    fluency
Reflexes: decreased righting reflex, absent ankle reflexes, postural instability
Sensory: presbyacusis or diminished high-frequency hearing
    Presbyopia due to decreased lens elasticity
    Olfactory system deterioration
    Vertigo
    Decreased upward gaze
Gait/balance: stiffer, slower, forward flexed, unsteady, increased body sway
Sleep: fatigue, insomnia, increased naps, decrease in sleep stages 3 and 4

407. The answer is b. *(Tierney, pp 1126–1127.)* **Paget's disease of bone** (**osteitis deformans**) is a disorder in which normal bone is replaced by disorganized trabecular bone. Patients may be asymptomatic but may present with increased hat size (skull enlargement), hearing loss (involvement of the ossicles of the inner ear), facial pain, headache, backache, leg pain, growth of the lower extremities (one leg may be longer than the other), tibial bowing, and increased blood flow to the involved areas of bone growth. Alkaline phosphatase may be elevated, and a bone scan will detect the lesions. A complication of Paget's disease is osteosarcoma (<1%).

408. The answer is d. *(Tierney, pp 58–59.)* **Femoral neck fractures** are common in the elderly and occur more frequently in women than in men. Ninety percent are due to minor trauma secondary to falls. **Displaced fractures** cause pain and inability to walk. The involved extremity is often shorter, slightly externally rotated, and abducted.

409. The answer is c. *(Tierney, pp 373–374.)* The patient most likely has **cardiac syncope,** which results from a sudden reduction in cardiac output usually caused by an arrhythmia. Patients with **vasovagal** or **neurocardiogenic syncope** (common fainting) present with bradycardia and hypotension due to activation of the parasympathetic nervous system. Patients with **carotid sinus syncope** can initiate symptoms by turning the head to one side, wearing a tight shirt collar, or shaving over the carotid artery. The **subclavian steal syndrome** (transient vertebrobasilar ischemia) occurs with exercise of the upper extremities. When a subclavian artery is occluded and the patient exercises the upper arms, blood is stolen by the ipsilateral vertebral artery from the contralateral vertebral artery bypassing the subclavian artery (reversal of flow). Patients may have a decreased radial pulse amplitude, lower blood pressure in the affected arm, and syncope.

410. The answer is d. *(Tierney, pp 58–59.)* Risk factors for **falls** in the elderly are reduced visual acuity, reduced hearing, vestibular dysfunction, peripheral neuropathy, dementia, musculoskeletal disorders, foot disorders (bunions, **edema**), postural hypotension, alcohol use, and medications (diuretics, sedatives, benzodiazepines, antidepressants, antihypertensives, antiarrhythmics, anticonvulsants).

411. The answer is a. *(Tierney, pp 1334–1335.)* Secondary bacterial infection may be a complication of **acute influenza.** The common pathogens are *Streptococcus pneumoniae, Staphylococcus aureus,* and *Haemophilus influenzae.* Often, the patient experiences improvement in the influenza symptoms prior to the development of the bacterial pneumonia. A sputum Gram stain or sputum culture is often helpful because patients may have a primary influenza viral pneumonia (the most common complication of influenza) or a mixed viral-bacterial pneumonia.

412. The answer is b. *(Tierney, pp 1035–1037.)* The patient most likely has depression. The mnemonic for depression is **SIGE CAPS.**

S = **S**leep problems
I = decreased **I**nterest in life
G = **G**uilt feelings
E = lowered **E**nergy level
C = decreased **C**oncentration
A = decreased **A**ppetite
P = **P**sychomotor retardation/agitation
S = **S**uicidal ideation

413. The answer is b. *(Tierney, p 51.)* Patients who are unable to perform IADLs may be aided by a chore worker, a day care program, a boarding home, or an assisted living situation. Once patients are unable to perform ADLs, they usually **require a nursing home** level of care or a full-time caregiver at home. An elderly patient's decline in function in response to disease usually follows the same pattern. **Hygiene or bathing are lost first,** followed by dressing, toileting, ambulating (transferring), and eating. Recovery usually occurs in the reverse order.

414–416. The answers are 414-a, 415-a, 416-c. *(Seidel, p 583.)* Normal **postvoid residual urine volume** (**PVR**) is less than 50 mL, and normal bladder capacity is 400 to 600 mL. Patients with stroke and BPH have **urge incontinence** or **detrusor overactivity.** Patients with parkinsonism and dementia may also develop urge incontinence. Patients complain of urinary incontinence (sometimes of large volume) following a sudden urge to urinate. The patient senses the need to void at below normal volumes (<200 mL), and the bladder is unable to tolerate normal bladder capacity. **Overflow incontinence** is caused by (1) an acontractile bladder (diabetes or spinal cord injury), (2) anatomic obstruction (BPH), and (3) **detrusor-sphincter dyssynergy** or **neurogenic bladder** (multiple sclerosis and spinal cord lesions). Often, a tense, smooth, and round mass (overdistended bladder) will be palpated on abdominal exam and the bladder can be percussed (a lower percussion note than the surrounding air-filled intestines). Patients with overflow incontinence often have leakage of small amounts of urine and calculated PVRs of more than 100 mL. **Stress incontinence** is characterized by the loss of small amounts of urine during activities that increase abdominal pressure, such as coughing, laughing, sneezing, and exercising. **Functional incontinence** is often due to the combination of cognitive impairment and immobility. The urinary tract is intact in functional incontinence.

Infectious Diseases

Questions

DIRECTIONS: Each item below contains a question followed by suggested responses. Select the **one best** response to each question.

417. A 25-year-old heterosexual man develops a urethral discharge and dysuria five days after having unprotected sexual intercourse with a new partner. Physical examination reveals meatal erythema. There are no penile lesions and no inguinal lymphadenopathy. A purulent urethral discharge is evident. Gram stain of the discharge reveals neutrophils and intracellular gram-negative diplococci, and the patient is treated for *Neisseria gonorrhoeae*. Two weeks after antibiotic therapy (ceftriaxone intramuscular injection), the patient returns with a clear urethral discharge and dysuria. Gram stain reveals many neutrophils but no organisms. Which of the following is the most likely diagnosis?

a. Resistant strain of *N. gonorrhoeae*
b. Lymphogranuloma venereum
c. Chancroid
d. *Chlamydia trachomatis* urethritis
e. Syphilis infection

418. A 41-year-old woman presents with a maculopapular rash on her soles and palms. Both the VDRL (RPR) and FTA-ABS are positive. Two hours after being treated with penicillin, the patient develops fever, chills, myalgias, tachypnea, tachycardia, and a leukocytosis. Which of the following is the most likely diagnosis?

a. Neurosyphilis
b. Tertiary syphilis
c. Jarisch-Herxheimer reaction
d. Rocky Mountain spotted fever
e. Endocarditis

419. A 26-year-old woman presents with disseminated gonorrhea. She has a past medical history significant for meningococcal meningitis when she was 19 years old. Which of the following complement deficiencies is the most likely cause of her recurrent infections?

a. C2
b. C3
c. C3, C4
d. C5, C6, C7, C8, C9
e. C1q, C1r, C1s

420. A 19-year-old previously healthy college student presents with a five-day history of fever, generalized malaise, and sore throat. He denies cough. He does not use illicit drugs and uses condoms with his one sexual partner. He has been vaccinated against hepatitis B. On physical examination the patient appears jaundiced and has a temperature of 38.7°C (101.7°F). The pharynx is erythematous but has no exudate. There is bilateral tender cervical lymphadenopathy. Liver size is 14 cm in the midclavicular line (MCL), and the spleen tip is palpable 2 cm below the left costal margin. The white blood cell count is elevated, and many atypical forms are reported. Which of the following is the most likely diagnosis?

a. Drug-induced hepatitis
b. Mononucleosis syndrome
c. Hepatitis B infection
d. Hepatitis C infection
e. *Mycoplasma pneumoniae*

421. A neonate develops meningitis, and you suspect that the responsible organism was acquired during passage through the birth canal. Which of the following organisms is most likely responsible for the neonate's illness?

a. *Staphylococcus aureus*
b. *Pseudomonas*
c. *Rubeola*
d. *Listeria monocytogenes*
e. *Salmonella*

422. A 23-year-old man presents with the acute onset of fever, skin lesions that are papular and erythematous with a hemorrhagic and necrotic center, joint pain, and an acute tenosynovitis of the dorsum of his left foot. He has no past medical history and takes no medications. He does not smoke, drink alcohol, or use illicit drugs. On physical examination, the patient has a temperature of 39.1°C (102.4°F). Passive flexion and extension of the left great toe causes severe pain over the dorsum of the midfoot and ankle. Which of the following is the most likely diagnosis?

a. de Quervain's tenosynovitis
b. Reiter's syndrome
c. Acute gouty attack
d. Disseminated gonococcal infection
e. Still's disease

423. A 52-year-old man presents with fever and leukocytosis. He has splinter hemorrhages and a holosystolic murmur that radiates to the axilla. Transesophageal echocardiogram demonstrates several vegetations located on the mitral valve; there is moderate mitral regurgitation. Blood culture bottles continuously reveal no growth of organisms. Which of the following may be the causal agent of the endocarditis?

a. *Staphylococcus aureus*
b. *Campylobacter jejuni*
c. *Vibrio parahaemolyticus*
d. *Haemophilus aphrophilus*
e. *Streptococcus viridans*

424. A 40-year-old gardener presents with painless papules that appeared following a puncture wound from a rose thorn a few weeks earlier. Physical examination reveals a chain of erythematous nodules along the dorsal aspect of the arm. Which of the following is the most likely diagnosis?

a. Coccidioidomycosis
b. Sporotrichosis
c. Blastomycosis
d. Cutaneous larva migrans
e. Histoplasmosis

425. An ill-looking 58-year-old man with a 20-year history of diabetes mellitus presents with severe pain and swelling of his right arm that started two days ago after some minor trauma. He has a temperature of 39.8°C (103.6°F). Examination of the arm reveals a 13-cm area of dark red epidermal induration. Large bullae filled with purple fluid are seen in the center of the wound. Some parts of the wound are friable and appear black in color. Crepitus is felt with palpation of the arm. Laboratory data reveal a leukocytosis and an elevated serum creatinine phosphokinase. Which of the following is the most likely diagnosis?

a. Erysipelas
b. Folliculitis
c. Cellulitis
d. Necrotizing fasciitis
e. Fournier's gangrene

426. A 54-year-old man presents with a two-week history of headache, fever, chills, and night sweats. He complains of myalgias and easy fatigability. He has just returned from a business trip to Africa and the Middle East. Before the trip, the patient received immunizations against poliomyelitis, hepatitis A, hepatitis B, and dengue fever. Throughout the trip, he took chloroquine prophylaxis against malaria. On physical examination, the patient has a temperature of 39.5°C (103.2°F) and is diaphoretic. There is no neck stiffness, photophobia, or lymphadenopathy. Heart and lung examinations are normal. There is mild splenomegaly. Which of the following is the most likely diagnosis in this patient?

a. Malaria
b. Tuberculosis
c. Mononucleosis
d. Trypanosomiasis
e. Toxoplasmosis

427. A 68-year-old man with endocarditis and bacteremia from *Streptococcus bovis* infection may have a high incidence of which of the following malignancies?

a. Prostate cancer
b. Pancreatic cancer
c. Lymphoma
d. Colon cancer
e. Lung cancer

428. A 19-year-old college student has had a lump in the left supraclavicular area for over three weeks. He denies fever, chills, and night sweats. He has no recent weight loss. The lymph node appeared after a recent upper respiratory tract infection. Physical examination is remarkable for a 2-cm left supraclavicular node that is nontender, rubbery, and freely movable. He has no hepatosplenomegaly or other lymphadenopathy. Complete blood count and chest radiograph are normal. Which of the following is the most appropriate next step in diagnosis?

a. Bone marrow aspirate
b. CT scan of the chest
c. Lymph node biopsy
d. Observation for a total of six weeks
e. Indirect laryngoscopy
f. CT scan of the neck

429. A 35-year-old woman presents with fever, diarrhea, and right upper quadrant pain. She recently returned from a two-month business trip in Mexico. Physical examination reveals no jaundice. She has point tenderness over the liver and has a positive FOBT. CT scan of the abdomen reveals several oval lesions in the liver. Which of the following is the most likely diagnosis in this patient?

a. Hepatitis A infection
b. Hepatocellular carcinoma
c. Metastatic liver disease
d. *Entamoeba histolytica*
e. *Campylobacter jejuni*
f. *Salmonella*

430. A 46-year-old woman with a history of sinusitis presents with a severe headache. She complains of neck stiffness and photophobia. On physical examination she has a temperature of 39.7°C (103.4°F). Blood pressure is normal, and heart rate is 110 beats per minute. She has a normal funduscopic examination and no focal neurologic deficit. She has nuchal rigidity. Brudzinski's and Kernig's signs are positive. Which of the following is the most likely diagnosis?

a. Migraine headache
b. Cluster headache
c. Torticollis
d. Bacterial meningitis
e. Cysticercosis
f. Fever of unknown origin

431. A 16-year-old boy is bitten on the leg by a neighbor's dog. The dog is healthy and has proof of a rabies vaccination. The next day, the patient develops a cellulitis at the site of the bite, accompanied by a purulent, foul-smelling discharge. There is unilateral inguinal lymphadenopathy. Which of the following organisms is most likely responsible for the patient's symptoms?

a. Rabies virus
b. *Pasteurella multocida*
c. *Aeromonas hydrophila*
d. *Pseudomonas aeruginosa*
e. *Vibrio parahaemolyticus*

432. A 41-year-old woman develops abdominal cramps and diarrhea two hours after eating fried rice. Physical examination is normal except for some mild abdominal tenderness with palpation. Examination of the stool reveals no fecal leukocytes. Which of the following is the most likely etiology for the symptoms?

a. *Shigella*
b. *Salmonella*
c. *Vibrio cholerae*
d. *Bacillus cereus*
e. *Staphylococcus aureus*
f. *Vibrio parahaemolyticus*

433. A 33-year-old man presents with diarrhea and weight loss. He denies chills and night sweats but has low-grade fevers. He has no recent travel history. He has no lymphadenopathy; abdominal examination is normal. His stool is negative for blood but positive for leukocytes. Which of the following is the most likely pathogen?

a. *Vibrio cholerae*
b. *Giardia lamblia*
c. *Campylobacter jejuni*
d. *Clostridium perfringens*
e. *Aeromonas hydrophila*
f. *Cryptosporidium*
g. Rotovirus
h. Norwalk virus

434. A 47-year-old patient with a history of glucose-6-phosphate dehydrogenase deficiency will be traveling throughout Europe and Africa. He presents to your office seeking advice regarding immunization and disease prevention. This patient's underlying disease affords him protection against which of the following?

a. *Rickettsia typhi*
b. *Borrelia burgdorferi*
c. *Plasmodium falciparum*
d. Hantavirus
e. Monkeypox virus

435. A 52-year-old woman presents to the emergency room five hours after eating some grouper at a seafood restaurant while on vacation in Hawaii. She has abdominal cramps, nausea, vomiting, and watery diarrhea. She also complains of tingling and numbness of her lips and extremities. Physical examination reveals a fine tremor and some mild ataxia. Which of the following is the most likely diagnosis in this patient?

a. Ciguatera poisoning
b. Scromboid poisoning
c. Traveler's diarrhea
d. Pseudomembranous colitis
e. *Mycobacterium marinum*

436. A 34-year-old woman was recently told by another physician that her blood test was positive for *Helicobacter pylori*. She completed a course of medication but is concerned about this finding. This patient is at risk for which of the following?

a. Squamous cell carcinoma of the esophagus
b. Adenocarcinoma of the esophagus
c. Barrett's esophagus
d. Gastroesophageal reflux disease
e. Mucosa-associated tissue lymphomas (MALT)
f. Non-Hodgkin's lymphoma of the small intestine

437. A 22-year-old woman with sickle cell disease presents with a painful pretibial ulcer. Physical examination reveals the presence of purulent material draining from the wound site. The patient has a low-grade fever. Radiographs reveal soft tissue swelling and a periosteal reaction. Which of the following is the most likely pathogen responsible for the symptoms?

a. *Staphylococcus epidermis*
b. *Salmonella*
c. *Shigella*
d. *Streptococcus pyogenes*
e. *Mycobacterium tuberculosis*

DIRECTIONS: Each group of questions below consists of lettered options followed by a set of numbered items. For each numbered item, select the **one** lettered option with which it is **most** closely associated. Each lettered option may be used once, more than once, or not at all.

Questions 438–441

For each patient with symptoms, select the most likely responsible pathogen.

a. *Giardia lamblia*
b. *Trichinella*
c. *Chlamydia psittaci*
d. *Acanthamoeba castellanii*
e. *Brucella*
f. *Clostridium tetani*
g. *Cysticercus*

438. A 41-year-old man presents with periorbital edema, myalgias, and eosinophilia three weeks after eating some undercooked pork at an outdoor restaurant.

439. A 19-year-old college student develops a keratitis thought to be secondary to use of disposable soft contact lenses.

440. A 22-year-old veterinary student develops fever, myalgias, joint pain, and headache. He has lymphadenopathy and hepatosplenomegaly. A murmur is heard on auscultation of the heart.

441. A 28-year-old immigrant from Mexico is brought to the emergency room because of new onset of seizures. CT scan of the head reveals several discrete calcified densities throughout the frontal lobe, brainstem, and cerebellum.

Questions 442–443

For each patient with neurologic symptoms, select the most likely diagnosis.

a. Toxoplasmosis
b. Cryptococcal meningitis
c. Progressive multifocal leukoencephalopathy (PML)
d. HIV dementia

442. A 37-year-old woman with HIV presents with headache, irritability, and confusion. Funduscopic examination reveals bilateral papilledema. India ink smear of the spinal fluid is positive.

443. A 47-year-old woman with HIV presents with new right-sided arm and leg weakness. CT scan of the head reveals multiple ring-enhancing lesions located in both hemispheres and involving the basal ganglia and corticomedullary junction.

Infectious Diseases

Answers

417. The answer is d. (*Tierney, pp 1382–1384.*) The patient has **gonococcal urethritis** (Gram stain is a sensitive and specific method of making the diagnosis) and concomitant **C. trachomatis** infection. Patients require treatment for the gonococcal infection (usually ceftriaxone intramuscularly) and doxycycline or a macrolide for eradication of the chlamydial infection. Gonococcal resistance to penicillin and tetracycline (but not to ceftriaxone) has developed. Patients with **lymphogranuloma venereum** (*C. trachomatis*) present with inguinal buboes. Patients with **chancroid** (*Haemophilus ducreyi*) present with a painful genital ulcer. **Primary syphilis** is characterized by a painless chancre that appears 21 days after exposure and disappears in three to six weeks.

418. The answer is c. (*Tierney, pp 1394–1397.*) The **Jarisch-Herxheimer reaction** is a dramatic flulike reaction that occurs within two hours of syphilis treatment. It may occur in patients with primary, secondary, or early latent syphilis and is thought to be secondary to the massive destruction of spirochetes and the formation of inflammatory mediators (**tumor necrosis factor**). The **Venereal Disease Research Laboratory** (**VDRL**) **rapid plasma reagin** (**RPR**) is a nonspecific screening test for syphilis and reverts to negative with treatment. The **fluorescent treponemal antibody absorption** (**FTA-ABS**) is a sensitive and specific diagnostic test and will remain positive for life. The rash of **Rocky Mountain spotted fever** begins in the palms and soles and spreads centrally; the disease may be confirmed by the **Weil-Felix test.**

419. The answer is d. (*Tierney, p 829.*) Patients deficient in complement components **C5, C6, C7, C8,** and **C9** are susceptible to gonococcemia and meningococcemia infections due to an inability to mount a bactericidal response to these organisms.

420. The answer is b. (*Tierney, pp 1312–1313.*) The patient's symptomatology is most consistent with **mononucleosis.** A monospot test (**IgM or**

heterophile test) must be ordered to confirm the diagnosis of EBV mononucleosis syndrome. If the heterophile test is negative, the most likely etiology of the mononucleosis is CMV. **Atypical lymphocytes** may be seen transiently in EBV, CMV, toxoplasmosis, drug reactions, viral hepatitis, rubella, mumps, and rubeola. Mononucleosis is transmitted through saliva.

421. The answer is d. *(Tierney, p 1364.)* Organisms of the female genital tract may be acquired during passage through the birth canal and may cause meningitis in neonates. These organisms include *L. monocytogenes,* group B β-hemolytic streptococci, and gram-negative rods such as *Escherichia coli.* Neonates may develop infections outside the birth canal, namely *Salmonella, S. aureus, Proteus,* and *Pseudomonas,* from contact with contaminated persons or articles after birth. The **TORCHES** organisms (**TO**xoplasmosis, **R**ubella, **C**ytomegalovirus, **HE**rpes simplex, **S**yphilis) and HIV (human immunodeficiency syndrome) are other intrauterine-acquired infections.

422. The answer is d. *(Tierney, p 1382.)* **Disseminated gonococcal infection** is the leading cause of bacterial arthritis in young adults. This disease often starts as an early **tenosynovitis-dermatitis syndrome,** which is often followed by a septic arthritis. Tenosynovitis is most commonly seen over the dorsum of the hand, wrist, ankle, or knee. **de Quervain's synovitis** is a chronic inflammation of the common sheath of the abductor pollicis longus and extensor pollicis brevis tendons due to repetitive use and causes marked pain and tenderness in the region of the anatomic snuffbox. In **Reiter's syndrome,** patients develop an inflammatory arthritis after an episode of urethritis, dysentery, or cervicitis. It is more common in males than in females, and HLA-B27 is present in more than 60% of patients. Other findings in Reiter's syndrome include conjunctivitis, circinate balanitis (superficial ulcer on the glans penis), and keratoderma blennorrhagica (papules on the soles of the feet). Patients with **Still's disease** present with a salmon rash, symmetrical joint involvement, and hepatosplenomegaly.

423. The answer is d. *(Tierney, p 1365.)* Specific gram-negative organisms are slow growing (fastidious) and require carbon dioxide for growth. Blood cultures may take 30 days to become positive. These organisms are often referred to as the **HACEK** organisms (**H**aemophilus parainfluenzae,

Haemophilus aphrophilus, Actinobacillus actinomycetemcomitans, Cardiobacterium hominis, Eikenella corrodens, and **Kingella** *kingae).*

424. The answer is b. *(Fitzpatrick, pp 731–732.)* The occupational history and cutaneous skin findings are consistent with **sporotrichosis.** The mycotic organism *Sporothrix schenckii* is found in soil. The lesion begins as a painless nodule that eventually becomes fixed and necrotic. After a few weeks, multiple nodules develop along the lymphatic channels, causing a chronic nodular lymphangitis. **Blastomycosis** is endemic in the southeastern United States and may be found in agricultural workers but is characterized by pulmonary symptoms. Skin lesions are usually ulcerated, hyperkeratotic, and verrucous. **Histoplasmosis** is transmitted through bird and bat droppings and is endemic in the Ohio and Mississippi River valleys of the United States. Agricultural workers and others involved in outdoor activities, including cave explorers, are at risk for outbreaks. An acute pulmonary infection typically precedes the skin lesions. **Coccidioidomycosis** is caused by a soil saprophyte endemic to the arid San Joaquin Valley of the United States (Arizona, California, and western Texas). Patients present with respiratory symptoms and skin lesions such as **erythema nodosum.**

425. The answer is d. *(Tierney, p 1352.)* **Necrotizing fasciitis** is a painful and rapidly spreading infection of the fascia of muscle. It often begins at the site of nonpenetrating minor trauma and is usually due to *Streptococcus pyogenes,* although infections may be polymicrobial. Toxicity is severe, and patients require immediate surgical exploration to deep fascia and muscle and subsequent debridement. Crepitus (crackling of the skin due to small bubbles of air moving through the tissues) may be felt in necrotizing fasciitis due to the presence of gas-producing organisms (*Clostridium perfringens*). Necrotizing fasciitis that leaks into the peritoneum is called **Fournier's gangrene. Cellulitis** is an acute inflammatory condition of the skin that causes erythema, pain, and localized swelling. Cellulitis is well demarcated from normal skin. **Erysipelas** is a painful superficial cellulitis of the face. **Folliculitis** is typically due to *Staphylococcus aureus;* patients present with pustules of the hair follicles.

426. The answer is a. *(Tierney, pp 1436–1438.)* **Chloroquine-resistant malaria** is an increasing problem because *Plasmodium vivax* and falciparum malaria may be multidrug resistant. Because of the increasing spread and intensity of plasmodium resistance, the Centers for Disease Control and Prevention recommends a weekly dose of mefloquine for all travelers. Chemoprophylaxis is never entirely reliable, and malaria must always be considered in the differential diagnosis of fever in patients who have traveled to endemic areas. **Trypanosomiasis,** caused by the protozoan *Trypanosoma cruzi*, is a parasite found only in the Americas. Patients present with **Romaña's sign** (unilateral and painless edema of the periocular tissues) and cardiomyopathy (**Chagas disease**). Patients with toxoplasmosis who are immunocompetent are generally asymptomatic and have self-limiting disease.

427. The answer is d. *(Tierney, p 1352.)* For unknown reasons, patients with **S. *bovis* bacteremia** have a high incidence of **colon carcinoma** (and perhaps upper gastrointestinal malignancies as well) and require colonoscopy.

428. The answer is c. *(Seidel, p 239.)* **Cancerous nodes** are usually nontender. The more tender the node, the more likely it is to be due to inflammation. The harder and more discrete the node, the more likely it is to be malignant. A **left supraclavicular node,** since it is located at the end of the thoracic duct, is a clue to gastrointestinal or thoracic malignancy. A **sentinel node** or **Virchow's node** is a firm supraclavicular node. The patient should have a lymph node biopsy.

429. The answer is d. *(Tierney, pp 1417–1419.)* **E. *histolytica*** is the third most common cause of death by parasites worldwide (after schistosomiasis and malaria). Endemic areas include Mexico, India, Central America, South America, tropical Asia, and Africa. Patients may present with fever, right upper quadrant pain, and stools that are FOBT positive. There is no eosinophilia, but alkaline phosphatase is often elevated. Abdominal radiographs (CT scan or MRI) typically show the abscesses.

430. The answer is d. *(Seidel, p 800.)* The patient demonstrates signs of meningeal irritation. She has nuchal rigidity, a positive **Brudzinski's sign** (involuntary flexion of the hips and knees when flexing the neck), and a positive **Kernig's sign** (flexing the hip and knee when the patient is supine, then straightening out the leg, causes resistance and back pain). Other signs of meningitis include headache, photophobia, seizures, and altered mental status. Patients with meningitis (<1%) rarely have papilledema secondary to increased intracranial pressure. Risk factors for meningitis include sinusitis, ear infection, and sick contacts. **Fever of unknown origin (FUO)** is defined as a fever of lower than 38.3°C (101°F) for three weeks that remains undiagnosed after one week of aggressive investigation.

431. The answer is b. *(Tierney, pp 1253–1254.)* Dogs are responsible for 80% of animal bites; organisms include *P. multocida, Eikenella corrodens,* and *Capnocytophaga canimorsus* (**formerly called DF-2**). *A. hydrophila* is the organism seen in bite wounds from alligators and other aquatic animals. **Rabies** is an acute viral disease of the central nervous system and is transmitted by infected dogs, cats, skunks, foxes, raccoons, mongooses, wolves, and bats. *P. aeruginosa* may cause a variety of skin lesions, such as hot tub folliculitis and ecthyma gangrenosum. *V. parahaemolyticus* is an organism found in undercooked shellfish; patients present with diarrhea.

432. The answer is d. *(Tierney, pp 1256–1259.)* The incubation period for both **S. aureus** and **B. cereus** is one to two hours after eating. *B. cereus* toxicity is often due to eating fried (**the toxin is heat-stable**) or uncooked rice. *S. aureus* toxicity is usually due to eating ham, poultry, potato or egg salad, mayonnaise, or cream pastries. All the other organisms require an incubation period of more than 16 hours. *V.* **cholerae** toxicity is due to eating shellfish and causes an inflammatory (presence of fecal leukocytes) diarrhea. *V. parahaemolyticus* toxicity is due to eating mollusks and crustaceans and causes dysentery (production of cytotoxins, bacterial invasion, and destruction of intestinal mucosal cells). *Salmonella* toxicity is due to eating beef, poultry, eggs, or dairy products and causes a watery diarrhea. *Shigella* causes dysentery and can be present in potato or egg salad, lettuce, or raw vegetables.

433. The answer is c. *(Tierney, pp 1256–1259.)* Pathogens that may cause an **inflammatory diarrhea** and produce **fecal leukocytes** include *Shigella, Salmonella, C. jejuni, Yersinia enterocolitica, Clostridium difficile, Vibrio parahaemolyticus,* enterohemorrhagic *Escherichia coli,* and enteroinvasive *E. coli.*

434. The answer is c. *(Tierney, p 474.)* The geographic distribution of **glucose-6-phosphate dehydrogenase (G6PD) deficiency,** sickle cell disease, sickle cell trait, and thalassemia resembles that of malaria, and having one of these disorders affords protection against *P. falciparum.*

435. The answer is a. *(Tierney, pp 1585–1586.)* The most likely pathogen responsible for the symptoms is **ciguatera poison,** which is found in the Caribbean, Hawaii, and Florida and is associated with consumption of carnivorous reef fish such as grouper or barracuda. **Scromboid poisoning** is associated with consumption of tuna, mackerel, and dolphin; patients present with flushing, headache, dizziness, palpitations, nausea, diarrhea, and vomiting (due to histidine release). **Traveler's diarrhea** is predominantly due to enterotoxigenic *Escherichia coli;* patients develop the symptoms within three to five days of arriving in a tropical area. **Pseudomembranous colitis** is a nosocomial infection due to *Clostridium difficile;* patients often have a previous history of antibiotic use. **M. marinum** is an organism of swimming pools and fish tanks that produces a pustule or nodule at the site of minor trauma.

436. The answer is e. *(Tierney, pp 527–528.)* **H. pylori** is associated with gastritis, duodenal ulcer, gastric ulcer, non-Hodgkin's gastric lymphoma, adenocarcinoma of the stomach, and mucosa-associated tissue lymphomas (**MALT**).

437. The answer is b. *(Tierney, pp 830–832.)* **Osteomyelitis** is usually a polymicrobial infection, but *S. aureus* is the pathogen in over 50% of all cases. Patients with sickle cell disease are at risk of developing *Salmonella* **osteomyelitis** (>50% of all cases). **Pott's disease** is spinal tuberculosis; it usually involves the upper thoracic vertebral bodies.

438–441. The answers are 438-b, 439-d, 440-e, 441-g. *(Tierney, pp 1480–1481.)* **Trichinosis** is caused by the ingestion of infected pork products. Patients present with abdominal pain, diarrhea, a maculopapular rash, periorbital edema, myositis (especially of the extraocular muscles), eosinophilia, and myocarditis. **A. castellanii** is associated with contact lens usage. **Brucellosis** is transmitted through infected milk or raw meat or inhaled during contact with animals (i.e., by slaughterhouse workers, veterinarians, and farmers). Patients present with fever, chills, ophthalmoplegia, joint pain, skin rash, lymphadenopathy, hepatosplenomegaly, cardiac murmur, endocarditis, and meningitis. **Cysticercosis** is associated with the pork tapeworm (***Taenia solium***); patients commonly present with neurologic manifestations, such as seizures and signs of increased intracranial pressure. CT scan of the head often shows the multiple calcified lesions of varying size common in neurocysticercosis. **G. lamblia** may be asymptomatic or may cause severe diarrhea and malabsorption. Transmission is usually waterborne (i.e., camping sites, sewers, reservoirs), since the cysts survive both cold water and routine chlorination. **C. psittaci** is associated with bird exposure; patients present with fever, cough, chest pain, dyspnea, pleural effusion, pleural rub, pericardial effusion, and pneumonia. Patients with **C. tetani** present with an infected wound, muscle spasms, and increased muscle tone, especially of the masseter muscles (**lockjaw**).

442–443. The answers are 442-b, 443-a. (*Tierney, pp 1491–1492.*) Patients with HIV may develop **cryptococcal meningitis.** Patients present with headache, irritability, confusion, ataxia, blurred vision, papilledema, and cranial nerve palsies. Fever and neck stiffness are rare. India ink smear of the spinal fluid will demonstrate the encapsulated yeast. Lesions of **toxoplasmosis** are usually multiple and ring-enhancing (lymphomas in HIV patients may also be multiple and ring-enhancing, so this description is not pathognomonic for toxoplasmosis). **PML** is a progressive disorder due to **JC virus.** The disorder is one of demyelination; patients present with visual deficits, mental impairment, and motor deficits. CT scan or MRI may show the hypodense, nonenhancing white-matter lesions. Patients with **HIV dementia** present with apathy, hyperreflexia, clumsiness, weakness, ataxia, and loss of memory.

Obstetrics and Gynecology

Questions

DIRECTIONS: Each item below contains a question followed by suggested responses. Select the **one best** response to each question.

444. A 23-year-old woman presents with fever and bilateral lower quadrant abdominal pain for two days. She complains of the onset of a mucopurulent vaginal discharge with her menses, which she states is yellowish in color. She has a new sexual partner and uses a nonbarrier method of contraception. Her temperature is 39.5°C (103.2°F). She has bilateral lower quadrant tenderness with palpation, and pelvic examination reveals cervical and adnexal motion tenderness. A mass is palpable in the left adnexa. Which of the following is the most likely diagnosis?

a. Fitz-Hugh–Curtis syndrome
b. Pelvic inflammatory disease
c. Perihepatitis
d. Acute inflammation of Bartholin's gland
e. Chancroid

445. A 37-year-old woman in her thirty-second week of gestation (G2P1) presents with a seizure. She has been healthy and does not smoke cigarettes, drink alcohol, or use illicit drugs. She has been poorly compliant in receiving her prenatal care. Physical examination reveals a blood pressure of 150/95 mmHg. The patient's face and hands appear edematous. Other than the patient being postictal (confused and disoriented after the seizure), the neurologic examination is normal. The urinalysis reveals proteinuria. The rest of the patient's laboratory data are normal. Which of the following is the most likely diagnosis?

a. HELLP syndrome
b. Preeclampsia
c. Eclampsia
d. Essential hypertension
e. Primary seizure disorder

446. A 20-year-old woman presents with the sudden onset of severe lower abdominal pain that radiates to her left shoulder. She has some vaginal bleeding now, but her last menstrual period was six weeks ago. She has no history of sexually transmitted diseases and has never been pregnant. She uses condoms inconsistently, about 50% of the time, with her partner of 18 months. She denies dysuria or frequency. On physical examination, blood pressure is 100/70 mmHg, heart rate is 100 beats per minute, and temperature is normal. Abdominal exam reveals tenderness and rebound in the left lower quadrant. Adler's sign is positive. Pelvic examination reveals a boggy and poorly delineated mass in the left adnexa. The patient's abdominal pain worsens upon slight movement of the cervix. Which of the following is the most likely diagnosis?

a. Pelvic inflammatory disease
b. Pyelonephritis
c. Appendicitis
d. Ectopic pregnancy
e. Ruptured corpus luteum cyst

447. A 53-year old G2P2 woman complains of irregular, prolonged, and heavy menstrual bleeding. She thinks she is going through menopause and has occasional hot flashes and palpitations. She has no weight loss. She has never taken oral contraceptives or hormone therapy. Her last Pap smear two years ago was normal. Pelvic examination reveals blood at the cervical os but is otherwise normal. Which of the following is the most appropriate next step in management?

a. Repeat Pap smear
b. Colposcopy
c. Hormone replacement therapy
d. Endometrial sampling
e. Reassurance
f. Follow-up reexamination in six months

448. A 24-year-old woman, G3P2, presents with the chief complaint of some lower abdominal pain accompanied by a small amount of vaginal bleeding. She is 16 weeks' pregnant and has been healthy throughout the pregnancy. She does not smoke cigarettes, drink alcohol, or use illicit drugs. Abdominal examination is normal. Pelvic examination reveals that the internal cervical os is closed. Which of the following is the most likely diagnosis?

a. Complete abortion
b. Incomplete abortion
c. Threatened abortion
d. Inevitable abortion
e. Missed abortion

449. A 42-year-old woman, G2P2, presents with the chief complaint of severe bilateral breast pain that seems to be worse around the time of menses. Physical examination reveals bilateral breast tenderness with palpation. Multiple lumps are palpated in both breasts. Mammogram reveals dense bilateral breast tissue. Which of the following is the most likely diagnosis in this patient?

a. Fibroadenoma
b. Fibrocystic disease
c. Paget's disease
d. Mastitis
e. Mammary duct ectasia

450. A 32-year-old woman in her third trimester presents with painless and profuse bright red vaginal bleeding. Pelvic examination is deferred. Transvaginal ultrasonography reveals an abnormally positioned placenta. Which of the following is the most likely diagnosis?

a. Placenta accreta
b. Placenta previa
c. Abruptio placentae
d. Bloody show
e. Vasa previa

451. A 52-year-old woman complains of recurrent episodes in which she becomes extremely hot and diaphoretic. During these episodes, she becomes anxious and feels like her heart is racing. Each episode lasts approximately five minutes. The episodes are so intense that she must put on the air conditioner or open a window until the episode resolves. Hot weather and stress often precipitate the symptoms. The episodes seem to be worse at night. The patient further states that she has been amenorrheic for 12 months and has recently begun experiencing vaginal dryness and dyspareunia. Physical examination is normal. Which of the following is the most likely diagnosis?

a. Depression
b. Menopause
c. Hypothyroidism
d. Somatization
e. Personality disorder

452. A 30-year-old woman in her thirty-sixth week of gestation (G1P0) presents with a platelet count of 85,000/μL. She has no complaints of easy bruisability or mucosal bleeding and feels healthy. She has no past illnesses and takes no medications. She has no family history of bleeding problems. Laboratory data reveal a normal complete blood count, prothrombin time, and partial thromboplastin time. Liver enzymes and urinalysis are normal. Peripheral blood smear reveals normal morphology of red blood cells and platelets. Which of the following is the most likely diagnosis?

a. Idiopathic thrombocytopenic purpura (ITP)
b. Pseudothrombocytopenia
c. Gestational thrombocytopenia
d. HELLP syndrome
e. Thrombotic thrombocytopenic purpura (TTP)
f. Hemolytic-uremic syndrome (HUS)

453. As you are performing the external portion of a pelvic examination, you palpate a warm, fluctuant mass that is unilateral in the posterolateral portion of the labia majora. The patient states that palpation is painful. The surrounding tissue is inflamed and edematous. Which of the following is the most likely diagnosis?

a. Bartholin's cyst
b. Bartholin's abscess
c. Rectocele
d. Cystocele
e. Genital herpes

454. A 64-year-old woman presents with vaginal bleeding similar to spotting that has occurred daily for one month. Her last menses was at age 50 and she has been healthy her entire life. She denies fever, weight loss, or abdominal pain. Physical examination is normal. Which of the following is the most likely diagnosis?

a. Atrophic vaginitis
b. Endometriosis
c. Uterine leiomyoma
d. Endometrial carcinoma
e. Polycystic ovarian syndrome

455. A 29-year-old woman in her first trimester presents with painless profuse vaginal bleeding. Her blood pressure is 130/90 mmHg. She has facial and hand edema. Pelvic examination reveals a 24-week-sized uterus. Urinalysis reveals proteinuria. Which of the following is the most likely diagnosis?

a. Placenta previa
b. Abruptio placenta
c. Hydatidiform mole
d. Normal pregnancy
e. Multiple-gestation pregnancy

456. A 23-year-old woman presents to your office for a prenatal visit. She has not received any previous prenatal care and does not know the date of her last menstrual period. On physical examination, the fundal height is palpated to be at the level of the umbilicus. Which of the following is the estimated number of weeks of gestation?

a. 10
b. 15
c. 20
d. 25
e. 30

DIRECTIONS: Each group of questions below consists of lettered options followed by a set of numbered items. For each numbered item, select the **one** lettered option with which it is **most** closely associated. Each lettered option may be used once, more than once, or not at all.

Questions 457–459

For each patient with a vaginal finding, select the most likely causative organism.

a. *Trichomonas vaginalis*
b. *Neisseria gonorrhoeae*
c. *Gardnerella vaginalis*
d. *Candida albicans*
e. *Chlamydia trachomatis*
f. *Enterobius vermicularis*

457. A 19-year-old woman presents with a malodorous, watery, gray-colored vaginal discharge. Clue cells are visible on wet-mount preparation, and there is a fishy odor to the discharge when mixed with potassium hydroxide (KOH).

458. A 35-year-old woman presents with vaginal itching. Examination reveals strawberry patches or petechiae on the cervix and vaginal mucosa and a frothy green-colored discharge. A pear-shaped organism is visible on wet-mount preparation.

459. A 31-year-old woman presents with vaginal burning and a white, cheeselike vaginal discharge. Pseudohyphae are visible with a KOH preparation.

Questions 460–464

For each patient with a breast finding, select the most likely diagnosis.

a. Breast cancer
b. Paget's disease of the breast
c. Inflammatory breast carcinoma
d. Intraductal papilloma
e. Fibroadenoma

460. A 25-year-old woman presents with a palpable breast mass that has well-defined margins and is moveable.

461. A 50-year-old woman presents with a hard, circumscribed, fixed, edematous breast mass. The overlying skin has a peau d'orange (orange peel) appearance.

462. A 52-year-old woman presents with bloody discharge from her right nipple. She has no palpable breast mass.

463. A 36-year-old woman has erythema and a visible erysipeloid margin of her left breast. The involved area is warm and tender to palpation.

464. A 39-year-old woman presents with eczematoid changes of her left breast, which occasionally itches, burns, oozes an exudate, and bleeds.

Obstetrics and Gynecology

Answers

444. The answer is b. (*Tierney, pp 718–719.*) The patient most likely has **pelvic inflammatory disease** (**PID**) due to *Neisseria gonorrhoeae.* Infections typically occur during menstruation, and patients complain of abdominal pain and yellow mucopurulent vaginal discharge. Spread of the gonococci (or, in some cases, *Chlamydia*) into the upper abdomen may cause a perihepatitis, or **Fitz-Hugh–Curtis syndrome;** patients will complain of upper abdominal pain and may have an audible **hepatic rub.** Acute inflammation of Bartholin's gland (an infected duct) would be visible in the labium majus. **Chancroid** is due to *Haemophilus ducreyi;* patients typically present with a painful ulcer that bleeds easily.

445. The answer is c. (*Tierney, pp 747–749.*) **Preeclampsia** is defined as hypertension, proteinuria (>300 mg/24 h), and/or nondependent edema of the face and hands. **Risk factors** for preeclampsia include African American race, nulliparity, multiple gestations, extremes of age (<15 or >35), chronic hypertension, and a family history positive for preeclampsia. **Eclampsia** is defined as seizures in a patient with preeclampsia. The cure for preeclampsia/eclampsia is delivery. Magnesium sulfate is often used for seizure prophylaxis and management. The **HELLP syndrome** (**H**emolysis, **E**levated **L**iver enzymes, **L**ow **P**latelets) is a variant of preeclampsia.

446. The answer is d. (*Tierney, pp 745–746.*) The incidence of **ectopic pregnancy** (outside the uterine cavity) is 1 in 100 pregnancies. Risk factors include previous history of PID or ectopic pregnancy, use of an intrauterine device (IUD), DES exposure, and prior pelvic surgery. Patients present with abdominal pain that may radiate to the shoulder (indicating irritation of the diaphragm from the hemoperitoneum), vaginal bleeding, cervical motion tenderness (CMT), and the presence of a boggy and poorly delineated pelvic mass one to eight weeks after a missed period. The patient may have other symptoms of pregnancy, such as nausea, vomiting, and breast tenderness. If the ectopic pregnancy ruptures, the patient may present with signs of shock. **Adler's sign** is the presence of fixed abdominal tenderness on turning the patient and may be seen in ectopic pregnancy. A ruptured corpus luteum cyst causes a tender ovary but no palpable mass. PID causes fever and bilateral lower quadrant pain and tenderness. Appendicitis involves right-sided pain. Pelvic examination is typically normal in appendicitis and pyelonephritis.

447. The answer is d. *(Seidel, p 641.)* The patient has **menometrorrhagia**, which is prolonged and heavy menstrual bleeding that occurs at irregular intervals. Even though this may be seen with menopause, an endometrial sampling is necessary to exclude endometrial carcinoma. **Menorrhagia** is excessive or prolonged menses. **Metrorrhagia** or intermenstrual bleeding occurs at any time between menstrual periods. **Polymenorrhea** is increased frequency of menstruation, and oligomenorrhea is scanty menstruation.

448. The answer is c. *(Tierney, p 744.)* **Threatened abortion, incomplete abortion, complete abortion,** and **inevitable abortion** all present with vaginal bleeding and occur at **less than 20 weeks** of gestation. Patients with **threatened abortion** complain of abdominal pain and vaginal bleeding. The membranes remain intact and no products of conception are expelled. The internal cervical os is closed and the fetus is viable. The internal cervical os is open and some products of conception are expelled in **incomplete abortion.** In **complete abortion,** all products of conception are expelled and the internal cervical os is closed. **Inevitable abortion** is when the membranes rupture, the internal cervical os is open, and no products of conception are expelled. Patients complain of abdominal cramps in inevitable abortion. **Missed abortion** is retained fetal tissue with no cardiac activity in a uterus that is not growing. There is no vaginal bleeding, no products of conception are expelled, and the internal cervical os is closed.

449. The answer is b. *(Seidel, pp 519–524.)* Women between the ages of 30 and 55 may develop benign cyst formation of the breasts or **fibrocystic breast disease.** Patients typically state that the symptoms worsen premenstrually or as they approach menopause (**decreased progesterone**). Physical examination often reveals bilateral lumpy and tender breasts. Mammography shows dense breast tissue. **Mastitis** is most common in lactating breasts and is usually secondary to *Staphylococcus aureus* infection.

The breast is warm, tender, swollen, and erythematous. **Mammary duct ectasia** is a nonmalignant condition that affects menopausal women. The subareolar ducts become blocked with debris, causing pain, inflammation, nipple discharge, and retraction of the nipple. A **fibroadenoma** is a benign neoplasm found in young women. They are usually round, rubbery, moveable, and nontender.

450. The answer is b. *(Tierney, p 750.)* **Placenta previa** and **abruptio placenta** are the two most common causes of third-trimester bleeding. **Placenta previa** is abnormal implantation of placenta near or at the cervical os, and may be total, partial, marginal, or low-lying. **Risk factors** for placenta previa include advanced maternal age, multiparity, smoking history, and prior cesarean section. Patients present at 30 weeks of gestation with painless vaginal bleeding. There is no fetal distress. Vaginal examination is contraindicated, and sonogram is required to make the diagnosis. **Abruptio placentae** is premature separation of a normally implanted placenta. Patients present with painful (unremitting abdominal and back pain) vaginal bleeding, and there is fetal distress. **Risk factors** for abruptio placentae include advanced maternal age, multiparity, diabetes, hypertension, tobacco use, alcohol use, and cocaine use. **Placenta accreta** is a placenta that adheres to the myometrium without an intervening decidual layer; it is associated with postpartum hemorrhage. In **vasa previa,** the fetal vessels associated with the cord traverse the lower uterine segment and present in advance of the fetal presenting part, causing rapid bleeding when disrupted during labor. **Bloody show** is a blood-tinged vaginal discharge that occurs when the cervix is dilated and the onset of labor is imminent.

451. The answer is b. *(Tierney, pp 736–737.)* The patient is presenting with symptoms of normal **menopause,** which may include hot flashes, urinary frequency, dysuria, urinary incontinence, vaginal dryness, vaginal itchiness, and dyspareunia. Patients also have amenorrhea. Patients may become anxious or depressed during this time, but there is no evidence that personality or mood changes are due to menopause.

452. The answer is c. *(Tierney, pp 747–748.)* **Gestational thrombocytopenia** develops in the last trimester of pregnancy (in 8% of pregnant women) and is reversible after delivery. It is difficult to differentiate between gestational thrombocytopenia and ITP, but ITP will persist after delivery. The **HELLP** (**H**emolysis, **E**levated **L**iver enzymes, **L**ow **P**latelet count) syndrome, a variant of preeclampsia, is unlikely in this patient with no evidence of hemolysis and normal liver enzymes. Immediate delivery is the treatment for HELLP syndrome. **Pseudothrombocytopenia** occurs when platelets aggregate in laboratory test tubes, giving falsely decreased platelet counts. Careful inspection of the peripheral smear will show the aggregates. TTP is unlikely, since the patient does not have the pentad of symptoms seen in 40% of patients (**FAT R.N.** = **F**ever, **A**utoimmune hemolytic anemia, **T**hrombocytopenia, **R**enal disease, **N**eurologic disease). **HUS** presents with three of the five symptoms seen in TTP (**RAT** = **R**enal disease, **A**utoimmune hemolytic anemia, and **T**hrombocytopenia). TTP and HUS are unlikely in this patient without kidney involvement.

453. The answer is b. (*Seidel, pp 638–640.*) Obstruction of the main duct of **Bartholin's gland** results in retention of secretions (cyst) and secondary infection (abscess). Abscesses are generally painful to palpation, hot to the touch, and fluctuant. A **rectocele** is a weakness in the fascia of the posterior vaginal wall in which the rectum appears as a bulging mass. A **cystocele** is a protrusion of the bladder into the anterior vaginal wall. Asking the patient to bear down will enhance these protrusions and make them more easily seen.

454. The answer is a. (*Tierney, p 706.*) The most common cause of postmenopausal vaginal bleeding is **atrophic vaginitis** (with or without trauma). **Endometriosis** is the most common cause of infertility; patients present with dyspareunia (painful intercourse), abnormal vaginal bleeding, and pelvic pain. **Uterine leiomyomas** (uterine fibroids) change in size with the menstrual cycle but regress in size during menopause. Often, the fibroid is palpable on pelvic examination. Polycystic ovarian syndrome (**Stein-Leventhal syndrome**) affects younger women (age 15 to 30). The etiology of polycystic ovary syndrome is unknown; patients present with amenorrhea, obesity, hirsutism, and infertility. All postmenopausal women with vaginal bleeding require a **biopsy** to rule out endometrial carcinoma.

455. The answer is c. (*Tierney, pp 749–750.*) Malignant gestational trophoblastic neoplasms include the tumors of **hydatidiform mole, invasive mole,** and **choriocarcinoma.** These tumors arise from **fetal tissue,** not maternal tissue. Patients present with first-trimester vaginal bleeding and signs of preeclampsia (pathognomonic for hydatidiform mole). Typically, patients have increased β-**hCG titers** (greater than expected for gestational age) and rapid enlargement of the uterus (greater than anticipated by dates) with absence of fetal heart sounds and structures. The **cluster of grapes** appearance of the mole makes it easily identifiable on gross examination (**snowstorm** appearance on ultrasonography). Rarely, patients with hydatidiform moles may present with **hyperthyroidism** due to the production of thyrotropin by the molar tissue.

456. The answer is c. *(Seidel, p 623.)* At 20 weeks of pregnancy, fundal height is at the level of the umbilicus. Part of the obstetrics and gynecology history should include **GPAL** (**G**eorgia **P**ower **A**nd **L**ight): **G**ravida, **P**ara, **A**bortions, and **L**iving children.

457–459. The answers are 457-c, 458-a, 459-d. *(Tierney, pp 707–709.)* **G. vaginalis** (the most common cause of vaginitis) causes a profuse, malodorous discharge. Wet-mount preparation will demonstrate clue cells (epithelial cells with adherent bacteria that cause their borders to be irregular), and a KOH preparation will reveal the discharge to have a **fishy odor** (**positive sniff or whiff test**). **Candida** produces a thick, white, cottage-cheese-appearing discharge, and KOH preparation will reveal the characteristic **pseudohyphae.** Ten percent of patients with **Trichomonas** will have a **strawberry-appearing** cervix or vaginal mucosa. The vaginal discharge may be green and is often described as frothy. The trichomonal flagellates are characteristically motile and pear-shaped. A vaginal discharge with leukocytes but no organisms is characteristic of *Chlamydia. E. vermicularis* (pinworms) may cause pruritus of the perineum. The diagnosis is made by applying scotch tape to the perineum, then to a slide; looking microscopically will reveal the characteristic double-walled ova of the parasite.

460–464. The answers are 460-e, 461-a, 462-d, 463-c, 464-b. *(Tierney, pp 679–685.)* Most **breast cancers** present in the upper outer quadrant of the breast; patients may present with a hard, circumscribed mass that is fixed to the skin or deep muscle. Cancer may be nodular with indistinct borders. Patients may also have nipple edema or retraction. A woman under the age of 30 years presenting with a mobile breast mass that has well-defined borders most likely has a fibroadenoma. However, breast cancer must still be ruled out since clinical exam and even mammography are not sufficient to exclude the diagnosis. **Intraductal papilloma** is a benign tumor; patients often present with a bloody discharge from the nipple in the absence of a breast mass. Patients who present with an erythematous and warm breast (which eventually becomes indurated and firm) may have **inflammatory breast carcinoma.** Patients with **Paget's disease** classically present with eczematoid changes in the nipple (i.e., itching, oozing, and bleeding), all of which occur over a relatively long period of time. Mammography may be negative, and biopsy is required to make the diagnosis.

Pediatrics and Neonatology

Questions

DIRECTIONS: Each item below contains a question followed by suggested responses. Select the **one best** response to each question.

465. An 18-month-old boy is brought to the pediatrician because of progressively worsening episodes of cyanosis. The child has moments when he turns blue and becomes dyspneic. During these episodes the child becomes irritable and remains in a squatting position. Physical examination reveals a small and thin child with clubbing of the fingers and toes. Lungs are normal. Heart auscultation reveals a right ventricular (RV) lift and a grade 3/4 harsh systolic ejection murmur at the upper left sternal border. Which of the following is the most likely diagnosis?

a. Transposition of the great vessels (TOGV)
b. Tetralogy of Fallot (TOF)
c. Truncus arteriosus
d. Tricuspid atresia
e. Total anomalous pulmonary venous return

466. A 3-year-old boy is brought to the emergency room with lethargy, irritability, and ataxia. The child often complains of diffuse abdominal pain and is constipated. On physical examination, the tongue size is normal but a black line is visible along the gingiva. Peripheral smear reveals basophilic stippling of the red blood cells. Which of the following is the most likely diagnosis?

a. Porphyria
b. Kernicterus
c. Fragile X syndrome
d. Lead poisoning
e. Cretinism

467. A grammar school is going to start screening children for scoliosis and has asked for your recommendations regarding testing. Which of the following is the most appropriate screening test for this purpose?

a. Growth charts
b. Lateral radiograph of the thoracic spine
c. Forward bending test
d. MRI of the thoracic spine
e. Ortolani test

468. A 4-year-old boy is brought to the emergency room complaining of left ear pain that awakened him from sleep. The child has no past medical history and has been in good health. During the physical examination, the child is irritable and often tugs at his left ear. His temperature is 38.6°C (101.5°F), and he has no lymphadenopathy. The left tympanic membrane is bulging and erythematous. Which of the following is the most likely diagnosis?

a. Perforation of the eardrum
b. Serous otitis media
c. Acute otitis media
d. Acute mastoiditis
e. Foreign body in the ear

469. The mother of an 11-month-old infant is concerned because her child is easily startled by slight noise and cannot sit alone without assistance. On physical examination, the child does not seem to respond to visual cues and is extremely hypotonic. Funduscopic examination reveals a macular cherry red spot. Which of the following is the most likely diagnosis?

a. Pompe's disease
b. Tay-Sachs disease
c. Adrenoleukodystrophy
d. Phenylketonuria
e. Cerebral palsy
f. Dandy-Walker malformation

470. A 2-year-old boy presents with a barking cough and fever. The cough started suddenly in the middle of the night. On physical examination, the patient's temperature is 38.6°C (101.5°F), and he appears frightened and anxious. He has a heart rate of 160 beats per minute and a respiratory rate of 36 breaths per minute. His breathing is labored, and he is using his accessory muscles of respiration. Marked inspiratory stridor is audible. Lung examination is unremarkable. Which of the following is the most likely diagnosis?

a. Epiglottitis
b. Peritonsillar abscess
c. Croup
d. Asthma
e. Bronchiolitis

471. A 2-year-old boy is having difficulty breathing. The mother states that he has had a cough since birth and that this visit to the emergency room is one of many for her sickly son. The neonatal history reveals that the boy did not defecate for some time after delivery. The growth chart reveals that the child is in the fifth percentile. Which of the following is the most helpful test to order in this patient?

a. HIV antibody test
b. Sweat test
c. Urine toxicology screen
d. Lead level
e. MRI of the head

472. A 6-year-old girl is brought to your office by her parents, who believe that the child has been having brief episodes of unresponsiveness with fluttering of the eyelids and lip smacking. The child's schoolteacher has recently sent home a note stating that the girl is "daydreaming" in class and is often inattentive. Physical examination is normal, but at least twice during the examination, the child appears to look blank or be dazed for 20 to 30 seconds. Which of the following is the most likely diagnosis?

a. Atonic seizure
b. Absence seizure
c. Neonatal seizure
d. Focal seizure
e. Tardive dyskinesia
f. Psychomotor seizure

473. A 6-week-old girl is constantly coughing. She is afebrile and began coughing about 10 days ago with increasing regularity. Delivery was uncomplicated, but when the girl was 10 days old a mild conjunctivitis developed, which responded well to topical antibiotics. On physical examination, respiratory rate is 55 breaths per minute, and the infant is breathing by using the accessory muscles of respiration. Lung auscultation reveals bilateral diffuse crackles. A chest radiograph reveals a bilateral diffuse interstitial infiltrate. Which of the following is the most likely diagnosis?

a. Chlamydial pneumonia
b. Pertussis
c. Respiratory syncytial viral (RSV) pneumonia
d. Foreign body aspiration
e. *Pneumocystis carinii* pneumonia (PCP)

474. A mother brings her infant son to your office for a well-baby checkup. On physical examination, you see that the boy's optic fundus is positive for a white reflex. Which of the following is the most likely cause of the white reflex?

a. Retinoblastoma
b. Retinocerebellar angioma
c. Choroidal angioma
d. Primary congenital glaucoma
e. Papilledema

475. A 9-month-old child is brought to the emergency room by her parents. They report that the child has been irritable for the last several days and progressively lethargic. The infant vomited several times in the car on the way to the hospital. The parents state that the infant has not previously been ill. They deny any history of trauma or accidental ingestion of medication or poisons. On physical examination, the child is lethargic and difficult to arouse. Her vital signs are normal. There is no evidence of external trauma, but retinal hemorrhages are visible on funduscopic examination. Her fontanel is bulging. Which of the following is the most likely diagnosis?

a. Bacterial meningitis
b. Oligodendroglioma
c. DiGeorge's syndrome
d. Fetal alcohol syndrome
e. Shaken baby syndrome

476. A 4-hour-old full-term newborn had been doing well until the staff in the nursery attempted to feed her. The girl became cyanotic during the feeding challenge but improved with crying when the attempt to feed was discontinued. Which of the following is the most likely diagnosis?

a. Hyaline membrane disease
b. Choanal atresia
c. Meconium aspiration
d. Tracheal-esophageal fistula
e. Tracheomalacia

477. A 10-year-old girl presents with several light brown maculae, each greater than 1 cm in diameter, on her trunk. Physical examination reveals axillary freckling and firm subcutaneous masses. Which of the following is the most likely diagnosis?

a. Von Hippel-Lindau syndrome
b. Tuberous sclerosis
c. Meningioma
d. Craniopharyngioma
e. Neurofibromatosis type 1

478. An 8-year-old girl presents with the acute onset of swelling of her hands, feet, legs, and face. Her past medical history is significant for a recent upper respiratory tract infection. Physical examination reveals normal vital signs. The patient has clear lungs but has pitting edema up to her sacrum. Heart examination is normal. Urinalysis reveals severe proteinuria (4+). Which of the following is the most likely diagnosis?

a. Rapidly progressive glomerulonephritis (RPGN)
b. Membranoproliferative glomerulonephritis (MPGN)
c. Minimal change disease
d. Focal glomerulosclerosis
e. Membranous nephropathy

479. A 3-year-old boy with a four-day history of upper respiratory tract infection presents to the emergency room for evaluation of pallor and fatigue. Physical examination reveals a pale child with normal vital signs. He has scattered petechiae on the chest and extremities and a palpable spleen tip. Laboratory data reveal a leukocytosis (white blood cell count of >30,000/μL). Hemoglobin is 7.4 gm/dL, and platelet count is 50,000/μL. The peripheral blood smear reveals the presence of blasts. Which of the following is the most likely diagnosis?

a. Acute lymphoblastic leukemia
b. Acute nonlymphocytic leukemia
c. Chronic lymphocytic leukemia
d. Acute myelogenous leukemia
e. Chronic myelogenous leukemia
f. Atypical lymphocytosis

480. Physical examination of a newborn female reveals that a posterior hip dislocation occurs when a posterior force is applied while flexing and adducting the hip. This positive maneuver for the diagnosis of congenital hip dislocation is called which of the following?

a. Ortolani maneuver
b. Trendelenburg's sign
c. Allis's sign
d. Barlow maneuver
e. Galeazzi's sign

481. A 7-year-old girl comes to the emergency room with fever, sore throat, and noisy breathing. She has no cough. On physical examination, she appears ill and speaks with a hoarse voice. She has obvious difficulty swallowing and is febrile, with a temperature of 39.9°C (103.8°F). Her pulse is 120 beats per minute and her respiratory rate is 18 breaths per minute. Her blood pressure is normal. She is drooling and prefers to remain in a sitting position, leaning forward with her mouth open. She has no palpable lymphadenopathy. Which of the following is the most likely diagnosis?

a. Exudative pharyngitis
b. Epiglottitis
c. Croup
d. Diphtheria
e. Peritonsillar abscess

482. A 4-month-old child is brought to the emergency room because of a swollen scrotum. On physical examination, the child is afebrile. The scrotum is distended but not taut. A mass is palpable that is firm, smooth, and nontender. The mass transilluminates with a penlight. Which of the following is the most likely diagnosis?

a. Inguinal hernia
b. Spermatocele
c. Varicocele
d. Hydrocele
e. Cryptorchidism

483. A 5-week-old infant is brought to the pediatrician for a well-baby visit. The mother states that the child has been healthy. Physical examination reveals no cyanosis and no clubbing. Palpation of the heart reveals a systolic thrill, and auscultation reveals a grade 4/6 pansystolic murmur heard best at the lower left sternal border. S_2 is loud but not split. Which of the following is the most likely diagnosis?

a. Atrial septal defect
b. Patent ductus arteriosus
c. Ventricular septal defect (VSD)
d. Eisenmenger's syndrome
e. Endocarditis

484. A 13-year-old boy, who has recently recovered from an upper respiratory tract infection, presents to the emergency room with lethargy, vomiting, and delirium. While being transported to the emergency room, the boy has a seizure. On physical examination, the child is jaundiced and has hepatomegaly. He has no focal deficits on neurologic examination but is comatose. Which of the following is the most likely diagnosis?

a. Reye's syndrome
b. Wilson's disease
c. West Nile encephalitis
d. Viral hepatitis
e. Botulism

485. A 1-year-old boy is brought to the emergency room because of the passage of several maroon-colored stools per rectum. Abdominal exam reveals normal bowel sounds and no masses. Which of the following is the most likely diagnosis?

a. Biliary atresia
b. Intussusception
c. Meckel's diverticulum
d. Zenker's diverticulum
e. Pyloric stenosis

486. A 9-year-old girl is brought into your office by her mother, who states that the daughter has been losing weight and having difficulty at school. The mother discovered some yellow-colored discharge on the child's underwear. On physical examination, you notice erythema of all parts of the patient's vulva and the vagina. There is some yellow discharge visible. Which of the following is the most likely diagnosis?

a. Müllerian duct tumor
b. Wolffian duct tumor
c. Dermatitis
d. Sexual abuse
e. Straddle injury

487. A 10-year-old child presents with a confluence of pustular and vesicular lesions on the hands and face, some of which have ruptured and expressed a serous exudate. They appear to be honey colored. A Tzanck preparation is negative for multinucleated giant cells, but a Gram stain is significant for gram-positive cocci. Which of the following is the most likely diagnosis?

a. Folliculitis
b. Kawasaki's disease
c. Staphylococcal scalded skin syndrome
d. Miliaria
e. Impetigo

488. A 2-year-old boy presents with progressive clumsiness and difficulty walking. Physical examination reveals that the child has large calves. He has difficulty walking on his toes and has a waddling gait. Gower maneuver is positive. Which of the following is the most likely diagnosis?

a. Becker muscular dystrophy
b. Myotonic dystrophy
c. Facioscapulohumeral dystrophy
d. Duchenne muscular dystrophy

489. A 6-year-old boy has a history of corneal opacities and relapsing polyneuropathy. Physical examination reveals the presence of large, orange-colored tonsils. The patient's serum cholesterol is low, but his triglyceride level is normal. Which of the following is the most likely diagnosis in this patient?

a. Malnutrition
b. Malabsorption
c. Exudative pharyngitis
d. HIV infection
e. Myeloproliferative disorder
f. Tangier disease

490. A 3-year-old child presents to the emergency room with dysuria and hematuria for one day. The mother states that the child has been losing weight and has been complaining of nausea and vomiting. Vital signs reveal a blood pressure of 135/85 mmHg and a temperature of 38.9°C (102°F). Palpation of the abdomen reveals a mass that extends to the left flank. Which of the following is the most likely diagnosis?

a. Neuroblastoma
b. Ewing's sarcoma
c. Wilms tumor
d. Rhabdomyosarcoma
e. Hodgkin's lymphoma

DIRECTIONS: Each group of questions below consists of lettered options followed by a set of numbered items. For each numbered item, select the **one** lettered option with which it is **most** closely associated. Each lettered option may be used once, more than once, or not at all.

Questions 491–492

For each child with a rash, select the most likely diagnosis.

a. Rubeola
b. Rubella
c. Varicella
d. Roseola

491. An 8-year-old child experiences a sudden onset of vesicles beginning first on the face and scalp and then spreading to the trunk and extremities. Some vesicles have evolved into pustules and crusts. The lesions are extremely pruritic. Two weeks ago, the child visited a nursing home on a school field trip.

492. A 1-year-old infant presents with a high fever for four days. Today the child is afebrile but developed a blanchable, maculopapular rash over the trunk and neck. The child appears remarkably well.

Pediatrics and Neonatology

Answers

465. The answer is b. *(Behrman, pp 1523–1528.)* The five congenital heart disorders listed in the answer (**the five T's**) cause right-to-left shunts and subsequent cyanosis. Tetralogy of Fallot is the most common type of cyanotic heart lesion and consists of **P**ulmonary stenosis, **R**VH, an **O**verriding aorta, and ventricular septal defect, or **V**SD (**PROV**). Children present with dyspnea, cyanosis after the neonatal period, irritability, easy fatigability, and retarded growth and development. Physical examination may reveal an RV lift, a murmur of VSD, and clubbing. The cyanosis of tetralogy is often relieved by increasing venous return to the heart by the knee-chest position (**squatting or tet spells**). Chest radiograph may reveal a **boot-shaped heart due to RVH.** Children with transposition of the great vessels (aorta connected to RV and pulmonary artery connected to LV), tricuspid atresia (no communication between RA and RV), truncus arteriosus (one great vessel arises from the heart to supply the arterial and pulmonary circulation), and total anomalous pulmonary venous return (blood drains into RA instead of LA) typically present with cyanosis in the neonatal period.

466. The answer is d. *(Behrman, pp 2358–2362.)* **Lead poisoning** produces a motor neuropathy and is associated with anemia, a gingival lead line, colicky abdominal pain, and basophilic stippling of red blood cells. Patients with **acute intermittent porphyria (AIP)** present with recurrent bouts of abdominal pain, confusion, and peripheral and cranial neuropathies. **Kernicterus** is accumulation of bilirubin in the newborn that may cause neuronal death and scarring. Children with **fragile X syndrome** present with mental retardation, large ears, and a prominent jaw. The triad of macroglossia, abdominal distention, and constipation is consistent with cretinism.

467. The answer is c. *(Behrman, pp 2280–2284.)* The presence of a hump or asymmetry when the patient bends forward is the hallmark of a **scoli-**

otic deformity. Radiographic evaluation is used to determine the degree of scoliosis but would not be a cost-effective screening test because films of the entire spine are required. The **Ortolani test** is used to identify congenital dislocation of the hip in an infant. While the patient is in the supine position, the examiner holds the legs with the thumbs against the inside of the knee and thigh and the fingers over the posterior aspect of the proximal femur. A click will be noted as the examiner applies anterior force to the femur and the hip is reduced into the acetabulum.

468. The answer is c. *(Behrman, pp 2138–2147.)* The most likely diagnosis in this patient is **acute bacterial otitis media.** A mucopurulent discharge in acute otitis media occurs only if the drum perforates; otherwise, the tympanic membrane is bulging and erythematous. The organisms responsible for this infection are *Haemophilus influenzae, Streptococcus pneumoniae,* and *Moraxella catarrhalis.* Adenopathy is usually absent in simple otitis media. **Perforations** of the eardrum may occur with infections, sudden changes in pressure, especially when diving, and trauma. **Serous otitis media** will cause the tympanic membrane to be retracted and scarred. **Acute mastoiditis** is caused by the breakdown of the thin bony partitions between the mastoid cells and occurs when an otitis media continues, often with few symptoms, despite adequate treatment. Patients have a continuous discharge through a perforation in the eardrum and complain of swelling, tenderness, and erythema over the mastoid bone.

469. The answer is b. *(Behrman, pp 2030–2032.)* **Tay-Sachs disease** is a progressive autosomal recessive disorder resulting from a deficiency of the enzyme hexosaminidase A with the subsequent storage of ganglioside in the lysosomes of the neurons. Infants present with hyperacusis (startling to sound), hypotonia, and delayed motor development. Funduscopic examination will reveal a **macular cherry red spot. Pompe's disease** is acid maltase deficiency; infants present with weakness and floppiness. **Adrenoleukodystrophy** is an inherited demyelinating disease of males resulting in an enzymatic defect in peroxisomes. Children present with behavioral problems, spasticity, deafness, visual loss, dementia, and brown skin pigmentation. **Phenylketonuria (PKU)** is an autosomal recessive disease in which neonates present with growth failure, seizures, and mental retardation. Patients are diagnosed by obtaining elevated phenylalanine levels during required screening. **Cerebral palsy (CP)** is a group of disorders in which patients present with motor deficits (intelligence may be spared) acquired in the prenatal or perinatal period because of an episode of hypoxemia, ischemia, or infection. There is midline cerebellar agenesis with a fourth ventricle cyst in the **Dandy-Walker malformation,** and this causes hydrocephalus.

470. The answer is c. *(Behrman, pp 1405–1406.)* **Croup** (acute laryngotracheobronchitis) occurs in the fall and winter months and is most often due to one of the **parainfluenzae viruses.** It occurs in boys more often than in girls, between the ages of 3 months and 5 years. The inflammation of croup is subglottic. Patients exhibit labored breathing, stridor, and use of the accessory muscles of respiration to assist breathing. Because of the viral etiology, temperature is typically less than 39.4°C (103°F), and peripheral white blood cell count is usually normal. An anteroposterior radiograph of the larynx will show subglottic narrowing, known as the **hourglass sign** or the **steeple sign. Epiglottitis** is most often caused by *Haemophilus influenzae* **type B.** It is seen in children between the ages of 2 and 7 and may cause life-threatening airway obstruction. Patients present with fever, dysphagia, muffled voice, inspiratory retractions, cyanosis, and drooling. To keep the airway open, patients with epiglottitis often sit in the **sniffing dog position.** The **thumbprint sign** is seen in a soft tissue lateral radiograph of the neck, but these films are rarely done because children require immediate protection of the airway with intubation. **Bronchiolitis** occurs in infants less than 6 months old and is most likely due to respiratory syncytial virus (RSV). There is characteristic hyperinflation of the lungs, and the infant appears anxious due to difficulty in expiration.

471. The answer is b. *(Behrman, pp 1437–1441.)* The child most likely has **cystic fibrosis (CF).** CF is a multisystemic autosomal recessive disorder that affects the sinuses, lower respiratory tract (bronchiectasis), exocrine function of the pancreas, intestinal function (deficiencies in fat-soluble **vitamins A, D, E,** and **K**), sweat glands, and urogenital tract (infertility). Patients have episodes of recurrent respiratory tract infections and a history of failure to thrive. Salt loss in sweat is distinctive. A **meconium ileus** (obstruction from hardened meconium) occurs in only 15% of all patients with CF and may be the first manifestation of CF. It is often pathognomonic for the disease. Respiratory infections are most often due to *Pseudomonas aeruginosa* and *Staphylococcus aureus.* The recurrent infections produce large amounts of mucus that cause obstructive lesions in the bronchi and bronchioles. Diagnosis is made by combining the clinical presentation with an abnormal sweat chloride value (>70 mmol/L).

472. The answer is b. *(Behrman, pp 1993–1997.)* **Absence seizure** (petit mal) occurs in children between the ages of 3 and 10 years and is characterized by numerous daily episodes of unresponsiveness, often associated with lip smacking, eye rolling, eyelid fluttering, or lip movement. **Atonic (astatic) seizures** are called **drop attacks;** patients experience a sudden loss of tone in postural muscles. **Neonatal seizures** are various forms of seizures that may be seen in the newborn. **Focal seizures (partial complex)** involve one part of the body and are not associated with loss of consciousness. These seizures can spread to involve adjacent areas of the body **(Jacksonian march)**. **Psychomotor seizures (temporal lobe)** are associated with automatisms (purposeless motor movements with altered consciousness). Lip smacking may be seen in tardive dyskinesia, but it is usually a consequence of the use of neuroleptics.

473. The answer is a. *(Behrman, pp 1432–1435.)* The clinical presentation is consistent with **chlamydial pneumonia,** which develops in 20% of infants born to women with chlamydia infections. Newborns will present within three months of birth with a week of persistent symptoms. The majority will have bilateral crackles on lung auscultation. Inclusion conjunctivitis and pneumonia are often a consequence of the perinatal infection. The etiologic agent (***Chlamydia trachomatis***) is found in up to 25% of pregnant women. **Pertussis,** or **whooping cough,** is a highly contagious infection and is unlikely to be mild on presentation. The word *pertussis* means "violent cough," and the disease is often called the **cough of 100 days** because of its chronic nature. The cough of pertussis is described as being paroxysmal and staccato in character, ending with a high-pitched inspiratory whoop. **Respiratory syncytial viral (RSV) pneumonia** presents like chlamydial pneumonia but with no history of conjunctivitis. Patients with RSV present with rhinorrhea and cough. Aspiration of a foreign body causes cyanosis, the abrupt onset of respiratory distress, stridor, intercostal retractions, wheezing, and asymmetric breath sounds.

474. The answer is a. *(Behrman, pp 1722–1723.)* **Retinoblastoma** causes a white reflex **(leukocoria)**. This is a life-threatening malignant tumor rarely seen in infants and children. Leukocoria may also be due to a cataract. **Retinocerebellar angiomatosis** is part of a rare autosomal dominant disease (**von Hippel-Lindau disease**); patients present with nystagmus, retinal detachment, cerebellar hemangioblastoma, intraabdominal cysts, and renal carcinoma. Choroidal angioma is found in **Sturge-Weber disease;** patients present with congenital glaucoma, cloudiness of the cornea, and marked enlargement of the eye at birth (buphthalmos). Infants with Sturge-Weber disease may also have facial angiomas. **Primary congenital glaucoma** is a condition of increased intraocular pressure caused by abnormal development of the aqueous drainage structures of the eye. In **papilledema,** the optic disc margins are bilaterally indistinct due to optic nerve swelling from increased intracranial pressure.

475. The answer is e. *(Behrman, p 123.)* Retinal hemorrhages with no evidence of external trauma, along with a history of irritability, lethargy, vomiting, and a bulging fontanel, suggest increased intracranial pressure from a chronic subdural hematoma or **shaken baby syndrome.** Increased head circumference is also suggestive of increased intracranial pressure. **DiGeorge's syndrome** is a congenital disorder; infants present with cardiac defects, tetany from hypocalcemia secondary to an underdeveloped parathyroid gland, facial abnormalities, and thymus gland maldevelopment causing an isolated T cell deficiency. **Oligodendroglioma** commonly involves the temporal lobe, and patients often present with seizures. **Fetal alcohol syndrome** is the number one cause of congenital malformations. Infants are born with developmental retardation and facial, heart, lung, and limb abnormalities.

476. The answer is b. *(Behrman, pp 1386–1387.)* **Choanal atresia** is a congenital nasal obstruction (due to a septum between the nose and pharynx). Newborns are obligate nose breathers, and any nasal obstruction may cause respiratory distress. In choanal atresia, the baby appears to be fine when crying (breathing through the mouth) but becomes cyanotic when crying stops. The incidence of this disorder is 1 in 2500 live births. Treatment consists of maintaining the airway (which may be achieved emergently by making a large hole in the pacifier), which allows the infant to mouth-breathe. Fifty percent of infants with choanal atresia have other congenital anomalies (**CHARGE syndrome** = **C**oloboma, **H**eart disease, **A**tresia choanae, **R**etarded growth, hypo**G**onadism, and **E**ar abnormalities). Newborns with **tracheal-esophageal (T-E) fistula** present within a few hours of birth with choking, cyanosis, and respiratory distress. **Hyaline membrane disease,** the most common cause of respiratory distress in the premature newborn, is a deficiency of surfactant causing severe respiratory distress, usually in premature newborns. **Meconium aspiration syndrome** occurs immediately upon birth and is associated with significant pulmonary morbidity. **Tracheomalacia** is a self-limited disorder that causes noisy breathing (wheezing or stridor) in infancy due to the lack of a rigid trachea.

477. The answer is e. (*Behrman, pp 2015–2019.*) Patients with **neurofibromatosis (NF) type 1** (classical or peripheral) typically present with multiple café au lait spots, axillary freckling, cutaneous neurofibromas, acoustic neuromas, neurilemomas, optic gliomas, **Lisch nodules** (hamartomas of the iris that appear as brown elevations), and skeletal abnormalities. Patients with **neurofibromatosis type 2** (central) present with bilateral acoustic neuromas and multiple meningiomas and rarely have café au lait spots. Neurofibromatosis is also called **von Recklinghausen's syndrome. Tuberous sclerosis (Bourneville's disease)** is a multisystem disease; patients present with skin lesions, benign tumors of the central nervous system, seizures, and mental retardation. **Von Hippel-Lindau (VHL) syndrome** is characterized by cerebellar hemangioblastoma, renal and pancreatic cysts, renal cell carcinoma, and retinal angiomatosis. The neurocutaneous syndromes (NF, VHL, and tuberous sclerosis) are all autosomal dominant disorders. **Meningioma** is a slow-growing benign tumor that arises from the leptomeningeal arachnoidal cells. **Craniopharyngioma** is a slow-growing cystic tumor arising from the pituitary; patients present with visual field defects and endocrine abnormalities.

478. The answer is c. (*Behrman, pp 1753–1757.*) **Nephrotic syndrome** is a clinical complex consisting of more than 3.0 g proteinuria in 24 hours, hypoalbuminemia, edema, hyperlipidemia, lipiduria, and hypercoagulability. **Minimal change disease (MCD)** accounts for 80% of nephrotic syndrome in children under the age of 16 and 20% of nephrotic syndrome in adults. Patients typically present with nephrosis and a benign urinary sediment. The etiology of MCD is unknown, but occasionally the syndrome develops after a respiratory tract infection or an immunization. Patients respond to steroids, and the prognosis is excellent. **RPGN** and **MPGN** are immunologically mediated diseases characterized by oliguria, subnephrotic proteinuria, edema, hematuria, red blood cell casts, and hypertension (acute nephritic syndrome).

479. The answer is a. *(Behrman, pp 1694–1696.)* **Acute lymphoblastic leukemia** (**ALL**) comprises 80% of all childhood leukemias (peak incidence is between 3 and 7 years of age). Most patients present with fatigue, mucosal bleeding, gum hypertrophy, and bone pain. Patients may present with an infection due to the severe neutropenia or with a dramatically high hyperleukocytosis. Physical examination is often remarkable for pallor, petechiae, purpura, mucous membrane bleeding, bone pain, generalized lymphadenopathy, and hepatosplenomegaly. The hallmark of ALL is pancytopenia with circulating blast cells on peripheral smear and bone marrow that is replaced by at least 30% blasts. **Acute nonlymphocytic leukemia** (**ANLL**), also called **acute myelogenous leukemia** (**AML**), is primarily a disease of adults. The **Auer rod** is pathognomonic of AML. **Atypical lymphocytosis** is seen in mononucleosis.

480. The answer is d. *(Behrman, pp 620, 2274.)* All newborns must be evaluated for **congenital hip dislocation,** but it is most commonly seen in females, firstborns, and breech presentations. The **Barlow test** (with the hip in 90° of flexion and maximum abduction, the femur is pushed down while trying to adduct the hip; this will dislocate an unstable hip joint) and Ortolani maneuver (thighs are abducted from the midline with anterior pressure on the greater trochanter; the femoral head is displaced anteriorly into the acetabulum and a soft click is produced) should be performed on all newborns. The **Ortolani test** is a maneuver to reduce a recently dislocated hip. Other maneuvers include **Trendelenburg's sign** (used in older children; a dip of the pelvis to the opposite side when the patient stands on the affected side or a waddling gait with bilateral dislocation of the hip) and **Allis's sign,** also called **Galeazzi's sign,** which is unequal heights of the knees (the dislocated side is lower) when the hips and knees are flexed.

481. The answer is b. *(Behrman, pp 1405–1407.)* **Epiglottitis** is a progressive cellulitis of the epiglottis and surrounding tissues due to *Haemophilus influenzae* type B in children (usual age is 2 to 7 years) or *Streptococcus pneumoniae* or *Staphylococcus aureus* in adults. Patients with epiglottitis have a high fever and complain of sore throat, drooling (inability to swallow secretions), dysphagia, odynophagia, and a muffled voice. The mnemonic to remember the symptoms of epiglottitis is the **four D's** (**D**rooling, **D**ysphagia, **D**yspnea, and **D**ysphonia). Posture is usually upright, leaning forward, and in children is called the **sniffing dog position.** Stridor (a loud, high-pitched sound) may also be present. The diagnosis of a **cherry red** epiglottis is confirmed by laryngoscopy. Patients with exudative pharyngitis due to group A *Streptococcus* present with fever and large, tender anterior cervical lymphadenopathy. **Peritonsillar abscess** (**quinsy**) occurs as a complication of bacterial tonsillitis and is the accumulation of pus between the tonsil and its bed. Patients complain of sore throat, unilateral otalgia, dysarthria, and trismus. On throat examination, an enlarged, medially displaced tonsil (abscess) is seen in the peritonsillar area and the uvula is displaced to the opposite side. A typical gray-white membranous exudate in the pharynx is consistent with diphtheria, but this infection is rare in North America.

482. The answer is d. (*Behrman, p 1820.*) **Hydrocele** is common in infancy; if the tunica vaginalis is not patent, the hydrocele will usually resolve in the first six months of life. A **spermatocele** does transilluminate, but it does not grow as large as a hydrocele and it remains localized as a cystic swelling on the epididymis. A **varicocele** is due to torsion of the pampiniform plexus that surrounds the spermatic cord. It usually occurs on the left side in boys or young men and is very painful. When palpated, a varicocele feels like a "bag of worms." **Cryptorchidism** is an undescended testis; the scrotum remains small, flat, and underdeveloped.

483. The answer is c. (*Behrman, pp 1508–1510, 1549–1551.*) The most common congenital heart abnormality is **VSD.** Small shunts may be asymptomatic, but large shunts may cause dyspnea, exercise intolerance, and congestive heart failure. Typically, patients have a loud P_2, a palpable thrill, and a pansystolic murmur. Small VSDs may close spontaneously, but others may progress to cause **Eisenmenger's syndrome** (pulmonary hypertension that leads to right heart failure and shunt reversal). Patients who develop Eisenmenger's syndrome (irreversible) are inoperable. The three congenital heart defects that cause left-to-right shunts are the **three D's** (VS**D**, AS**D**, and P**D**A). All three may cause Eisenmenger's syndrome. Endocarditis is a complication of VSD.

484. The answer is a. (*Behrman, p 2027.*) **Reye's syndrome** is an often fatal sequela to certain viral illnesses. Patients present with encephalopathy and fatty infiltration and dysfunction of the liver. Salicylates are suspected of potentiating this syndrome; however, they are not believed to be the primary cause of the syndrome because the illness may occur in the absence of salicylate use. The mortality rate in Reye's syndrome is 50%. Infants may become flaccid after eating **honey** due to the inhibition of acetylcholine release (from *Clostridium botulinum*), which causes botulism. **Botulism** bacillus is usually found in canned, smoked, or vacuum-packed foods. Patients present with dysphagia, dysphonia, visual disturbances, diplopia, ptosis, and fixed and dilated pupils. Patients with **Wilson's disease** have **Kayser-Fleischer rings** (yellow-brown) in the Descemet membrane and neuropsychiatric involvement. Identified in 1999, the **West Nile virus** is an arbovirus (anthropod-borne agent) that causes malaise, lethargy, sore throat, stiff neck, nausea, and vomiting. It progresses to stupor, convulsions, cranial nerve palsies, paralysis of extremities, and exaggerated deep tendon reflexes (signs of upper motor neuron disease).

485. The answer is c. *(Behrman, pp 1236–1237.)* **Meckel's diverticulum** rarely causes symptoms, but infants may present with the painless passage of maroon-colored stools. The diverticulum is a remnant of the omphalomesenteric duct and is the most common gastrointestinal tract congenital anomaly (2% of the population). It is usually 2 cm long within 2 ft of the ileocecal valve, and males (usually <2 years old) are affected two times more than females. It is made of two kinds of ectopic tissues (stomach and pancreas) and has two complications (bleeding and inflammation). The mnemonic for Meckel's diverticulum is called the **rule of 2's. Pyloric stenosis** is seen in newborns. Patients present with projectile vomiting, abdominal distention, and a palpable olive-sized mass in the right upper quadrant that appears after vomiting. Prominent peristaltic waves are often visible going from the left to the right side of the abdomen. **Intussusception** (one segment of the intestine prolapses into another) is the most common cause of obstruction in the first two years of life. Infants present with melena, abdominal pain, vomiting, and diarrhea mixed with mucus and blood, giving it a **red currant jelly** appearance. Often, a sausage-shaped mass is palpable in the upper midabdominal area. **Biliary atresia** is a congenital obstruction or absence of the bile duct system. Newborns (2 to 3 weeks old) present with light-colored stools, dark urine, hepatomegaly, pruritus, and jaundice. **Zenker's diverticulum** is a disorder of adults in which the pharyngeal mucosa protrudes through an area of weakness in the musculature proximal to the upper pharyngeal sphincter.

Patients present with halitosis from retention of food and saliva in the diverticulum.

486. The answer is d. *(Behrman, pp 126–128.)* The majority of victims of **sexual abuse** have no physical examination findings. Swelling and erythema of the vulvar tissue (genital trauma) should be a red flag for child abuse, especially if associated with bruising or a foul-smelling discharge. In addition to the anorectal and genitourinary problems, there can be significant behavioral changes, such as sexually provocative mannerisms, excessive masturbation, inappropriate sexual knowledge, enuresis, depression, social withdrawal, anxiety, school problems, and weight changes. A **straddle injury,** often from a bicycle seat, occurs over the symphysis pubis, whereas signs of sexual abuse are more posterior around the perineum.

487. The answer is e. *(Behrman, pp 2222–2225.)* **Impetigo,** which arises from minor superficial breaks in the skin, is caused by *Staphylococcus aureus* or β-hemolytic *Streptococcus* and usually occurs in children. It is a highly contagious epidermal rash characterized by vesicles, erosions, or ulcers that crust and appear golden-yellow and stuck on. **Folliculitis,** which is an infection of the upper portion of the hair follicle, may appear as an erythematous papule, pustule, erosion, or crust lesion and is usually due to *S. aureus.* In folliculitis due to hot tub use, the etiology is *Pseudomonas aeruginosa.* **Kawasaki's disease (KD)** or **mucocutaneous lymph node syndrome** is uncommon in children over the age of 8 years and is characterized by fever; a desquamating, edematous, blotchy-appearing mucocutaneous erythema; cervical lymphadenitis; and aneurysms of the coronary arteries. It is idiopathic. **Staphylococcal scalded skin syndrome (SSSS)** is most common in neonates during the first three months of life. It is a toxin-mediated epidermolytic disease characterized by tender erythema that wrinkles, resembling wet tissue paper. Bullous formation and desquamation may occur. Widespread detachment of the superficial layers of the epidermis resembles scalding. **Miliaria** or prickly heat is a burning and pruritic rash of infants localized to the upper extremities, the trunk, and the intertriginous areas. A **Tzanck smear** is most often used to diagnose herpesvirus.

488. The answer is d. *(Behrman, pp 2060–2069.)* Children with **Duchenne muscular dystrophy (DMD)** present between the ages of 2 and 6 years with fatigability, clumsiness, difficulty standing, difficulty walking on toes, pseudohypertrophy of the calf muscles, and a waddling gait. DMD results from a deficiency of dystrophin, while **Becker MD** is the result of abnormal dystrophin. Becker MD is less severe than DMD and occurs after the age of 5 years. Both Becker and Duchenne MD are X-linked myopathies. The autosomal dominant myopathies are myotonic dystrophy and facioscapulohumeral dystrophy. **Myotonic dystrophy** occurs in adolescence and is characterized by diminished facial movements, cataracts, testicular atrophy, and muscle weakness. **Facioscapulohumeral dystrophy** occurs between the ages of 10 and 20 years and is characterized by facial and shoulder girdle weakness. The **Gower maneuver** (pushing off with the hands when rising from the floor because of proximal muscle weakness) is positive in muscular dystrophy.

489. The answer is f. *(Behrman, p 457.)* **Tangier disease** is a rare inherited disorder of lipoprotein metabolism. Patients present with a low serum cholesterol level, virtually no HDL cholesterol, a normal or elevated triglyceride level, **orange-colored tonsils,** corneal opacities, and a relapsing polyneuropathy. The disorder does not lead to premature atherosclerosis, and treatment is not required.

490. The answer is c. *(Behrman, pp 1711–1714.)* The most common renal tumor in children is **Wilms tumor** or **nephroblastoma** (an embryonal tumor of renal origin). Children present with a painful abdominal mass, dysuria, polyuria, hematuria, weight loss, nausea, and vomiting. Physical examination typically reveals fever, hypertension, and an abdominal or flank mass. **Neuroblastoma** is a tumor of neural crest cell origin. Patients present with fever, anorexia, malaise, an abdominal mass, diarrhea, and neuromuscular symptoms. Physical examination may reveal fever, hypertension, abdominal distention, an abdominal mass, peripheral edema, and periorbital bruises. Both Wilms tumor and neuroblastoma are seen in children under 5 years old. Patients with **Hodgkin's lymphoma** usually present between the ages of 15 and 45 years or over the age of 60 years with the complaint of cervical lymphadenopathy. **Ewing's sarcoma** is a tumor predominantly of white children that involves the diaphyses of long bones. **Rhabdomyosarcoma** may occur anywhere in the body; symptoms depend on the location of the progressively enlarging mass.

491–492. The answers are 491-c, 492-d. *(Behrman, pp 1026–1033.)* **Rubella** (German measles or three-day measles) is a common childhood infection manifested by a characteristic exanthem and lymphadenopathy. **Rubeola,** or measles, is highly infectious and is characterized by fever, Conjunctivitis, Coryza, Cough (the **three C's**), and **Koplik spots.** It has a significant morbidity and mortality. Roseola (exanthem subitum) is a child-hood disease and is due to human herpesvirus type 6 and 7. It is charac-terized by high fever for several days before the skin lesions. Multiple blanchable macules and papules appear on the back as the fever resolves. Sequelae are rare. **Chickenpox** (varicella zoster virus) is characterized by crops of pruritic vesicles that evolve into pustules, crusts, and even scars. Most cases occur in young children and may be complicated by pneumo-nia or encephalitis. The incubation period is approximately 14 days. Pa-tients may remember an exposure to another child with chickenpox or to an older person with zoster.

Bonus Chapter: The Ten Toughest Physical Diagnosis Questions Ever Written

Questions

DIRECTIONS: Each item below contains a question followed by suggested responses. Select the **one best** response to each question.

1. A 42-year-old male was diagnosed with AIDS (acquired immunodeficiency syndrome) six years ago. His viral load is 200/μL, and his CD4 count is 199 cells/μL. He has been taking HAART (highly active antiretroviral treatment) since diagnosis and is compliant with his medications. For the last several months, he has been noticing peripheral muscle wasting and an increase in abdominal girth. He denies jaundice, fever, abdominal pain, nausea, vomiting, and diarrhea. He has no melena or hematochezia. On physical examination, the patient is afebrile; heart rate is 84 beats per minute and blood pressure is 110/70 mmHg. There is no jaundice or jugular venous distention (JVD); heart and lung examinations are normal. Abdominal examination reveals central obesity, normal bowel sounds, and no tenderness. Liver size is 14 cm in the midclavicular line (MCL); there is no splenomegaly. The patient has no caput medusa and no shifting dullness. There is no peripheral edema; there is skeletal atrophy. The patient is alert and oriented to person, place, and time and has no asterixis. There are no motor or sensory deficits. Which of the following is the most appropriate next step in diagnosis?

a. Liver biopsy
b. Ultrasound of the abdomen
c. CT scan of the abdomen
d. Cholesterol and triglyceride levels
e. Paracentesis
f. Repeat viral load
g. Repeat CD4 count

2. A 23-year-old woman presents to the emergency room with a four-day history of temperature spikes to 40.2°C (104.3°F), night sweats, and shaking chills. She has a sore throat and arthralgias but denies cough, shortness of breath, headache, neck stiffness, earache, and abdominal pain; she has no genitourinary symptoms. She develops a nonpruritic rash that appears with a temperature spike. On physical examination, the patient is febrile [38.3°C (101°F)] and has an evanescent salmon-colored rash located primarily over the chest and abdomen. Head, ear, eye, nose, and throat (HEENT) examination is normal except for some bilateral shoddy posterior cervical lymphadenopathy. Lungs, heart, abdomen, and joint examinations are normal. Laboratory data reveal a mild anemia and a white blood cell count of 40,000/μL. Iron levels are normal, but ferritin level is 600 ng/mL (normal female levels are 4 to 161 ng/mL). Chest radiograph, urine cultures, and blood cultures are normal. Which of the following is the most appropriate next step in management?

a. High-dose aspirin
b. Deferoxamine or chelating agent
c. Treatment for tuberculosis
d. Broad-spectrum antibiotics
e. High-dose prednisone
f. Antimalarial treatment

3. A 16-year-old girl has recently emigrated from Mexico with her family. Through an interpreter, the mother states that the teenager suddenly developed a fever to 38.9°C (102°F), chills, sore throat, malaise, and "breakbone" aching of the head, back, and extremities the day prior to the office visit. The patient denies earache, cough, abdominal pain, nausea, vomiting, diarrhea, and genitourinary complaints. The adolescent has never been sexually active. She has no pets and denies animal bites and ill contacts. Temperature is 39.2°C (102.5°F). When the blood pressure is taken, the "tourniquet sign" is positive. Additionally, she has conjunctival redness and a diffuse maculopapular blotching of the skin. The rest of the physical examination is normal. White blood cell (WBC) count is 2500/μL, and platelet count is 55×10^3/μL. The rest of the laboratory data are normal. Which of the following is the most likely diagnosis?

a. Malaria (*Plasmodium falciparum*)
b. Yellow fever
c. Influenza
d. Dengue fever
e. Hantavirus
f. Colorado tick fever

4. A 31-year-old high school teacher presents to your office with a three-day history of cough productive of greenish-colored sputum. The patient has been feeling feverish but denies chills, night sweats, shortness of breath, and chest pain. Past medical history is remarkable for seven episodes of otitis media in childhood, three episodes of sinusitis, four episodes of pharyngitis, two episodes of bronchitis, and two previous episodes of pneumonia over the last 10 years. The patient denies tobacco use, alcohol abuse, and illicit drug use. She has no recent travel history and no ill contacts. On physical examination, she has a temperature of 38.9°C (102°F); pulse oximetry shows a saturation of 98% on room air. Respiratory rate is 18 breaths per minute, and the patient is in no distress. She has bronchophony and crackles at the right base; there is no clubbing. Laboratory data reveal a leukocytosis with bandemia; chest radiograph is positive for a right lower lobe alveolar infiltrate. HIV test is nonreactive. Which of the following is the most appropriate next step in diagnosis?

a. CD4 and CD8 counts
b. Serum immunoglobulin levels
c. Purified protein derivative (PPD) skin test
d. Bone marrow biopsy
e. Abdominal fat aspiration
f. Bronchoscopy with transbronchial biopsy

5. A 19-year-old man presents with muscle aches and fatigue for several weeks. He denies fever, chills, night sweats, and weight loss. He has no sore throat, cough, chest pain, shortness of breath, abdominal pain, nausea, vomiting, diarrhea, or genitourinary complaints. He has no rashes, weakness, incontinence, gait disturbance, or sensory deficits. He does not use tobacco, drink alcohol, or use illicit drugs. He has no past illnesses, no recent travel, and no ill contacts. He takes no medications or herbal medicines. His diet consists of milk shakes, hamburgers, and french fries with extra salt added; he works as a cashier in a fast-food restaurant. The patient is afebrile, with normal blood pressure and pulse and no orthostatic changes. HEENT, heart, lung, and abdominal exams are normal. Musculoskeletal examination reveals no muscle tenderness or atrophy. There are no neurologic deficits. Chvostek's sign is positive. Laboratory data show a normal WBC count and differential, normal platelets and no anemia. His basic metabolic profile reveals a sodium of 142 meq/L, potassium of 2.1 meq/L, chloride of 88 meq/L, and a bicarbonate of 29 meq/L. His blood urea nitrogen (BUN) and creatinine are normal. Calcium and phosphorus levels are normal; magnesium level is 0.8 mg/dL. Urinalysis is unremarkable. Electrocardiogram shows a normal QT interval and diffuse u waves. The potassium and magnesium are replaced, and the patient becomes asymptomatic; u waves on EKG resolve. Which of the following is the most likely diagnosis?

a. Liddle's syndrome
b. Dehydration
c. Rhabdomyolysis
d. Bartter's syndrome
e. Gitelman's syndrome

6. A 49-year-old man was diagnosed with multiple myeloma four years ago. He has had an indolent course with low serum myeloma protein levels and has not required antitumor therapy. Over the last several months, he has noticed gynecomastia and has experienced intermittent erectile dysfunction. He has had excessive hair growth over his chest and back. Vital signs are normal. Hypertrichosis and clubbing are evident. There are no visual field cuts. Nontender, freely moveable lymphadenopathy is present in the posterior cervical, submandibular, submental, and inguinal chains. There is bilateral gynecomastia but no galactorrhea. Heart and lung examinations are normal. Abdominal exam shows hepatosplenomegaly. There is testicular atrophy and 1+ pretibial edema. Neurologic exam reveals decreased loss of pinprick sensation and weakness of the lower extremities. Cranial nerves are intact. Laboratory data are normal except for hyperprolactinemia and hyperglycemia. Which of the following is the most likely diagnosis?

a. Castleman's disease
b. Rosai-Dorfman disease
c. GRFoma
d. POEMS syndrome
e. Acute disseminated encephalomyelitis (ADEM)

7. A 47-year-old woman is started on warfarin for paroxysmal atrial fibrillation. After seven days of therapy, she develops sharply demarcated, erythematous lesions that are purpuric and indurated. Hemorrhagic bullae and eschar formation are evident over some of the lesions located over the breasts, thighs, and buttocks. Which of the following mechanisms best explains the etiology of the findings?

a. Protein S deficiency
b. Protein C deficiency
c. Antithrombin III deficiency
d. Lupus anticoagulant
e. Anticardiolipin antibody syndrome

8. A 32-year-old church pastor presents with the chief complaint of "first morning" reddish brown urine for three weeks and a three-day history of slowly progressive right-sided vision loss. He has no past medical history and takes no medications. He denies trauma, fever, chills, night sweats, and weight loss. He has no back pain, abdominal pain, dysuria, or frequency. He does not smoke cigarettes, drink alcohol, or use illicit drugs. Family history is unremarkable. On physical examination, vital signs are normal. Pupils are equal and reactive to light, and extraocular muscle movements are intact. Vision in the left eye is 20/20; vision in the right eye is limited to seeing fingers (patient reports that his vision one year ago was 20/20 bilaterally). Funduscopic examination is remarkable for a retina with a "blood and thunder" appearance. Lungs, heart, abdomen, and genitalia are normal. There is no costovertebral angle (CVA) tenderness. Rectal examination is fecal occult blood test (FOBT) negative, and the prostate gland is normal. Laboratory data are consistent with a normochromic normocytic anemia; there is leukopenia and thrombocytopenia. Peripheral smear shows schistocytes; leukocyte alkaline phosphatase level is decreased. BUN and creatinine are normal, but there is blood in the urine by dipstick but not microscopically. Bone marrow biopsy is consistent with erythroid hyperplasia. Which of the following is the most appropriate next step in diagnosis?

a. Ham test
b. Sucrose lysis test
c. Serum lysis test
d. LDH level
e. CD59 protein
f. Serum iron level

9. A 5-month-old female infant is brought to your office by anxious parents for abnormal hand movements, which started several days ago. The parents at first thought that the movements were "cute" because they appeared as though their daughter was wringing her hands. There has been no loss of consciousness, fever, vomiting, or seizure activity. Although the child has never been ill and was a normal vaginal delivery, the parents sense that their daughter has poor language skills and is not as socially interactive compared to other children in her age group. They thought it might be secondary to shyness, which she would "grow out of." On physical examination, the child is afebrile and is breathing normally. Head circumference is reduced (twentieth percentile), but height and weight are normal. There is no cyanosis or neck stiffness. Heart, lung, and abdominal examinations are normal. The child has no neurological deficits. Which of the following is the most likely diagnosis?

a. Asperger's syndrome
b. Oppositional defiant disorder
c. Autism
d. Attention deficit hyperactive disorder (ADHD)
e. Childhood schizophrenia
f. Rett's disorder
g. Conduct disorder
h. Pervasive developmental disorder (NOS)

10. A 41-year-old woman presents with a five-day history of a 4-cm linear lesion of her right breast. She complains that the breast is painful, tender, and swollen. She denies fever, chills, and weight loss. The patient is G2P2 (children are 11 and 9 years old), and her last menstrual period was seven days ago. She does not think she can be pregnant, since she and her husband practice birth control. The patient had a mammogram five months ago, which was normal. There is no family history of breast cancer. She does not use tobacco, alcohol, or illicit drugs. She denies trauma. Physical examination is remarkable for a cordlike subcutaneous 4-cm lesion of the right breast that is fibrous and tender to palpation. The breast is swollen and tender; the nipple is normal. There is no erythema or lymphadenopathy. There are no other masses palpable. Which of the following is the most appropriate next step in management?

a. Anticoagulation with heparin
b. Nonsteroidal anti-inflammatory drugs
c. Oral antibiotics for 10 to 14 days
d. Schedule for repeat mammography
e. *BRCA1* and *BRCA2* genetic testing
f. Oral prednisone for 10 to 14 days
g. Schedule for fine needle aspiration

Bonus Chapter: The Ten Toughest Physical Diagnosis Questions Ever Written

Answers

1. The answer is d. *(Tierney, p 1297.)* The patient is experiencing changes in body fat composition (i.e., abdominal obesity and skeletal wasting) due to protease inhibitors. Protease inhibitor and nucleoside analogue use have been associated with a constellation of abnormalities including elevated cholesterol and triglyceride levels, insulin resistance, and diabetes mellitus. The abnormalities in cholesterol levels, triglyceride levels, and body fat composition are changes referred to as **lipodystrophy.** The correct answer is to order cholesterol and triglyceride levels; if necessary, you must treat with pravastatin or atorvastatin (**lovastatin and simvastatin should be avoided because of their interactions with protease inhibitors**). Similar changes in body habitus have been reported in patients with HIV who have never been treated with these medications.

2. The answer is a. *(Tierney, p 807.)* The patient requires high-dose aspirin (1 g three times a day) or an NSAID for treatment of **adult Still's disease.** Still's disease is considered a **variant of rheumatoid arthritis** in which high-spiking fevers are the predominant presenting symptom rather than joint disease. Patients are usually between 20 and 30 years of age. Fevers can be as high as 40.5°C (105°F) and are accompanied by the **classic salmon-colored evanescent truncal rash,** shaking chills, and night sweats. It is not uncommon for fevers to plunge to several degrees below normal intermittently. The fever pattern strongly suggests the diagnosis. Patients may have lymphadenopathy and pericardial effusions. Joint symptoms are mild in the beginning, but a destructive arthritis develops months later. Patients may have anemia, prominent leukocytosis, and **very high ferritin levels** (no known etiology). Half of patients require high-dose prednisone, but aspirin is typically given first. A third of patients have recurrent episodes.

3. The answer is d. (*Tierney, pp 1329–1333.*) **Dengue fever** is due to a flavivirus transmitted by the bite of an Aedes mosquito. Worldwide there are approximately 100 million cases of dengue; several hundred thousand will go on to develop **dengue hemorrhagic fever.** The incubation period is usually 7 to 10 days. Dengue fever's presentation is nonspecific and may range from no symptoms to severe hemorrhagic shock. Patients will complain of high fevers, chills, sore throat, a diffuse maculopapular rash, and "**breakbone**" head, back, and extremity pain. Thrombocytopenia may cause a positive "**tourniquet sign**" in which petechiae develop when the blood pressure cuff is inflated. IgM and IgG ELISA tests usually confirm the diagnosis; treatment is supportive. **Yellow fever** is also a flavivirus more endemic in Africa and South America. Patients (who are usually adult male, due to work habits) may have retroorbital pain, photophobia, leukopenia, proteinuria, and abnormal liver function tests. A positive **Faget's sign** (**fever with bradycardia**) is often seen in patients with yellow fever. Patients with **hantavirus** often present with a pulmonary syndrome that leads to acute respiratory distress syndrome (ARDS). **Colorado tick fever** is usually benign and is self-limited. Influenza is usually accompanied by a nonproductive cough and coryza. Patients with **malaria** due to *P. falciparum* will have profuse sweating, abdominal cramps, vomiting, diarrhea, hemolytic anemia, dark urine ("**blackwater fever**"), splenomegaly, and central nervous system involvement.

4. The answer is b. (*Tierney, pp 771–772.*) The patient most likely has **common variable immunodeficiency syndrome,** which is a defect in terminal differentiation of B cells with absent plasma cells and deficient synthesis of secreted antibody. Patients present with recurrent sinopulmonary infections secondary to humoral immune deficiency (**panhypogammaglobulinemia**). Patients may also have diarrhea, malabsorption, hepatosplenomegaly, protein-losing enteropathy, and a spruelike syndrome. Paradoxically, there may be an increase in autoimmune diseases (20%); there is also an increase in B cell neoplasms (lymphomas) as well as gastric and skin cancers. Diagnosis is confirmed by the demonstration of defects in antibody production. Infections must be treated aggressively with antibiotics; monthly maintenance therapy with intravenous immunoglobulin should be considered in all patients (need to follow serum IgG trough levels). **Abdominal fat aspiration** may be done to diagnose **amyloidosis** (sensitivity of 80%).

5. The answer is e. *(Goldman, p 749.)* The patient has **Gitelman's syndrome** (a variant of Bartter's syndrome) due to a gene defect in the distal convoluted tubule Na-Cl cotransporter (a distal tubule disorder). Patients present with muscle aches, cramps, fatigue, and **salt craving.** It is important to ask patients about adding extra salt or eating high-salt-content foods to determine salt craving. Patients with Gitelman's will have a metabolic alkalosis, hypokalemia, hypomagnesemia, and hypocalciuria (with normal serum calcium levels). In this case, the positive **Chvostek's sign** is due to **hypomagnesemia** and not hypocalcemia. **Bartter's syndrome** is a genetic defect affecting channels in the medullary thick ascending limb of Henle's loop. Patients have a metabolic alkalosis, hypokalemia, hypomagnesemia, and hypocalcemia (positive Chvostek's sign). Patients with Bartter's syndrome present in childhood (there is evidence of growth failure), while patients with Gitelman's syndrome present in early adulthood. **Liddle's syndrome** is a rare inherited tubular disorder causing distal nephron hyperfunction and is characterized by alkalosis, hypokalemia and hypertension. The patient has no blood (false positive dipstick) in the urine to suggest rhabdomyolysis and no orthostatic changes to suggest dehydration. An electrocardiogram with **u waves** is consistent with hypokalemia; hypomagnesemia may cause **prolongation of the QT interval.**

6. The answer is d. *(Goldman, p 1191.)* The features of **POEMS syndrome** (**osteosclerotic myeloma** or **Crow-Fukase syndrome**) are **P**olyneuropathy, **O**rganomegaly, **E**ndocrinopathy, **M**-protein, and **S**kin changes. Besides the progressive sensorimotor neuropathy, patients present with lymphadenopathy and organomegaly. Skin changes consist of hypertrichosis, hyperpigmentation, skin thickening, and digital clubbing. Endocrine manifestations may include type 2 diabetes, amenorrhea, erectile dysfunction, adrenal insufficiency, hypothyroidism, and hyperprolactinemia. The pathogenesis of POEMS syndrome is unknown but is probably related to high-circulating cytokine levels. Treatment of the multiple myeloma may result in improvement of manifestations. Patients with **Castleman's disease** present with localized or disseminated lymphadenopathy, anemia, fever, malaise, weight loss, and polyclonal hypergammaglobulinemia. The condition has been associated with an overproduction of interleukin 6 most likely caused by human herpesvirus type 8. Patients with disseminated disease are treated with steroids. **Rosai-Dorfman disease** is a nonprogressive self-limited disease found in children and young adults;

patients present with bulky lymphadenopathy. **Acute disseminated encephalomyelitis** (**ADEM**) is associated with antecedent smallpox, measles, chicken pox, or rabies immunization; patients present with sensory loss, hemiplegia, quadriplegia, and brainstem involvement. A **GRFoma** is an endocrine tumor that secretes excessive amounts of GRF, which causes acromegaly.

7. The answer is b. *(Tierney, p 513.)* The rare reaction of **warfarin-induced skin necrosis** occurs in patients with **protein C deficiency** between the third and tenth days of therapy with warfarin derivatives. Protein C is a vitamin K–dependent protein that has a shorter half-life than the other coagulation proteins. Warfarin creates a vitamin K–independent state and will transiently deplete protein C before it leads to anticoagulation. Without protein C, there is a hypercoagulable state, and thrombosis of the skin vessels leads to what is known as warfarin-induced necrosis. The development of the syndrome is unrelated to drug dose or underlying condition. The most common areas for the skin necrosis are **thighs, buttocks, and breasts** (the reaction is more common in **women**). Using heparin for five to seven days until warfarin induces anticoagulation can prevent the syndrome. Warfarin-induced necrosis is treated with heparin and vitamin K. Protein C concentrates may be helpful in patients with known protein C deficiency. The course is not altered by discontinuation of warfarin after onset of the eruption.

8. The answer is e. *(Goldman, pp 1018–1019.)* The most common manifestations of **paroxysmal nocturnal hemoglobinuria** (**PNH**) are hemolytic anemia, venous thrombosis, and defective hematopoiesis acquired at the stem cell level. Patients have evidence of intravascular hemolysis, that is, hemoglobinuria and hemosiderinuria; they often have leukopenia and thrombocytopenia (further reflection of impaired hematopoiesis). The activation of complement indirectly stimulates platelet aggregation and hypercoagulability, which leads to thrombosis (in this case, retinal vein thrombosis). Bone marrow may appear normocellular. For many years, the diagnosis of PNH depended upon demonstrating red blood cell (RBC) lysis after complement activation by either acid (**Ham test**) or by reduction in ionic strength (**sucrose lysis test**), but these have been replaced by analysis of complement defense proteins (either CD59 or DAF). These proteins block complement activation on the cell surface, and if absent, RBCs will be sensitive to complement lysis and have a tendency for platelets to abnormally initiate clotting. The Ham and sucrose lysis tests are no longer reliable. Hemoglobinuria (as well as myoglobinuria) should not be confused with hematuria. A urine microscopy that reveals more than 3 RBCs/HPF would support the diagnosis of hematuria.

9. The answer is f. (*Behrman, pp 93–94.*) Females are more likely than males to present with **Rett's disorder,** an X-linked dominant disorder with a prevalence of 1/10,000 (males usually die at birth). Clinical features include reduced head circumference (microcephaly), loss of social relatedness, stereotyped hand movements ("hand wringing"), impaired language function, scoliosis, and impaired mental functioning. Children are approximately five months of age at the time of diagnosis. Children with **autism** have severe deficits in social responsiveness and interpersonal relationships. Speech and language development are abnormal; children often demonstrate peculiarities, such as ritualized behaviors, rigidity, and lack of interest in age-typical activities. Children may lack attention to the primary caregiver's face and fail to respond to voices. Most autistic children function at the mentally retarded level. Onset is usually in early childhood, and more boys than girls are affected. Children with **Asperger's syndrome** (also more common in males) are of normal intelligence but are considered to be "odd children." They have a limited ability to appreciate social nuances, they display motor clumsiness, and they have eccentric interests. Children with **childhood schizophrenia** have hallucinations and delusions. Thought content is bizarre and morbid; speech is rambling and illogical. **Attention deficit hyperactive disorder** (**ADHD**) is characterized by distractibility, short attention span, and impulsiveness. Children may engage in aimless activity and display hyperactive behavior at home and on the playground, in the classroom (this is usually where it is first recognized), and even in the doctor's office. The disorder is more common in boys than in girls. **Oppositional defiant disorder** is characterized by persistent disobedience and opposition to authority figures, especially in the home. However, children still respect the basic rights of others, and age-appropriate societal rules and behavior are not violated. Before puberty, the disorder is more frequently found in males than in females; after puberty, the ratio evens out. The typical child with **conduct disorder** is a boy with academic difficulties who is constantly fighting, running away, throwing tantrums, and in general is defiant of authority. With increasing age, truancy, vandalism, fire setting, theft, sexual promiscuity, substance abuse, and other criminal behaviors may occur. **Pervasive developmental disorder** (**PDD**) denotes a group of disorders with the common findings of impairment of socialization skills and characteristic behavioral abnormalities. Patients may also have speech and language deficits. PDD may be autistic, nonautistic (i.e., Rett's disorder), or NOS (not otherwise specified).

10. The answer is b. (*Tierney, pp 455–456.*) The patient has **Mondor's disease,** or thrombophlebitis of the subcutaneous veins of the anterolateral thoracoabdominal wall. It is a self-limited disease that responds to nonsteroidal anti-inflammatory drugs (NSAIDs). Mondor's disease is more common in women but may be seen in men. It is associated with breast cancer; yearly mammograms are recommended.

High-Yield Facts

DERMATOLOGY

- Morphologic warning signs of **MELANOMA:**
  mnemonic: **ABCD**

  Asymmetry
  Border
  Color variation
  Diameter increase

- Possible causes of **ACANTHOSIS NIGRICANS:**
  mnemonic: **PAID COb**

  Polycystic ovarian disease
  Acromegaly
  Insulin resistance
  Diabetes mellitus
  Cancer (colon, stomach)
  Obesity

- Possible cause of migratory necrolytic erythema: **GLUCAGONOMA**

- Possible cause of acrodermatitis enteropathica: **ZINC DEFICIENCY**

- Precursor lesion of squamous cell carcinoma of the skin: **ACTINIC KERATOSIS**

- Precursor lesion of melanoma: **DYSPLASTIC NEVUS**

- **ERYTHEMA NODOSUM** associated conditions:
  mnemonic: **BUMP SIS**

  Behçet syndrome, **B**irth control pills (BCPs)
  Ulcerative colitis
  ***M**ycobacterium tuberculosis* (MTB)
  Parasites
  Sarcoidosis, **S**ulfonamides
  Inflammatory bowel disease (IBD)
  Streptococcal and fungal infections

- **ERYTHEMA CHRONICUM MIGRANS (ECM):** Lyme disease

- **ERYTHEMA MIGRANS LINGUALIS:** geographic tongue (erythema migrans of the tongue)
- **ERYTHEMA MARGINATUM:** rheumatic fever
- **ERYTHEMA MULTIFORME:** Stevens-Johnson syndrome, sulfonamides, NSAIDs, Dilantin
- **PITYRIASIS ROSEA:** initial lesion "herald patch"; other lesions follow a "Christmas tree" pattern
- Ice-pick-like pitting of the nails: specific for **PSORIASIS**
- **NAIL CLUBBING:**
  Lung diseases: lung cancer, chronic bronchitis (not emphysema), TB, bronchiectasis, hypoxemia due to pulmonary shunts
  GI diseases: IBD (Crohn's disease/ulcerative colitis), cirrhosis
  Cardiac diseases: infective endocarditis, cardiogenic shunts
  Hypertrophic pulmonary osteoarthropathy (HPO)
  Pregnancy
  Amyloidosis

HEENT

- **ARGYLL ROBERTSON PUPILS:** pupils constrict only in response to accommodation but not to light
  mnemonic: **SAD**
  　　　　　　Tertiary **S**yphilis
  　　　　　　Alcoholism (Wernicke's encephalopathy)
  　　　　　　Diabetes
- **MARCUS GUNN PUPIL:** seen in **OPTIC NEURITIS, CENTRAL RETINAL ARTERY OCCLUSION**
- **BLUE SCLERAS:** hallmark of **OSTEOGENESIS IMPERFECTA**
- Most common causes of **PAPILLEDEMA:**
  Conditions associated with increased intracranial pressure:
  mnemonic: **HAM TIP**
  　　　　　　Hematoma
  　　　　　　Abscesses
  　　　　　　Meningitis
  　　　　　　Tumors
  　　　　　　Intracranial hemorrhages
  　　　　　　Pseudotumor cerebri

- **BULLOUS MYRINGITIS:**
  Pathognomonic for *Mycoplasma pneumoniae* infection
  May occur in Ramsay Hunt's syndrome
  Viral and bacterial infections
- **WEBER TEST:** base of vibrating fork over the midline of the SKULL
  In CONDUCTIVE hearing loss: Weber's sign lateralizes to the bad ear
  In SENSORINEURAL loss: Weber's sign lateralizes to the good ear
- **RINNE TEST:** base of vibrating tuning fork over the MASTOID
  In CONDUCTIVE defect: Normal bone conduction
                             Impaired air conduction
  In SENSORINEURAL loss: Air and bone conduction are equally affected
                             Air conduction lasts longer than bone conduction

RESPIRATORY DISEASES

- **SADDLE NOSE DEFORMITY:**
  mnemonic: **CRoWS**
  Cocaine abuse
  Relapsing polychondritis
  Wegener's granulomatosis
  Syphilis
- Criteria for **ALLERGIC BRONCHOPULMONARY ASPERGILLOSIS (ABPA):**
  mnemonic: **ESCAPE A** (escape ABPA)
  Eosinophilia
  Skin reactivity to *Aspergillus* antigen
  Central bronchiectasis
  Asthma
  Pulmonary infiltrates
  Elevated serum IgE levels
  Antibodies to *Aspergillus* antigen

- The most sensitive physical sign of **PULMONARY EMBOLISM:** sinus tachycardia
- Livedo reticularis + shortness of breath following fracture of femur: **FAT EMBOLI**
- **B**lue **b**loater: chronic **b**ronchitis
- Pink puffer: **EMPHYSEMA**

	Chest Examination Physical Findings:			
Disease	**Trachea**	**Fremitus**	**Percussion**	**Breath Sounds**
Pleural effusion (large)	Shifted to opposite side	Decreased	Dull	Decreased
Consolidation (pneumonia)	Midline	Increased	Dull	Bronchial
Pneumothorax	Shifted to opposite side	Decreased	Hyperresonant	Decreased
Atelectasis	Shifted to same side	Decreased	Dull	Decreased
Emphysema	Midline	Decreased	Hyperresonant	Decreased

CARDIOLOGY

- Jones criteria:

  mnemonic: **FEAR CASES**

Minor Criteria*	**Major Criteria***
Fever	**C**arditis
ECG changes (PR prolonged)	Migratory **A**rthritis
Arthralgias	**S**ydenham's chorea
Reactant, acute phase	**E**rythema marginatum
	Subcutaneous nodules

*To fulfill the Jones criteria, either 2 major criteria or 1 major and 2 minor criteria plus evidence of an antecedent streptococcal infection is required.

- Tumor plop: **ATRIAL MYXOMA**
- **AORTIC REGURGITATION:** Corrigan pulse, water hammer pulse, "pistol shot" femoral sound, Duroziez's sign, (+) Hill's sign (BP in thigh 20 mmHg higher than arm BP), Quincke pulses, Austin Flint murmur
- Continuous machinery murmur: **PATENT DUCTUS ARTERIOSUS**
- Mnemonic for the four auscultatory sites: **APT. M** or **A**ll **P**eople **T**ry **M**ushrooms

> **A**ortic (2 RICS)
> **P**ulmonic (2 LICS)
> **T**ricuspid (4 LICS)
> **M**itral (5 LICS)

- **BACTERIAL ENDOCARDITIS:** Roth spots, splinter hemorrhages, Janeway lesions (nontender), Osler nodes (painful)
- Systolic ejection murmur with a THRILL ON THE UPPER LEFT STERNAL BORDER: **PULMONIC STENOSIS**
- Holosystolic murmur with a THRILL ON THE LOWER LEFT STERNAL BORDER: **VSD**
- Holosystolic murmur best heard on the apex, radiating to the AXILLA: **MITRAL REGURGITATION**
- Systolic murmur along with LSB THRILL RADIATING TO THE RIGHT SIDE OF THE NECK: **AORTIC STENOSIS**
- Midsystolic click with late systolic murmur: **MITRAL VALVE PROLAPSE**
- Opening snap, loud S_1, diastolic rumble, atrial fibrillation: **MITRAL STENOSIS**
- Pericardial knock: **CONSTRICTIVE PERICARDITIS**
- **ATRIAL FLUTTER:** "sawtooth" pattern on ECG
- **ATRIAL FIBRILLATION:** "irregularly irregular" pulse, absent P waves, and irregular baseline on ECG

Important Pulse Patterns	
Pulsus alternans:	Cardiac tamponade
Pulsus bisferiens:	Aortic regurgitation and HCM/IHSS
Pulsus paradoxus:	Cardiac tamponade, asthma, constrictive pericarditis
Pulsus tardus:	Aortic stenosis

Heart Sounds	
Midsystolic click:	MVP
Opening snap:	Mitral/tricuspid stenosis
Pericardial knock:	Constrictive pericarditis
Pericardial friction rub:	Pericarditis

First Heart Sound	
Loud	**Soft**
Mitral stenosis	Mitral regurgitation
Short PR interval (WPW)	Long PR interval
Left atrial myxoma	LBBB
MVP with regurgitation	AR, TR

Second Heart Sound:			
Wide Split	**Narrow or Paradoxical**	**Fixed Split**	**Summary**
1. RBBB	1. **L**BBB	1. ASD	Fixed split = ASD (the only 1)
2. MR, VSD	2. **H**TN		Narrow/paradoxical **LHAIM**
3. RV volume overload (l-r shunt)	3. **A**ortic stenosis		All others have a wide split
4. RV pressure overload (PS, PAH)	4. **I**HSS		
	5. Acute **M**I		

GASTROENTEROLOGY

- **CHARCOT TRIAD:** indicates acute cholangitis in 70% of cases
  1. Biliary pain
  2. Jaundice
  3. Fever (with chills and rigor)

- **RAYNOLD'S PENTAD:** positive in only 10% of patients with cholangitis
  1–3. Charcot triad
  4. Mental confusion
  5. Refractory sepsis manifested by hypotension
- Common **MANEUVERS/SIGNS** and their associations:
  Cullen's sign, Turner's sign: hemorrhagic pancreatitis
  Murphy's sign: acute cholecystitis
  Caput medusae: liver cirrhosis
  Courvoisier gallbladder: cancer of the biliary tract or pancreatic head
  Kehr's sign: splenic rupture
  Obturator test, reverse psoas maneuver: retrocecal appendicitis
  Markle's sign (jar tenderness): specific for peritonitis
  Succussion splash: intestinal obstruction or gastric dilatation
- Bedside maneuvers to detect **ASCITES:**
  Inspection for bulging flanks
  Percussion for flank dullness
  Puddle sign
  Shifting dullness maneuver
  Fluid wave maneuver
- Best clues to make a diagnosis of **ASCITES:**
  Focused history (history of liver disease)
  Recent weight gain
  Ankle edema
  Increased abdominal girth
- Causes of CIRRHOSIS:
  mnemonic: **ABCDEF**
      Alpha 1-antitrypsin deficiency
      Budd-Chiari syndrome, hepatitis B
      Hepatitis **C**, **C**opper overload
      Drugs
      Ethanol
      Fe overload

- Physical findings seen in **HEMOCHROMATOSIS:**
  Bronzed skin pigmentation (sun-exposed areas)
  Hepatomegaly with or without cirrhosis
  Degenerative arthritis of the hands and fingers (proximal PIPs)
  Testicular atrophy
- Irreversible complications of **HEMOCHROMATOSIS** (despite therapy):
  Arthropathy
  Hypogonadism
  Cirrhosis

NEPHROLOGY

- Causes of **HIGH ANION GAP ACIDOSIS:**
  mnemonic: **C MUDPILES**
  - **C**yanide
  - **M**ethanol
  - **U**remia
  - **D**iabetic ketoacidosis
  - **P**araldehyde
  - **I**soniazid, Iron
  - **L**actic acidosis
  - **E**thylene glycol, **E**thanol
  - **S**alicylates, **S**tarvation
- Causes of **NON–ANION GAP ACIDOSIS** (hyperchloremia):
  mnemonic: **USED CARP**
  - **U**reteroenterostomy
  - **S**pironolactone
  - **E**xpansion acidosis (saline)
  - **D**iarrhea
  - **C**arbonic anhydrase inhibitors, **C**yclosporine
  - **A**miloride: **A**ddison's disease
  - **R**enal tubular acidosis
  - **P**ancreatic fistula, **P**entamidine

- Causes of **HEMATURIA:**
  mnemonic: **SWITCH GPS**

  Stones, **S**ickle cell disease, **S**cleroderma, **S**LE, **S**ulfonamides

  Wegener's granulomatosis

  Infections, **I**nstrumentation, **I**atrogenic, **I**nterstitial nephritis

  Trauma, **T**B, **T**umor, **T**TP, **T**ubulointerstitial disease

  Cryoglobulinemia, **C**yclophosphamide

  Hemolytic uremic syndrome, **H**enoch-Schönlein purpura, **H**emophilia

  Goodpasture's disease

  Papillary necrosis, **P**olycystic kidney disease, **P**olyarteritis nodosa

  Schistosomiasis, **S**ponge disease (medullary)

- Most common organisms responsible for **URINARY TRACT INFECTIONS (UTIs):**
  mnemonic: **SEEK PP**

  Serratia marcescens

  Escherichia coli

  Enterobacter cloacae

  Klebsiella

  Proteus mirabilis

  Pseudomonas aeruginosa

ENDOCRINOLOGY

- Complications of **ACROMEGALY:**

  Sleep apnea syndrome

  Carpal tunnel syndrome

  CHF (LVH)

  Increased risk of colon cancer

  Increased risk of osteoarthritis

  Hypertension

- **BITEMPORAL HEMIANOPSIA**   vs.   **HOMONYMOUS HEMIANOPSIA**

  Etiologies:

  Craniopharyngioma
  Aneurysm
  Pituitary tumor

  Occipital lesions secondary to AIDS, herpes, tumor

- **SYNDROME OF INAPPROPRIATE ADH SECRETION (SIADH)**   vs.   **DIABETES INSIPIDUS (DI)**

  Decreased serum sodium
  Increased urine osmolality
  Increased urine sodium

  Increased serum sodium
  Decreased urine osmolality

- **TSH:** single best test of thyroid function

- Lid lag and stare: most important physical findings to suggest **GRAVES' DISEASE**

- Delayed deep tendon reflexes (DTRs): most important physical finding in **HYPOTHYROIDISM**

- **CHVOSTEK'S** and **TROUSSEAU'S SIGNS:** suggest hypocalcemia

- **POLYCYSTIC OVARIAN DISEASE (Stein-Leventhal syndrome, PCOD):** amenorrhea, obesity, hirsutism, elevated LH:FSH ratio (>3)

MEN I (Wermer Syndrome)	MEN 2A (Sipple Syndrome)	MEN 2B
PPP	**PPT**	**PNT**
Pituitary adenoma	**P**arathyroid hyperplasia	**P**heochromocytoma
Pancreatic islet cell tumor	**P**heochromocytoma	**N**euromas
Parathyroid hyperplasia	Medullary **T**hyroid cancer	Medullary **T**hyroid cancer

- A man with gynecomastia + small testes + tall stature + female hair distribution: think **KLINEFELTER'S SYNDROME**

- A patient with pigmented mucosa of the gums + hypokalemia + pigmentation of skin creases: think **ADDISON'S DISEASE**

- Hypogonadism + anosmia: **KALLMANN'S SYNDROME**
- **PHEOCHROMOCYTOMA:** rule of 10's: bilateral, malignant, extra-adrenal, familial, children

HEMATOLOGY AND ONCOLOGY

- Purpuric rash + abdominal pain + glomerulonephritis in a child/young patient: **HENOCH-SCHÖNLEIN PURPURA (HSP):**

  mnemonic: **AGAR**

  Abdominal pain

  Glomerulonephritis

  Arthralgia

  Rash

- Purpura (livedo reticularis) after a coronary angiogram: think **CHOLES-TEROL ATHEROEMBOLIC DISEASE**
- Purpura (livedo reticularis) + hepatitis B + abdominal pain after meals + footdrop + HTN: think **POLYARTERITIS NODOSA**
- **THROMBOTIC THROMBOCYTOPENIC PURPURA (TTP):**

  mnemonic: **FAT RN**

  Pentad:

  1. **F**ever
  2. Microangiopathic hemolytic **A**nemia (+) schistocytes
  3. **T**hrombocytopenia
  4. **R**enal abnormalities
  5. **N**eurologic abnormalities (confusion, aphasia, headache, coma, seizures)

- **HEMOLYTIC UREMIC SYNDROME (HUS):**

  mnemonic: **RAT**

  Renal failure

  Microangiopathic hemolytic **A**nemia

  Thrombocytopenia

- The FAT RN has TTP and her HUS has a RAT

- TTP and HUS both have:
  1. Normal coagulation tests (normal PT/PTT)
  2. Elevated LDH
- HUS is similar to TTP, except that it only affects the RENAL system
- For patients with chronic low-grade lymphoproliferative disorders for years who develop new lymphadenopathy, consider transformation to a high-grade lymphoma.
- Patients with **ACUTE LEUKEMIAS** usually present with low to normal WBC, whereas patients with **CHRONIC LEUKEMIAS** may present with splenomegaly and high WBC

More Common Peripheral Smears and Genetic Markers

- Smudge cells (mature lymphocytes): chronic lymphocytic leukemia
- Auer rods: acute myelogenous leukemia/promyelocytic leukemia
- Reed-Sternberg cells: Hodgkin's disease
- Burr cells: uremia, DIC
- Spur cells: liver disease, DIC
- Reactive lymphocytes: infectious mononucleosis
- "Fried egg" appearance of cells that are TRAP (+): hairy cell leukemia
- Target cells: liver disease, iron deficiency, thalassemia
- Helmet cells: traumatic hemolysis, DIC
- Polychromasia and spherocytosis: implies autoimmune hemolytic anemia
- Young patients with unexplained pancytopenia: consider paroxysmal nocturnal hemoglobinuria
- Philadelphia chromosome t(9;22)/bcr-abl gene: chronic myelogenous leukemia
- Bite cells/Heinz bodies: think glucose-6-phosphate dehydrogenase (G6PD) deficiency

Iron-Deficiency Anemia vs. Anemia of Chronic Disease:

IRON	Decreased	Decreased
FERRITIN	Decreased	Increased
TIBC	Increased	Decreased

- **LEAD POISONING** signs:
  mnemonic: **LEAD**
  Lead lines in gingiva
  Erythrocyte stippling
  Abdominal pain
  Drop (foot, wrist)

- Causes of **HYPERCALCEMIA:**
  mnemonic: **CHIMPANZEES**
  Calcium supplements
  Hyperparathyroidism
  Iatrogenic (thiazides), **I**mmobility
  Milk-alkali syndrome
  Paget's disease
  Addison's disease/**A**cromegaly
  Neoplasm
  Zollinger-Ellison syndrome (MEN 1)
  Excess vitamin A
  Excess vitamin D
  Sarcoidosis

RHEUMATOLOGY

- **CHURG-STRAUSS SYNDROME:**
  mnemonic: **RAVE**
  Rhinitis
  Asthma
  Vasculitis
  Eosinophilia

- **BEHÇET SYNDROME:**

  mnemonic: **PGOES**

  Pathergy

  Genital ulcers (recurrent)

  Oral ulcers (recurrent aphthous ulcers)

  Eye lesions (uveitis)

  Skin lesions (erythema nodosum, vasculitis)

- **DRUGS THAT MAY INDUCE LUPUS (SLE):**

  mnemonic: **Be HIPP DAQ**

  Beta blockers

  Hydralazine

  Isoniazid

  Procainamide

  Phenothiazine

  Dilantin

  Aldomet

  Quinidine

- **REITER'S SYNDROME:**

  mnemonic: **CUBA**

  Conjunctivitis ("can't see")

  Urethritis ("can't pee")

  Balanitis

  Arthritis ("can't bend my knees")

- **SAUSAGE-SHAPED DIGITS:**

  mnemonic: **RAP** (rap those digits)

  Reiter's syndrome

  Ankylosing spondylitis

  Psoriatic arthritis

- "Ice pick"-like pitting of the nails: specific for **PSORIASIS**

- **STILL'S DISEASE (adult onset)** vs. **FELTY'S SYNDROME**
  Rheumatoid arthritis   Rheumatoid arthritis
  Splenomegaly   Splenomegaly
  Leukocytosis   Neutropenia
  Rash (salmon colored)
  Fever

NEUROLOGY

- Cranial nerves involved in Ramsay Hunt's syndrome: seventh and eighth CN

- Facial palsy + herpes zoster of the face: think Ramsay Hunt's syndrome

- Third cranial nerve palsy + pupil sparing: think diabetes or hypertension

- Third cranial nerve palsy + dilated pupil: think compression by a tumor or aneurysm

- Third cranial nerve palsy + fifth nerve palsy: think tumor/aneurysm/thrombosis in the cavernous sinus

- Triad of **NORMAL PRESSURE HYDROCEPHALUS:** weird, wet, and wobbly

  1. Altered mentation/dementia ("weird")

  2. Urinary incontinence ("wet")

  3. Ataxic gait ("wobbly")

- **WERNICKE'S ENCEPHALOPATHY:**

  mnemonic: Wernicke's **COAt**

          Confusion

          Ophthalmoplegia

          Ataxia

- Korsakoff's psychosis: confusion, confabulation, antegrade and retrograde amnesia

- Triad of niacin deficiency/pellagra: **D**ementia, **D**ermatitis, **D**iarrhea (**triple D**)

- **CLASSIC MIGRAINE:**

  mnemonic: **A POUND**

    Aura

    Pulsatile

    One-day duration

    Unilateral

    Nausea

    Interferes with **D**aily activities

- Eye examination: all the eye muscles are supplied by CN3 (cranial nerve 3) except LR6 SO4

  LR6: lateral rectus/CN6

  SO4: superior oblique/CN4

- **CLAWHAND DEFORMITY:** ulnar nerve paralysis
- **WRISTDROP:** radial nerve palsy
- **CARPAL TUNNEL SYNDROME:** median nerve compression

Brain Tumors:	
Adults	**Children**
Supratentorial	Infratentorial
1. Astrocytoma	1. Medulloblastoma
2. Meningioma	2. Astrocytoma
3. Pituitary	3. Ependymoma

- **METASTASIS TO THE BRAIN:**

  mnemonic: **L**ots of **B**ad **S**tuff **K**ills **G**lia (**LBSKG**)

    Lung

    Breast

    Skin

    Kidney

    GI

GERIATRICS

- **ACTIVITIES OF DAILY LIVING (ADLs):**

  mnemonic: **DEATH**

  Dressing

  Eating

  Ambulating

  Toileting

  Hygiene

- **INSTRUMENTAL ACTIVITIES OF DAILY LIVING (IADLs):**

  mnemonic: **SHAFT**

  Shopping

  Housekeeping

  Accounting

  Food preparation

  Transportation

- **COMMON CAUSES OF ACUTE URINARY INCONTINENCE:**

  mnemonic: **DRIP**

  Delirium

  Restricted mobility

  Impaction

  Polyuria

- **COMMON CAUSES OF CHRONIC URINARY INCONTINENCE:**

  mnemonic: **DIAPPERS**

  Delirium

  Infection

  Atrophy (postmenopausal)

  Pharmacologic

  Psychogenic

  Endocrine

  Restricted mobility

  Stool impaction

- **COMMON SYMPTOMS OF DEPRESSION IN THE ELDERLY:**
  mnemonic: **PAGE SICS** or **SIGE CAPS**

  Psychomotor retardation/agitation

  Appetite loss

  Guilt feelings

  Lowered **E**nergy level

  Sleep problems

  Decreased **I**nterest in life

  Decreased **C**oncentration

  Suicidal ideation

- **COMMON CAUSES OF VISUAL LOSS IN THE ELDERLY:**
  1. Macular degeneration
  2. Cataracts
  3. Glaucoma
  4. Diabetes mellitus

OBSTETRICS AND GYNECOLOGY

- **PREECLAMPSIA:**
  mnemonic: **HEP**

  Triad: 1. **H**ypertension (>140/90)

              2. **E**dema

              3. **P**roteinuria (>0.5g in 24 h)

- **ECLAMPSIA:** preeclampsia (HEP) + seizures

- **HELLP SYNDROME:**

  Hemolysis

  ELevated liver enzymes

  Low **P**latelets

- **PLACENTA PREVIA:** sudden, painless vaginal bleeding in the third trimester

- **ABRUPTIO PLACENTA:**
  Premature separation of the placenta with unremitting abdominal (uterine) and low back pain
  Visible or concealed bleeding in the third trimester
- **CONDYLOMA LATA:** flat warts that are lesions of secondary syphilis
- **CONDYLOMA ACUMINATA:** genital warts caused by human papillomavirus (HPV)
- Purulent-appearing cervical discharge: harbinger of **PURULENT CERVICITIS**
- **CHANDELIER SIGN** or cervical motion tenderness: indicator of **PELVIC INFLAMMATORY DISEASE**
- **CHADWICK'S SIGN:** bluish-violet appearance of the cervix or vagina
  Sign of PREGNANCY that appears after the seventh week of pregnancy
  May also be associated with a PELVIC TUMOR
- **GOODELL'S SIGN:** softening of the cervix associated with pregnancy; occurs at about the eighth week of gestation
- **HEGAR SIGN:** softening of the uterus at the junction between the cervix and the fundus; occurs in the first trimester of pregnancy
- Differential diagnosis of **ADNEXAL TENDERNESS:**
  Ectopic pregnancy
  Tuboovarian abscess
  Ovarian cysts
  Endometriomas
  Appendicitis

PEDIATRICS

- **TETRALOGY OF FALLOT:**
  mnemonic: **PROVe**
  >   **P**ulmonic stenosis (PS)
  >   **R**ight ventricular hypertrophy (RVH)
  >   **O**verriding aorta
  >   **Ve**ntricular septal defect (VSD)

- **CONGENITAL RIGHT-TO-LEFT SHUNTS:**
  mnemonic: **Five T's**
  - **T**etralogy of Fallot
  - **T**ransportation of great vessels
  - **T**ricuspid atresia
  - **T**otal anomalous pulmonary venous return
  - **T**runcus arteriosus
- **CONGENITAL LEFT-TO-RIGHT SHUNTS:**
  mnemonic: **Three D's**
  - Ventricular septal **D**efect
  - Atrial septal **D**efect
  - Patent **D**uctus arteriosus
- The four **CARDINAL SIGNS OF CONGESTIVE HEART FAILURE** in small children
  1. Tachycardia
  2. Tachypnea with shallow respirations and retractions
  3. Cardiomegaly
  4. Hepatomegaly
- **VENTRICULAR SEPTAL DEFECT (VSD):** most common congenital heart disease
- Forced pharyngeal examination may precipitate acute airway obstruction in kids with **EPIGLOTTITIS** and should not be attempted in those who have stridor
- **INTUSSUSCEPTION:** sausage-shaped mass on abdominal exam and passage of "currant jelly" stools
- **INTRAUTERINE ACQUIRED INFECTIONS:**
  mnemonic: **TORCHES**
  - **T**oxoplasmosis
  - **R**ubella
  - **C**ytomegalovirus
  - **HE**rpes, **H**IV
  - **S**yphilis

Bibliography

Behrman RE et al: *Nelson's Book of Pediatrics*, 17/e. Philadelphia, Saunders, 2004.

Fitzpatrick TB et al: *Color Atlas and Synopsis of Clinical Dermatology*, 4/e. New York, McGraw-Hill, 2001.

Goldman L: *Cecil Textbook of Medicine*, 22/e. Philadelphia, Saunders, 2004.

Seidel HM et al: *Mosby's Guide to Physical Examination*, 5/e. St. Louis, MO, Mosby, 2003.

Tierney LM Jr, et al: *Current Medical Diagnosis and Treatment*, 44/e. New York, McGraw-Hill, 2005.

Index

Notes